Endocrine Diseases

Endocrine Diseases

Publisher: iConcept Press Ltd.
Cover design: Pineapple Design Ltd.
Interior design: iConcept Press Ltd.
Typesetting and copy editing: iConcept Press Ltd. and Pineapple Design Ltd.

ISBN: 978-1-922227-78-2

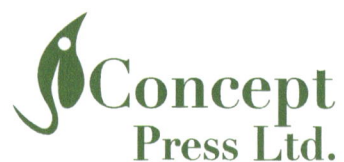

iConcept
Press Ltd.

www.iconceptpress.com

Contents

Maria Diakonova (*University of Toledo, USA*), Peter Oladimeji (*University of Toledo, USA*) and Leah Rider (*University of Toledo, USA*)

Virgilijus Beiša (*Vilnius University Hospital Santariskiu Clinics, Lithuania*)

Preface

Endocrine diseases are disorders of the endocrine system. The branch of medicine associated with endocrine disorders is known as endocrinology. Endocrine disorders can usually be divided into three categories: endocrine gland hyposecretion (leading to hormone deficiency), endocrine gland hypersecretion (leading to hormone excess) and tumours of endocrine glands. Endocrine disorders involve a mixed picture of hyposecretion and hypersecretion. *Endocrine Diseases* serves as an essential start to master the science and art of clinical practice and is going to discuss endocrine diseases.

There are totally 7 chapters in this book. Chapter 1 gives an outline of pancreatic cancer and reviews the biological character and clinical utility of prostate stem cell antigen (PSCA) in the context of pancreatic cancer. It is worth noting that pancreatic cancer is a highly fatal neoplasm and recent studies revealed involvement of PSCA in its carcinogenesis. Chapter 2 proposes a role for zinc transporters in cell signalling and glycaemic control in disease processes, especially insulin resistance and type 2 diabetes. It reveals an exciting role for these transporters as novel targets with utility for therapeutic intervention in the treatment of these diseases. Chapter 3 reviews the role of psychosocial factors including personality traits as well as stresses on the onset and clinical course of Graves' disease. In addition, this chapter also introduces the relationships between stress and other thyroid diseases including Hashimoto's thyroiditis, Plummer' disease and benign thyroid nodule. Chapter 4 summarizes the current and future clinical applications of ghrelin, the endogenous ligand of the growth hormone secretagogue-receptor type-1a (GHS-R1a), in various disorders. Major clinical applications of the available pharmacological tools modulating ghrelin action, in relation to their pharmacological targets, are also discussed.

Chapter 5 describes the regulatory mechanisms underlying the expression of the testis-specific gene PDHA2. Moreover, its somatic activation to correct pyruvate dehydrogenase complex deficiency caused by mutations in the paralog PDHA1 is discussed. Chapter 6 has linked prolactin and PAK1 as the JAK2 substrate to the stimulation of cyclin D1 promoter activity. The authors propose two PAK1-dependent mechanisms to activate cyclin D1 promoter activity: via nuclear translocation of tyrosyl-phosphorylated PAK1 and via formation of a Nck-PAK1 complex that sequesters PAK1 in the cytoplasm. Chapter 7 discusses the method of choice for adrenalectomy, depending on the size of the adrenal tumor.

Editing and publishing a book is never an easy task. Each chapter in this book has gone through a peer review, a selection and an editing process so as to guarantee its quality. Without the supports and contributions of the authors and reviewers, this book can never be able to complete. We would like to thank all of the authors in this book and all of the reviewers who participated in the reviewing process: Takashi Akamizu, Eman M. Alissa, Tao Cai, Jason S Carroll, Tai C. Chen, Ram Narayan Das, Sarinder K. Dhillon, Leonidas H. Duntas, Jia-Fu Feng, Renério Fráguas, M Julia García-Fuster, Tetsuaki Hirase, Naoki Hiroi,

Akio Inui, J. A. M. J. L. Janssen, Sang-Wook Kang, Noushin Khalili, Márta Korbonits, Carol A Lange, Ioannis Legakis, Job M.O, Rajat Maheshwari, Akira Miyajima, Mulchand S. Patel, Satyanarayana R. Pondugula, P. V. Pradeep, Evelyn H. Schlenker, Valeria Sibilia, Sheelu S. Siddiqi, Heather A. Simmons, Helena Soares, Sudhir Sukumar, Guang Sun, Xiaodong Sun, Junji Takaya, Giancarlo Vecchio, Erxi Wu, Weizhen Zhang and Yan Zhou. We hope that you, the reader, will find this book interesting and useful. Any advices please feel free and are always welcome to tell us.

iConcept Press Ltd
August 2014

Prostate Stem Cell Antigen and Pancreatic Cancer

Norihisa Saeki
Division of Genetics
National Cancer Center Research Institute, Japan
Corresponding author

Hiroe Ono
Division of Genetics
National Cancer Center Research Institute, Japan

1   Introduction

Pancreatic cancer is a highly fatal neoplasm and the fourth leading cause of cancer death in the United States. It is usually silent until the advanced stage, where it is recognized through symptoms that result from an invasion of tumor cells into the surrounding tissues, such as abdominal pain and obstructive jaundice, or through symptoms due to metastasis to distant organs. Even with a modern health-check system, it is difficult to recognize an early-stage tumor, as the small but highly malignant tumor cannot be detected by MRI or ultrasound imaging. Therefore, a sensitive and accurate blood marker is anticipated for utilization in patient screening. Recently, several candidate molecules for the blood marker have been reported, which include prostate stem cell antigen (PSCA). In this article, the biological character and clinical utility of PSCA are reviewed in the context of pancreatic cancer.

2   Pancreatic Cancer

2.1   Clinical Character of Pancreatic Cancer

The pancreas consists of mainly three types of cells: acinar cells secreting digestive enzymes, ductal cells forming ducts which transport the digestive enzymes to the duodenum, and islet cells secreting hormones such as insulin and glucagon. More than 85% of pancreatic tumors are of ductal cell origin (Basturk *et al.*, 2010). Therefore, ductal adenocarcinoma has actually become synonymous with pancreatic cancer. In this article, the term pancreatic cancer indicates ductal adenocarcinoma unless it is described with other particular histologic types.

Pancreatic cancer is the fourth leading cause of cancer death in the United States and 227,000 patients are estimated to die every year worldwide (See Vincent *et al.*, 2011 for review). Early-stage pancreatic cancer is usually silent until the patients have symptoms caused by invasion of cancer cells into surrounding tissues or metastasis to distant organs. In other words, most pancreatic cancer patients with symptoms have already reached the advanced stage. Typical symptoms are abdominal or mid-back pain, obstructive jaundice and weight loss. Tumors developed in the pancreatic head would be more susceptible to early diagnosis than those in the pancreatic tail, as the former often involve the common hepatic duct or the proximal side of the pancreatic duct in early stage, resulting in the development of recognizable symptoms such as obstructive jaundice. About 25% of patients with pancreatic cancer have diabetes mellitus at diagnosis and another 40% have impaired glucose tolerance, but the cause of these abnormalities in glucose tolerance is unknown (Chari *et al.*, 2008). New-onset diabetes in older people could suggest the development of pancreatic cancer.

Tri-phasic (i.e., arterial, late arterial, and venous phases) pancreatic-protocol CT is the best initial diagnostic test for pancreatic cancer, and optimum CT scans including 3-dimensional reconstruction have 80% accuracy for the prediction of resectability (Vincent *et al.*, 2011). Endoscopic ultrasound is also a highly reliable procedure for diagnosing pancreatic cancer, and, at the same time, fine-needle aspiration of the pancreatic mass could be performed to obtain cytological samples, with about 80% sensitivity for diagnosis (Harewood & Wiersema, 2002).

A complete cure can be obtained only by successful resection of the entire tumor mass by pancreatico-duodenectomy; however, for patients with surgically resected ductal adenocarcinoma of the pancreatic head, actuarial 5-year overall survival is about 20–25% (Vincent *et al.*, 2011). Adjuvant therapy is recommended for patients who undergo pancreatic resection with curative intent. The chemotherapeutic option for pancreatic cancer includes fluorouracil and gemcitabine, and several new regimens of chemotherapy have been clinically tried in comparison with gemcitabine, which includes erlotinib, a epidermal growth factor receptor inhibitor (Cao *et al.*, 2013). The efficacy of addition of radiation to chemotherapy is unproven and controversial.

2.2   Risk- and Genetic Susceptibility-Factors of Pancreatic Cancer

Risk factors of pancreatic cancer include smoking, family history of chronic pancreatitis, advancing age, male gender, diabetes mellitus, obesity, non-O blood group and occupational exposure to certain chemicals (Vincent *et al.*, 2011). Among the factors, cigarette smoking and family history are important. About 7–10% of pancreatic cancer patients have a family history (Petersen *et al.*, 2006), and the cancer is defined as familial pancreatic cancer if it occurs in families in which a pair of first-degree relatives have been diagnosed with a pancreatic tumor. First-degree relatives of individuals with familial pancreatic cancer are associated with a 9-fold increased risk of pancreatic cancer, and patients with familial pancreatic cancer have more precancerous lesions than those with sporadic pancreatic cancer (Klein *et al.*, 2004; Brune *et al.*, 2010). The risk of pancreatic cancer is also modestly increased in the case of sporadic pancreatic cancer. Other than that described above, alcohol consumption may also be a risk factor. One study revealed that alcohol consumption, specifically liquor consumption of 3 or more drinks per day, increases pancreatic cancer mortality independent of smoking (Gapstur *et al.*, 2011). Red meat intake, particularly meat cooked at high temperatures and associated with mutagens, was suggested to play a role in pancreatic cancer development (Stolzenberg-Solomon *et al.*, 2007). Intriguingly, recent meta-analyses showed an association between infection with *Helicobacter pylori* and the development of pancreatic cancer (Pooled adjusted odds ratio 1.38; 95% Confidence interval: 1.08-1.75; *P* value=0.009, Trikudanathan *et al.*, 2011).

Recently, several genomewide association studies (GWAS) using a single nucleotide polymorphism (SNP) as a genetic marker were conducted on a germline DNA sample set of a case-control cohort, to capture genes related to pancreatic cancer susceptibility. One study revealed an association between a SNP in the first intron of the ABO blood group gene and pancreatic cancer (Amundadottir *et al.*, 2009). The ABO gene encodes a glycosyltransferase that catalyzes the transfer of carbohydrates to the H antigen, forming the antigenic structure of the ABO blood groups. Although the reason for the association has not been uncovered, the result supports earlier epidemiologic evidence suggesting that people with blood group O may have a lower risk of pancreatic cancer than those with groups A or B. Another GWAS identified eight SNPs that map to three loci on chromosomes 13q22.1, 1q32.1 and 5p15.33 (Petersen *et al.*, 2010). Two correlated SNPs, rs9543325 and rs9564966, map to a 600-kb nongenic region between two genes, kruppel-like transcription factor-5 (*KLF5*) and *KLF12*, on chromosome 13q22.1. Five SNPs on 1q32.1 map to the *NR5A2* gene encoding nuclear receptor subfamily 5, group A, member 2. The NR5A2 protein is a nuclear receptor of the fushi tarazu (Ftz-F1) subfamily which is predominantly expressed in the exocrine gland of the pancreas, the liver, intestine and ovaries in an adult. It interacts with β–catenin to activate expression of cell-cycle genes (Botrugno *et al.*, 2004), which seems to be the reason for the correlation between the SNPs and pancreatic cancer. The one remaining SNP maps to 5p15.33, residing in intron 13 of *CLPTM1L* (encoding cleft lip and palate transmembrane 1-like). *CLPTM1L* is part of the *CLPTM1L-TERT* locus that includes *TERT* (encoding telomerase reverse transcriptase), which is only 23 kb distant from the gene. *CLPTM1L* is up-regulated in cisplatin-resistant cell lines and may play a role in apoptosis (Yamamoto *et al.*, 2001), while *TERT* encodes the catalytic subunit of telomerase, which is essential for maintaining telomere ends. This locus has been identified in a GWAS of a number of different cancers, including brain tumors, lung cancer, basal cell carcinoma and melanoma (Wang *et al.*, 2008;

McKay *et al.*, 2008; Rafner *et al.*, 2009; Stacey *et al.*, 2009; Shete *et al.*, 2009). There are 2 GWAS conducted on Asian population, which unveiled several other pancreatic cancer susceptibility loci (Low *et al.*, 2010; Wu *et al.*, 2012). However, the association of each locus was not replicated in the Caucasian population (Campa *et al.*, 2013). Association studies based on a candidate approach also disclosed an association of some genes with pancreatic cancer susceptibility, including cholecystokinin B receptor gene (Smith *et al.*, 2012), hypoxia-inducible factor-1α gene (Wang *et al.*, 2011) and *HNF1* gene encoding a homeobox transcription factor (Pierce & Ahsan, 2011).

2.3   Molecular Pathogenesis of Pancreatic Ductal Carcinoma

Pancreatic intraepithelial neoplasia (PanIN) is a major precursor lesion for pancreatic ductal carcinoma and the oncogenic molecular events occurring in its development have been well elucidated (Feldmann & Maitra, 2010). In accordance with the progression of the degree of histological atypism, PanIN is classified into three stages: PanIN-1 (with mild atypia), PanIN-2 (with moderate atypia) and PanIN-3 (carcinoma-in-situ), with PanIN-1 being further divided into PanIN-1A (flat lesion) and -1B (papillary lesion). The progression of PanIN is highly associated with a progressive accumulation of genetic aberration (Figure 1, Maitra *et al.*, 2003). Concordant with its pathogenesis, basically, pancreatic cancer develops in older people, and more than half of the population above the age of 65 has PanIN (Andea *et al.*, 2003).

The genetic events occur in a well-characterized sequence rather than in a random manner (Figure 1). In the early stage, *KRAS* activation resulting from a mutational event is important, as it was reported that an activating *KRAS* mutation resulted in the development of PanIN in transgenic mice (Hingorani *et al.*, 2003). Indeed, in humans, oncogenic mutations in *KRAS* were found in 36% of PanIN-1A, 44% of PanIN-1B and 87% of PanIN 2/3 lesions (Feldmann *et al.*, 2007). The *KRAS* activation initiates succeeding oncogenic signals: Raf/MEK/ERK pathway, PI3K/Akt pathway and Ral-GEF pathway. A recent study revealed that *WNK2* gene is down-regulated in PanIN via hypermethylation of its promoter (Dutruel *et al.*, 2013). As the gene encoding protein kinase is known to negatively regulate an activation of the MEK1/ERK pathway in cancer cells, its down-regulation may enhance activation of the pathway by KRAS. Loss of the *CDKN2A/p16* gene is observed in 30% of PanIN-1, 55% of PanIN-2 and 71% of PanIN-3 (Wilentz *et al.*, 1998). The gene encodes a cell-cycle checkpoint protein and its inactivation causes dysfunction in cell-cycle arrest in G2-S transition. Loss of *TP53* function was observed in 50–75% of pancreatic cancer (Feldmann *et al.*, 2007). Nuclear accumulation of TP53 protein reflects the mutational status of *TP53* and is observed in PanIN-3 (Maitra *et al.*, 2003). As *TP53* is involved in cell-cycle regulation and apoptosis induction, its inactivation is prone to promote carcinogenesis. *SMAD4* is one of the downstream molecules in TGF-beta cell growth inhibition signaling. *SMAD4* expression is intact in PanIN-1 and PanIN-2 lesions, but loss of *SMAD4* expression is observed in 31% of PanIN-3 lesions (Wilentz *et al.*, 2000). BRCA2 is also a tumor-suppressor, which is inactivated in the advanced stage (Goggins *et al.*, 2000). A genome-wide copy number analysis on individuals with a family history of pancreatic cancer revealed that somatic chromosomal copy number changes were identifiable in only 8 lesions of the 38 PanIN or intraductal papillary mucinous neoplasms (IPMN), and that only two precursor lesions had more than one somatic copy number alteration, while the overwhelming majority (~95%) of PanINs harbored *KRAS* mutations, suggesting that there is no one tumor suppressor gene locus consistently involved in initiating familial pancreatic neoplasia (Hong *et al.*, 2012). Another genome-wide copy number analysis on pancreatic ductal adenocarcinoma disclosed frequent gains of 1q, 2, 3, 5, 7p, 8q, 11, 14q and 17q (> or =78% of cases), and losses of 1p, 3p, 6, 9p, 13q, 14q, 17p and 18q (> or =44%), and the *SKAP2/SCAP2* gene (7p15.2), which belongs to the Src family kinases, was most frequently (63%)

amplified with a significant correlation between its DNA copy number and mRNA expression level (Harada *et al.*, 2008).

Recent exome sequencing revealed aberrations in axon guidance pathway genes (Biankin *et al.*, 2012). Notably, inactivation of SLIT/ROBO signaling was observed 20% of pancreatic ductal adenocarcinoma. It is suggested that SLIT/ROBO signaling modulates MET and WNT signaling activity through CDC42 and β–catenin, respectively. MET, a well-known proto-oncogene encoding a hepatocyte growth factor receptor with tyrosine-kinase activity, was known to have a role in a population of self-renewing cancer stem cells of pancreatic cancer (Li *et al.*, 2011), and it was recently reported that canonical Wnt signaling is required for pancreatic carcinogenesis (Zhang *et al.*, 2013a). Consequently, the loss of SLIT/ROBO signaling may promote pancreatic carcinogenesis. The exome sequencing was also performed by two other groups (Jones *et al.*, 2008; Murphy *et al.*, 2013). As a result of the 3 studies, 4 genes were listed as frequently mutated genes common to the 3 studies: *KRAS*, *TP53*, *SMAD4* and *ATM*.

MicroRNAs (miRNAs) are 18- to 22-nucleotide-long, noncoding RNAs. Accumulating evidence suggests that they are involved in an important biological process via regulation of gene expression. Three miRNAs, miR-21, miR-155 and miR-200, are frequently expressed in pancreatic cancer tissues and are supposed to have a significant role in carcinogenesis (Tang *et al.*, 2013). For example, miR-155 represses expression of TP53INP1 (P53 inducible nuclear protein) and prevents pancreatic cancer cells from apoptosis. The field of noncoding RNA is still progressing and will provide important knowledge about pancreatic carcinogenesis.

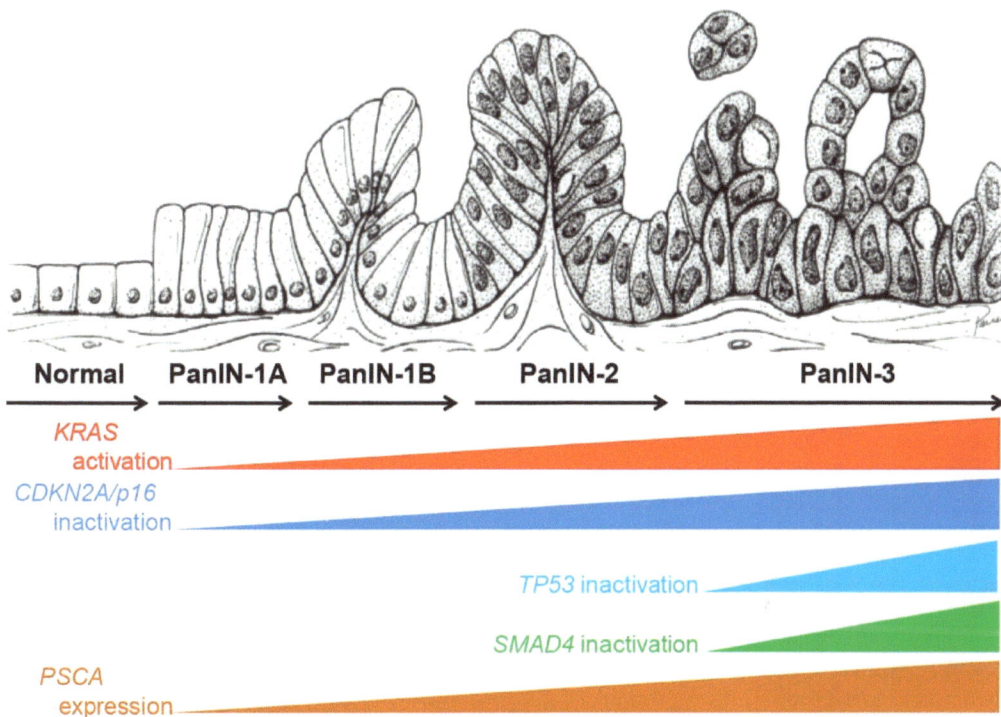

Figure 1: Development of pancreatic intraepithelial neoplasia (PanIN) and associated genetic changes. According to its histological atypism, PanIN is classified into three stages: PanIN-1 to -3. Aberrant expression of *PSCA* is started even in the early stage of carcinogenesis, in which *KRAS* activation is also identified, suggesting its contribution to carcinogenesis. (Adapted by permission from Macmillan Publishers: Modern Pathology (Maitra *et al.*, 2003), copyright 2003).

2.4   Pancreatic Neuroendocrine Tumor

Pancreatic neuroendcrine tumor (PanNET) is relatively rare and said to be 1-2% of all pancreatic neo-plasma (Asa, 2011). However, because of its clinically asymptomatic feature, it was reported that one of every five incidentally diagnosed pancreatic tumors is a PanNET, and up to 40% of all PanNETs are inci-dentally diagnosed, suggesting there may be more cases than the number diagnosed at hospitals (Zhang *et al.*, 2013b). PanNETs are of islet cell origin and known to release hormones such as insulin and glucagon, but 85% of them are non-functional (Franko *et al.*, 2010).

The genetic events that occur in PanNET carcinogenesis are totally different from those of ductal adenocarcinoma, and *KRAS* mutation is not actually observed. In brief, important in the carcinogenesis are gene alternations that result in activation of PI3K (phosphoinositide-3-kinase)/Akt (v-*akt* murine thy-moma viral oncogene) signaling and mTOR (mechanistic target of rapamycin serine/threonine kinase) pathway, and endothelial-independent islet cell survival (See Zhang *et al.*, 2013b for review). It was demonstrated that Akt activation was observed in many PanNET and that mutation in the genes of two inhibitory molecules for PI3K/Akt signaling, PTEN and TSC (tuberous sclerosis complex) was detected in 7.4 and 8.8%, respectively, of the PanNET cases (Ghayouri *et al.*, 2010; Krausch *at al.*, 2011; Krymskaya & Goncharova, 2009). Menin encoded by the *MEN1* gene promotes expression of 2 genes encoding cell cycle inhibitors, *CDKN1B* and *CDKN2C*, in the downstream of the PI3K/Akt signaling, and mutation in the *MEN1* was found in 44% of sporadic PanNETs (Jiao *et al.*, 2011). The mTOR pathway promotes cell survival, proliferation and motility and is activated in PanNETs (Zhou *et al.*, 2011).

3   Prostate Stem Cell Antigen

3.1   Contextual Expression of PSCA

Prostate stem cell antigen (PSCA) is a glycosylphosphatidylinositol (GPI)-anchored cell surface protein belonging to the Thy-1/Ly-6 family (Figure 2). It has123 amino acids and consists of an amino-terminal signal sequence, a carboxy-terminal guanosyl-phosphatidylinositol-anchoring sequence, and multiple N-glycosylation sites (Bahrenberg *et al.*, 2000). PSCA protein is detected between 10 and15 kDa molecular-weight markers in western blot analyses; however, PSCA protein with a larger size was also reported (Reiter *et al.*, 1998; Tanikawa *et al.*, 2012). Several antibodies were reported to be used in immunohisto-chemical analyses of PSCA (Gu *et al.*, 2000, Sakamoto *et al.*, 2008, Geiger *et al.*, 2011). Its expression in humans has been reported in the epithelia of prostate, urinary bladder, kidney, skin, esophagus, stomach, gallbladder and placenta (Reiter *et al.*, 1998; Bahrenberg *et al.*, 2000; Gu *et al.*, 2000; de Nooij-van Dalen *et al.*, 2003; Ono *et al.*, 2012a). *PSCA* expression was also observed in the telencephalon and peripheral ganglia of the nervous system in mice (Hruska *et al.*, 2009). Recently, its expression in islet cells of the normal pancreas was demonstrated by our groups (Ono *et al.*, 2012b), and will be described later in this article. Our knowledge about PSCA-expression sites in the human body is limited, and other cryptic ex-pression sites might be exhibited in the future.

Initially, *PSCA* was identified as a gene over-expressed in prostate cancer (Reiter *et al.*, 1998) and succeeding investigations revealed it is also up-regulated in urinary bladder cancer, renal cell carcinoma, pancreatic cancer, hydatidiform mole, ovarian mucinous tumor, glioma and lung cancer (Amara *et al.*, 2001; Elsamman *et al.*, 2006; Argani *et al.*, 2001; Feng *et al.*, 2008; Cao *et al.*, 2005; Geiger *et al.*, 2011; Kawaguchi *et al.*, 2010); however, it is down-regulated in esophageal, gastric and gallbladder cancers

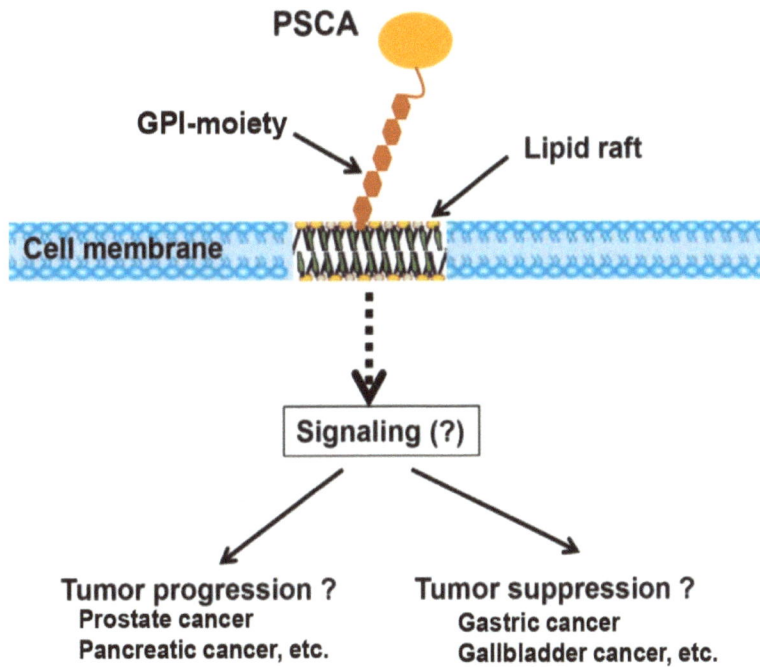

Figure 2: PSCA is a glycosylphosphatidylinositol (GPI)-anchored cell surface protein. It is thought to localize to lipid raft by its GPI moiety and be involved in subcellular signal transduction. However, molecules interacted with PSCA protein are yet to be identified.

(Bahrenberg *et al.*, 2000; Sakamoto *et al.*, 2008; Ono *et al.*, 2012a) (Table 1, Figures 3-5). It was identified as a gastric-cancer susceptibility gene by GWAS, for the first time, on the Japanese population (Sakamoto *et al.*, 2008), and the association between the gene and gastric cancer was replicated in other ethnic populations including Caucasian (Saeki *et al.*, 2013). It was also found as a bladder-cancer susceptibility gene by GWAS (Wu *et al.*, 2009). Intriguingly, a recent GWAS revealed an association of PSCA with duodenal ulcer, although it is not expressed in the duodenum (Tanikawa *et al.*, 2012).

Up-regulation	Down-regulation
Glioma (Geiger et al., 2011)	Esophageal squamous cancer (Bahrenberg et al., 2000)
Lung non-small cell carcinoma (Kawaguchi et al., 2010)	Gastric adenocarcinoma (Sakamoto et al., 2008)
	Gallbladder adenocarcinoma (Ono et al., 2012a)
Pancreatic ductal carcinoma (Argani et al., 2001)	
Prostate carcinoma (Reiter et al., 1998)	
Urinary bladder carcinoma (Amara et al., 2001)	
Renal cell carcinoma (Elamman et al., 2006)	
Ovarian mucinous tumor (Cao et al., 2005)	
Hydatidiform mole (Feng et al., 2008)	

Table 1: Expression status of PSCA in cancer.

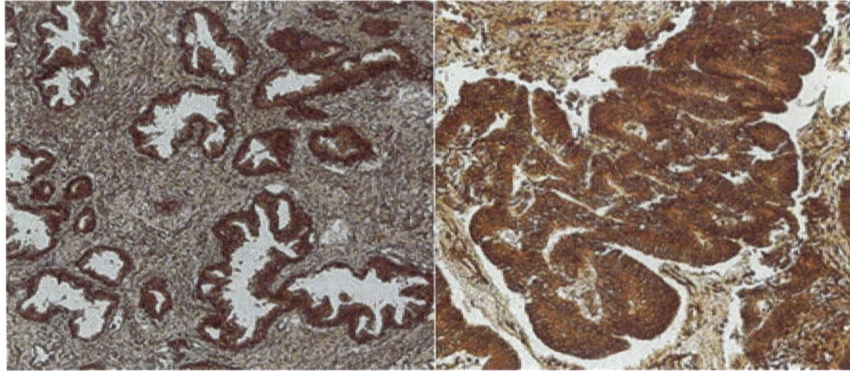

Figure 3: Immunohistochemistry showing PSCA expression (brown) in normal prostate gland (left panel) and its upregulation in prostate cancer (right). Immunohistochemistry was conducted using anti-PSCA antibody produced by our group and anti-mouse IgG antibody labeled with horseradish peroxidase. The localization of the antibodies was visualized using VECTASTAIN Universal Quick Kit (Vector Laboratories, Burlingame, CA, USA). Bar, 100µm.

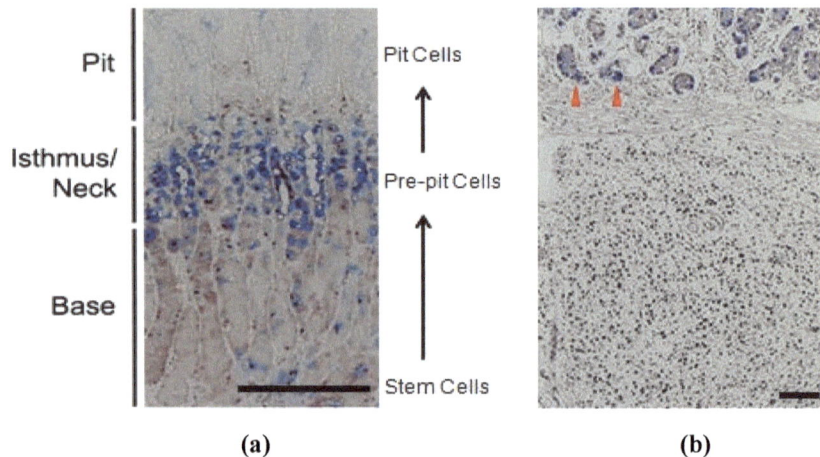

(a)   (b)

Figure 4: PSCA is expressed in the epithelium of gastric mucosa. (a) The gastric mucosa consists of 4 regions: base, neck, isthmus and pit, and stem cells at the base region differentiate to mature cells in gastric mucosa. PSCA (blue) is expressed in the middle portion of gastric mucosa, which harbors a pre-pit cell, a transit amplifying cell differentiating to pit cell. (b) PSCA is down-regulated in diffuse-type gastric cancer. Arrowheads indicate PSCA expression in normal gastric epithelial cells. Immunohistochemistry using anti-PSCA antibody produced by our group, double-stained with anti-PCNA (proliferating cell nuclear antigen) antibody (red). See Sakamoto *et al.*, 2008 for procedure details. Bar, 100µm.

As described above, PSCA shows a contextual expression pattern in normal and cancer tissues, but the regulatory mechanism of PSCA expression is almost unknown. It was reported that, in bladder carcinoma cell line RT112, PSCA expression was up-regulated by contact of the cells to a culture dish surface and resulted in an aggregation of cells, and also by phorbol ester, indicating that its expression is regulated by mechanisms related to the adhesion of epithelial cells (Bahrenberg *et al.*, 2001).

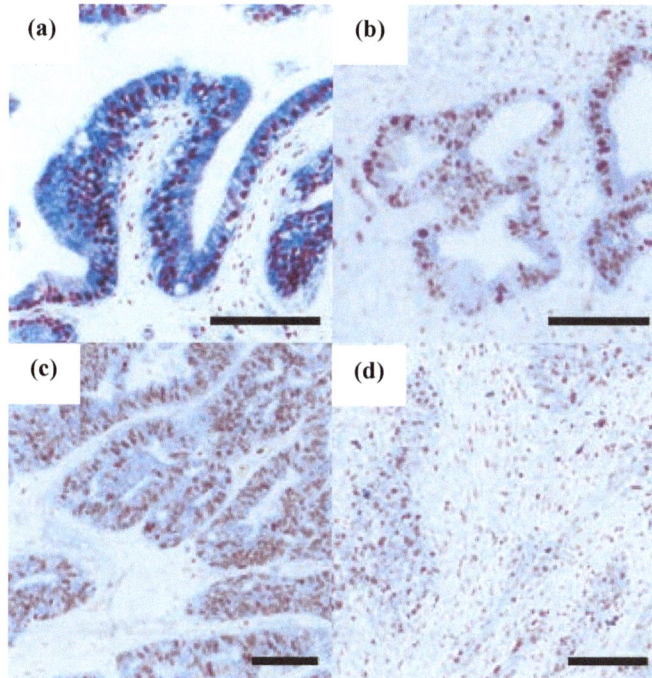

Figure 5: PSCA is down-regulated in gallbladder cancer. PSCA expression is observed in normal gallbladder epithelium (a) and it is down-regulated in well (b), moderately (c) and poorly (d) differentiated gallbladder carcinoma. Immunohistochemical double-staining for PSCA (blue) and PCNA (proliferating cell nuclear antigen, red). See Ono et al., 2012a for details of the study, and Sakamoto et al., 2008 for details of procedure.

Androgen seems to be involved in PSCA regulation, at least in the prostate epithelium, as an androgen responsive element was identified in its promoter region (Jain *et al.*, 2002) and transgenic mice introduced with *PSCA* promoter-driven GFP constructs exhibited GFP expression which was influenced by puberty, castration and androgen restoration (Watabe *et al.*, 2002). In humans, complete androgen ablation with bicalutamide and goserelin acetate decreased the number of PSCA-expressing cancer cells in 2/3 cases of prostate cancer (Zhigang & Wenlu, 2005). On the other hand, androgen-independent regulation is also suggested. 15-Lipooxygenase-2 (15-LOX2) is a human-specific, non-hem and iron-containing enzyme that metabolizes arachidonic acid to 15(S)-hydroxy-eicosatetraenoic acid, and transgenic expression of 15-LOX2 in mouse prostate resulted in age-dependent prostatic hyperplasia associated with expression of several stem or progenitor cell molecules, including Sca-1 and Psca (Suraneni *et al.*, 2010).

Intriguingly, it was also reported that PSCA is down-regulated in telomerase-transduced urothelial cells (Chapman *et al.*, 2008). DNA methylation was implicated as a mechanism of the down-regulation in gastric and gallbladder cancers (Ono *et al.*, 2012a).

3.2   Function of PSCA

Although the GPI-moiety is a common feature, the members of the GPI-anchored proteins have significant diversity in their structure and function (Chatterjee & Mayor, 2001) (Table 2). The GPI-anchored proteins lack a transmembrane domain and are thought to locate in lipid rafts, a special microdomain, enriched in specific proteins and lipids, of the surface of the outer cell membrane. In the lipid raft, the

GPI-moiety may have the capacity to transduce some signals across the cell membrane, and in fact, several studies demonstrated that cross-linking of the GPI-anchored proteins by antibodies elicit the signal transduction. A mouse monoclonal anti-PSCA antibody 1G8 inhibited tumor growth and metastasis, and prolonged the survival of mice that had been inoculated with human prostate cancer cell lines as xenografts, which is probably through inducing caspase-independent cell death of the cancer cells by cross-linking the proteins (Gu *et al.*, 2005). On the other hand, in chicken brain, Psca prevents a subpopulation of choroid cells from cell death by modulating a signaling pathway involving α7-containing nicotinic acetylcholine receptors (Hruska *et al.*, 2009). In addition, PSCA showed cell growth inhibition activity for gastric and gallbladder cancer cell lines, instead of cell death induction (Sakamoto *et al.,* 2008; Ono *et al.*, 2012a). In spite of its designation as stem cell antigen for its structural similarity to stem cell antigen 2 (SCA-2) (Reiter *et al.*, 1998), PSCA is expressed mainly in differentiating cells rather than in stem cells, which was revealed in a study on prostate and gastric epithelial cells (Tran *et al.*, 2002; Sakamoto *et al.*, 2008); however, PSCA expression can also be observed in mature or differentiated cells in gallbladder epithelium and pancreatic islet (Ono *et al.,* 2012a; Ono *et al.*, 2012b). Although PSCA is expressed in several tissues in the human body, a detailed expression pattern in the context of cell or tissue differentiation is not well elucidated in tissues other than prostate epithelium. It could be supposed that the pattern also depends on tissue type.

Function	GPI-proteins
Enzymes	Acetylcholinesterase (Roberts & Rosenberry, 1985)
	Alkaline phosphatase (Low & Finean, 1977)
	5′-nucleotidase (Zekri et al., 1989)
Adhesion molecules	Neural cell adhesion molecule (Powell et al., 1991)
	Contactin (Reid et al., 1994)
	Neurotrimin (Struyk et al., 1995)
Receptors	Folate receptor 1 (Rijnboutt et al., 1996)
	GDNF Family Receptor Alpha 1 (Treanor et al., 1996)
	Plasminogen Activator, Urokinase Receptor (Casey et al., 1994)
Surface antigens	Thy-1 cell surface antigen (Tse et al., 1985)
	CD48 (Korínek et al., 1999)
	Glypican 2 (Stipp et al., 1994)

Table 2: Functional diversity of GPI-anchored protein

Moreover, complicated as it is to understand its physiological significance, PSCA function seems to be contextual. The expression status of PSCA in cancer cells is dependent on the epithelium of their origin; up-regulated in prostate and urinary bladder cancers but down-regulated in esophageal and gastric cancers. This suggests that it could be oncogenic for some epithelial cells and also be a tumor suppressor for others. This contradiction may be related to the integrity of the cell polarity. One hypothesis is that PSCA basically has a role in regulation of cell proliferation and/or differentiation, which contributes to preventing a malignant transformation of the cells; but once the cell polarity is destroyed, it may act in tumor progression dependent on cell type. Mucin1 (*MUC1*), encoding a mucous protein in gastric mucous secreted by pit cells, is a good example. MUC1 is a membrane-bound protein (Bafna *et al.*, 2010). After being translated, a single MUC1 peptide is cleaved to N-terminal and C-terminal subunits, designated as MUC1-N and MUC1-C, respectively, but both the subunits are localized together to the cell membrane in the apical side of the epithelial cells. MUC1-C has a transmembrane domain and a cytoplasmic tail (CT) which is involved in subcellular signal transduction. On the other hand, MUC1-N present on the cell surface has multiple glycosylation sites and is thought to act in protection against many types of insults, after the front layer of defense by the secretary mucins in mucus. In a normal epithelium, MUC1 protein is localized to the apical side of the cells, which restricts interaction between MUC1 and other membrane proteins involved in signal transduction, and MUC1 is protective against environmental insults potentially leading to tumorigenesis. However, after significant epithelial damage, the cells lose their polarity and the membrane proteins change their distribution, which enables the membrane proteins to interact with MUC1 and finally results in eliciting MUC1's signaling promotional for cancer cell growth (Kufe, 2009).

On the other hand, it is worthwhile to consider the PSCA function in the immune system, as it is a membrane protein. One study revealed that down-regulation of *PSCA* using shRNA caused reduced cell proliferation of bladder cancer cell xenografts harbored in mice, and that the PSCA down-regulation in the bladder cancer cells resulted in up-regulation of genes involved in the interferon α/β signaling pathway as well as the Interleukin 1 signaling pathway *in vivo*, suggesting PSCA expressed in cancer cells counteracts a natural immune response through blocking the IFNα/β receptor (Marra *et al.*, 2010). PSCA may have a role in immune reaction in carcinogenesis such as immune escape and attack, in the context of the state and/or type of the cancer cells.

In conclusion, it is very likely that PSCA function is related to several subcellular signalings in the cells, depending on both the origin of the cells and their condition, i.e., normal or malignant. Psca knockout mice have been generated but these showed no abnormal phenotype except that the mice were susceptible to metastasis when implanted with cancer cell xenografts (Moore *et al.*, 2008).

4   PSCA and Pancreatic Cancer

4.1   PSCA is Expressed in Islet Cells but Not in Ductal Cells in Normal Pancreas

Recently, PSCA expression was observed in islet cells of the pancreas (Ono *et al.*, 2012b). Our immunohistochemical study revealed diffuse expression of PSCA in the islets (Figure 6). In our observation, acinar or ductal cells showed no PSCA expression.

This islet-restricted expression suggests some important role of PSCA in endocrine cells, which remains to be elucidated. Intriguingly, double staining with islet markers demonstrated that PSCA is expressed in all cell types in the islet: α (glucagon), β (insulin), δ (somatostatin) and PP (pancreatic polypeptide) cells (Figure 7). The expression common to these endocrine cells may suggest that PSCA has a role related to hormonal secretion, though a secretion-related function of PSCA has not been reported. It seems that PSCA itself has functional diversity dependent on cell type. The islet expression gives insight into the unrevealed function of PSCA. As mentioned above, PSCA is diffusely expressed in mature gallbladder epithelium, which consists of one layer of simple columner cells and has a simple function, *i.e.*, absorbing fluid and electrolytes to condense bile, suggesting PSCA may have a simple function in some epithelium rather than a complex function related to cell proliferation or differentiation.

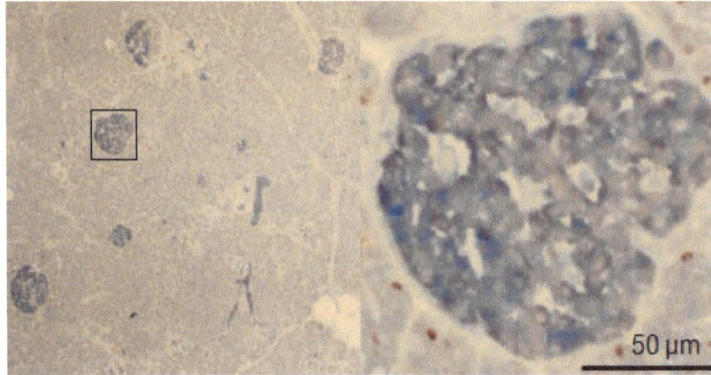

Figure 6: PSCA is expressed in islet cells but not in acinar or ductal cells. Imunnohistochemistry using anti-PSCA (blue) and anti-PCNA antibodies (red) shows diffuse PSCA signals in the islets suggesting it is expressed in multi-lineage of the islet cells. The right panel is a magnification of the islet demarcated in the left panel. (Adapted from Ono *et al.*, 2012b).

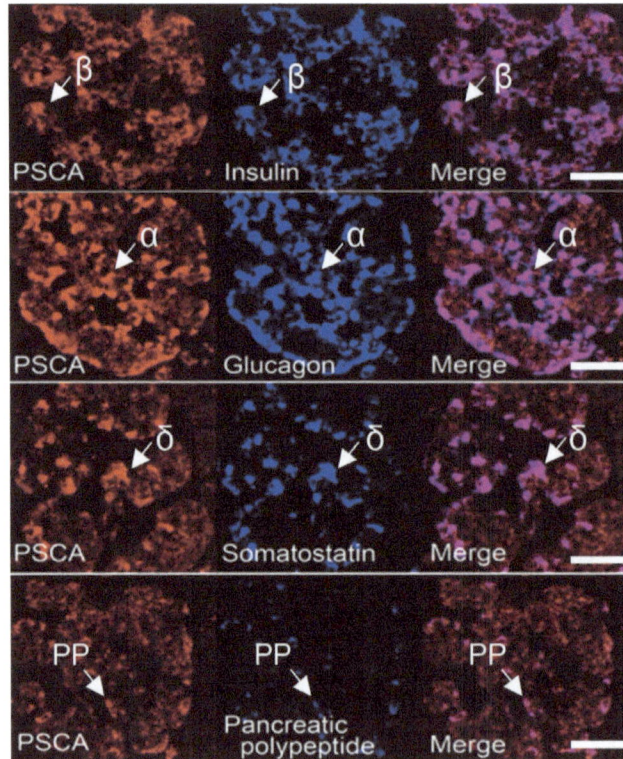

Figure 7: Fluorescent immunohistochemistry of PSCA (red) double-stained with islet cell markers (blue, glucagon for α cells, insulin for β, somatostatin for δ, pancreatic polypeptide for PP) exhibits PSCA expression in all the islet cell lineages (Arrows indicate representative staining of each type of cells). The β cells are numerous and situated in the central regions of the islets. The α cells are generally arranged around the periphery. The δ and PP cells are less numerous and do not display an obvious pattern of the arrangement (Klimstra *et al.*, 2007). Bar, 25μm. (Adapted from Ono *et al.*, 2012b).

The pancreatic expression was confirmed by detecting *PSCA* transcripts in RNA from pancreatic tissues. Intriguingly, in conducting an RNA ligase-mediated rapid amplification of 5' cDNA end procedure in order to elucidate the promoter region used for the pancreatic expression, we also detected a variant of the *PSCA* transcript, that encodes no protein (variant 2 in Figure 8a) (Ono 2012b). We extended the variant study to other tissues and their neoplastic lesions, which revealed that the non-coding variant is also expressed in stomach, gallbladder and their cancer cell lines (Figure 8b).

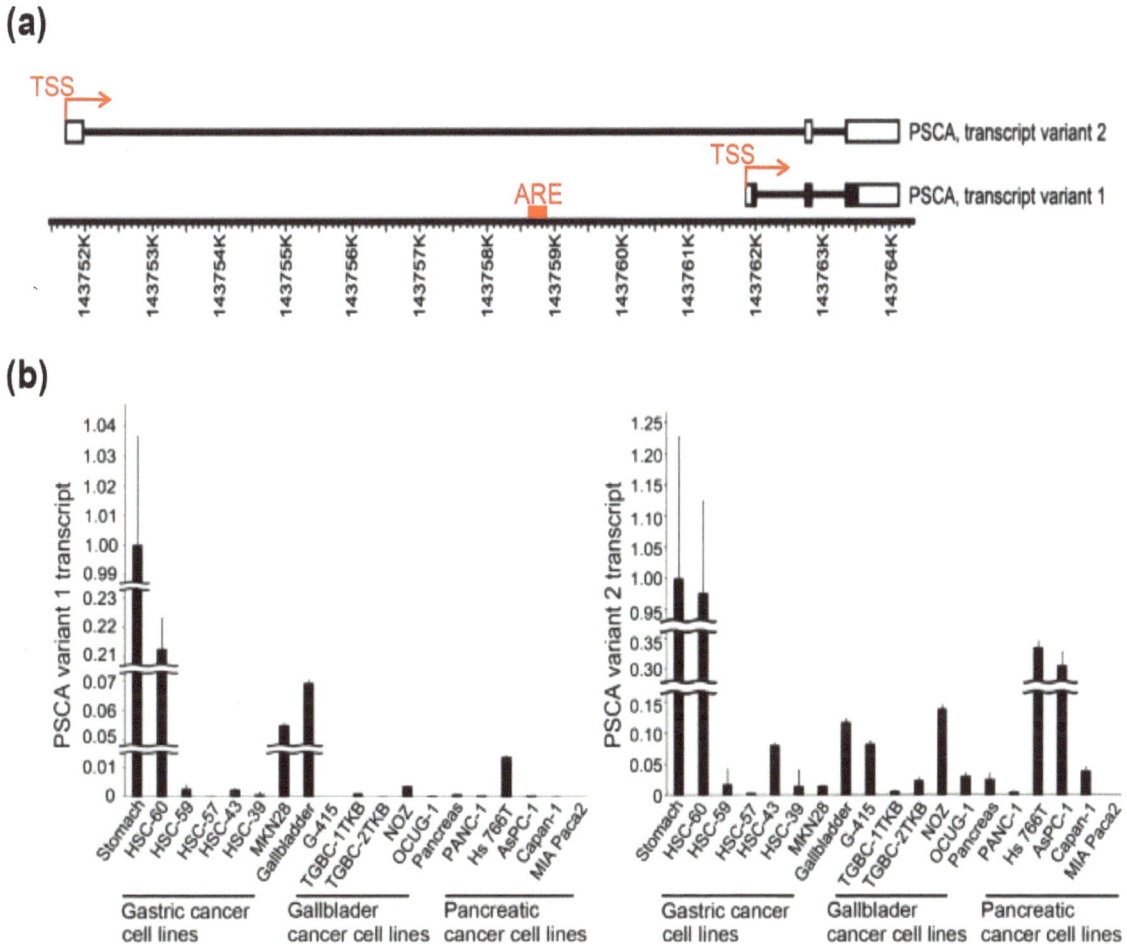

Figure 8: Expression of non-coding *PSCA* transcripts in pancreas, stomach, gallbladder and their cancer cell lines. (a) A schematic representation of the structure of the authentic (variant 1) and non-coding variant (variant 2). (b) Quantitative PCR detected variant 1 and 2 transcripts in gastric, gallbladder and pancreatic tissues and their cancer cell lines. TSS, transcription starting site. ARE, androgen responsive element. Quantitative RT-PCR was performed with gene expression assay using SYBR Premix Ex Taq II (Takara Bio Inc, Shiga, Japan), conducted in 40 cycles under a condition of 2 steps of temperature: 95°C for 5sec and 60°C for 30sec, by the ABI PRISM 7900HT Sequence Detection System. The relative transcript level was calculated using the Ct value of *GAPDH* transcript as reference. (Adapted from Ono *et al.*, 2012b).

The expression of the non-coding variant could have some important physiological function including moderation of *PSCA* expression. For example, the 3′ untranslated region (UTR) of variant 2, which is shared with variant 1, may act as a decoy in recognition by microRNA or other molecules. Intriguingly, variant 2 is a dominant *PSCA* transcript in some pancreatic and gallbladder cancer cell lines (Ono *et al.*, 2012b). The transcription start site (TSS) of variant 2 locates about 10-kb upstream to that of variant 1, which is even upstream to the androgen responsive element located about 3-kb upstream to the variant 1 TSS. This distance between the two TSS's suggests that transcription of the 2 variants is regulated by distinct promoters. It may be possible to hypothesize that variant 2 expressions may contribute to carcinogenesis in some tissues, like stomach and gallbladder, in which PSCA has a role in tumor suppression.

4.2   PSCA is Aberrantly Expressed in Pancreatic Cancer

PSCA expression in pancreatic cancer was reported for the first time by Argani *et al* (Argani *et al.*, 2001). They compared SAGE (serial analysis of gene expression) libraries derived from pancreatic adenocarcinoma to those derived from non-neoplastic pancreatic specimens and reported that *PSCA* was expressed in four of the six pancreatic cancer SAGE libraries but not in the libraries from normal pancreatic ductal cells. They also detected PSCA over-expression in 60% of primary pancreatic adenocarinoma by immunohistochemistry but not in 59 of 60 specimens from the adjacent non-neoplastic pancreas (Figure 9). Hypomethylation in the 5′ CpGs of the PSCA gene was suggested for the causal of the over-expression of PSCA in pancreatic cancer tissues and cell lines (Sato *et al.*, 2003).

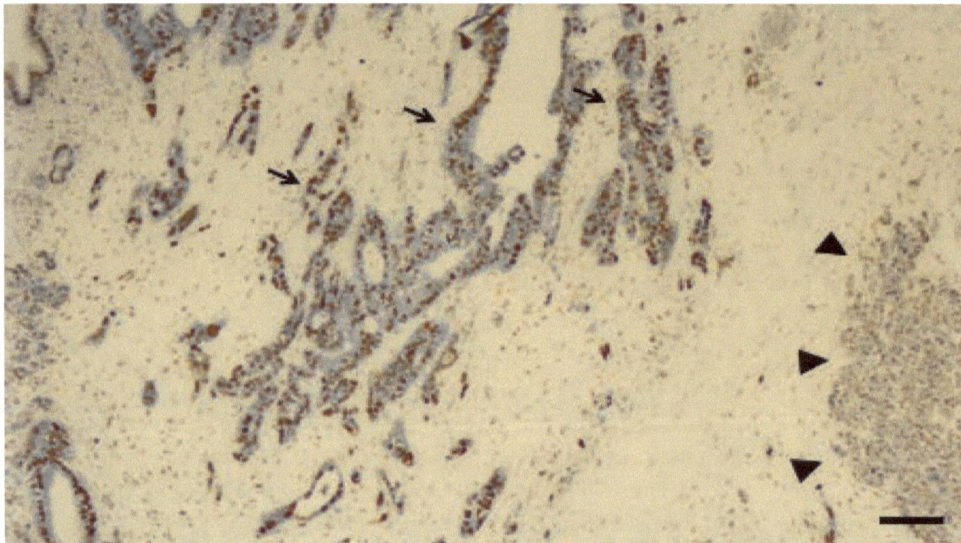

Figure 9: PSCA is up-regulated in pancreatic ductal carcinoma. PSCA expression is observed in cancer cells (arrows). Adjacent normal pancreatic ductal cells are weakly stained, probably as background signall (demarcated by arrowheads). Immunohistochemical double-stain for PSCA (blue) and PCNA (red). See Sakamoto et al., 2008 for details of procedure. Bar, 100μm.

4.3   PSCA is a Useful Marker in the Diagnosis of Pancreatic Cancer

There have been several reports on the utility of PSCA in diagnostic procedures for detecting pancreatic cancer cells. It was reported that the copy number of *PSCA* transcripts was significantly higher in the blood of patients with metastasis of pancreatic cancer (n=9) than in the blood of patients with benign pancreatic tissues (Grubbs *et al.*, 2006), and also that PSCA expression was present in the blood of 22 out of 47 (46.8%) patients with malignant tumors (11 pancreatic carcinoma, 8 gastric cancer, 15 colorectal carcinoma and 13 miscellaneous tumors), particularly in 7 out of 11 (63.6%) patients with pancreatic cancer (Lukyanchuk *et al.*, 2003). Tanaka et al. examined the plasma level of IgG antibodies reactive to 57 peptides encoded by *PSCA* and reported that the levels of IgGs reactive to each of the 10 different peptides were significantly higher in the plasma of pancreatic cancer patients than in that of patients with a non-neoplastic pancreatic lesion (Tanaka *et al.*, 2007). The 3 reports suggest that PSCA is a valuable biomarker in the blood for the diagnosis of pancreatic cancer. Fukushima *et al.* reported its usefulness in pathological examination and RT-PCR analyses to discriminate mucinous cystic neoplasms and non-neoplastic pseudocysts located in the pancreas (Fukushima *et al.*, 2004). PSCA was also reported as a useful marker in the cytological examination of pancreatic specimens obtained by fine-needle aspiration (sensitivity 84%, specificity 91%) (McCarthy *et al.*, 2003), and PSCA showed different expression pattern ($P \leq 0.001$), between benign and malignant pancreatic tissues, in RT-PCR analyses on pancreatic juice collected by intraoperative aspiration of the main pancreatic duct (Oliveira-Cunha *et al.*, 2011).

However, recently, the usefulness of PSCA in the diagnosis of pancreatic cancer was re-evaluated. The antibodies against five proteins, prostate stem cell antigen, fascin, 14-3-3 sigma, mesothelin and S100P (S100 calcium binding protein P), were studied for their utilization in immunohistochemistry on paraffin sections from cellblocks of the samples obtained by fine-needle aspiration, and as a result, S100P was revealed as the best diagnostic character showing 90% sensitivity and 67% specificity, while PSCA and 14-3-3 showed high sensitivity but zero specificity. Moreover, S100P correctly predicted six of seven cancers (Dim *et al.*, 2011). In another study which evaluated pancreatic tumor markers including PSCA, it was concluded that pVHL (von Hippel-Lindau tumor suppressor), maspin, S100P, and IMP-3 (insulin-like growth factor II mRNA-binding protein 3) constitute the best diagnostic panel of immunomarkers in both surgical and fine-needle aspiration specimens (Liu *et al.*, 2012). In this study, it was reported that strong background staining was frequently seen with PSCA. Thus, the specificity of the diagnosis by immunohistochemistry may depend on the quality of the antibodies. In conclusion, it seems that, although the result of immunohistochemistry-based procedures could be influenced by the quality of the antibody, RT-PCR-based examination is reliable in detecting pancreatic cancer cells in the tissue, blood and pancreatic juice, which may help early detection of pancreatic cancer in the human body.

4.4   PSCA is a Novel Target Molecule in the Treatment of Pancreatic Cancer

The effect of anti-PSCA antibodies has already been reported for pancreatic cancer xenografts in mice (Wente *et al.*, 2005). The anti-PSCA antibody 1G8, whose tumor-growth suppression effect was demonstrated on a prostate cancer xenograft model, was intraperitoneally applied to mice subcutaneously injected with Capan-1 pancreatic cancer cells, which showed its suppressive effect on tumor formation and tumor growth.

Moreover, the combination of AGS-1C4D4, a fully human monoclonal antibody to PSCA, and gemcitabine was studied in a randomized, phase II trial with 196 patients of metastatic pancreatic cancer (Wolpin *et al.*, 2013). In this study, the 6-month survival rate (SR) was 44.4% (95% Confidential interval

(CI), 31.9–57.5) in the gemcitabine arm and 60.9% (95% CI, 52.1–69.2) in the gemcitabine plus AGS-1C4D4 arm (P = 0.03), while the median survival was 5.5 versus 7.6 months and the response rate was 13.1% versus 21.6% in the two arms, respectively. The 6-month SR was 57.1% in the gemcitabine arm versus 79.5% in the gemcitabine plus AGS-1C4D4 arm among the PSCA-positive subgroup and 31.6% versus 46.2% among the PSCA-negative subgroup. However, among patients who received gemcitabine, the 6-month SR was higher among those with PSCA-positive tumors (57.1%) versus those with PSCA-negative tumors (31.6%), suggesting that tumor PSCA staining may also act as a prognostic marker, independent of treatment with AGS-1C4D4. The study concluded that the addition of AGS-1C4D4 to gemcitabine improved the 6-month SR among patients with previously untreated, metastatic pancreatic adenocarcinoma. This recent clinical trial suggested that additional administration of the anti-PSCA antibodies to chemotherapy reagents is a promising therapeutic strategy for metastatic pancreatic cancer. It is supposed that AGS-1C4D4 elicits an immunological response against cancer cells, as AGS-PSCA, a prototype of AGS-1C4D4, was found to induce antibody-dependent cell-mediated cytotoxicity and also to mediate complement-dependent cytotoxicity in PSCA-expressing prostate cancer xenografts in mice (Antonarakis *et al.*, 2012).

5   Concluding Remarks and Future Prospective

PSCA is aberrantly expressed in pancreatic ductal carcinoma, suggesting its usefulness in pancreatic cancer diagnosis. As it is up-regulated in other cancers, it will be useful if it is included as one of the tumor markers in blood examination for cancer screening. For precise evaluation of the utility of PSCA in immunohistochemical diagnosis, it seems that the best quality anti-PSCA antibody should be selected, and with it, a multi-institute study should be conducted. Several lines of evidence suggest that antibodies against PSCA have a therapeutic effect on cancer. However, the molecular mechanism of the PSCA function in carcinogenesis is almost unknown. Moreover, even its function in normal cells has not been unveiled yet, although it is expressed in a variety of the organs in the human body. In pancreatic cancer and some other cancers, PSCA is likely to have an onco-promoting function. This PSCA-related onco-promoting pathway as well as PSCA itself is supposed to be a strong candidate for a therapeutic target. To develop a novel therapeutic strategy for cancer, it is important to uncover the PSCA function in carcinogenesis at the molecular level. And it should be kept in mind that PSCA is expressed in normal tissues and that it is likely to function as a tumor-suppressor in some of the tissues. To avoid any undesirable events in a PSCA-targeted cancer therapy, it is also important to explore its expression sites in the human body and its function in those tissues. The authors believe that identification of molecules that interact with the PSCA protein will be the breakthrough in PSCA investigation. We are about to use PSCA as a therapeutic target in general medical practice but we know almost nothing about its function and significance in the body.

Acknowledgements

This study was supported by Grants-in-Aid for Scientific Research (KAKENHI) by the Japan Society for the Promotion of Science (No. 23501327) and partly by a grant from Japan Science and Technology Agency (JST).

References

Amara, N., Palapattu, G. S., Schrage, M., Gu, Z., Thomas, G. V., Dorey, F., Said, J. & Reiter, R. E. (2001). *Prostate stem cell antigen is overexpressed in human transitional cell carcinoma.* Cancer Research, 61, 4660–4665.

Amundadottir, L., Kraft, P., Stolzenberg-Solomon, R. Z., Fuchs, C. S., Petersen, G. M., Arslan, A. A., Bueno-de-Mesquita, H. B., Gross, M., Helzlsouer, K., Jacobs, E. J., LaCroix, A., Zheng, W., Albanes, D., Bamlet, W., Berg, C. D., Berrino, F., Bingham, S., Buring, J. E., Bracci, P. M., Canzian, F., Clavel-Chapelon, F., Clipp, S., Cotterchio, M., de Andrade, M., Duell, E. J., Fox, J. W. Jr., Gallinger, S., Gaziano, J. M., Giovannucci, E. L., Goggins, M., González, C. A., Hallmans, G., Hankinson, S. E., Hassan, M., Holly, E. A., Hunter, D. J., Hutchinson, A., Jackson, R., Jacobs, K. B., Jenab, M., Kaaks, R., Klein, A. P., Kooperberg, C., Kurtz, R. C., Li, D., Lynch, S. M., Mandelson, M., McWilliams, R. R., Mendelsohn, J. B., Michaud, D. S., Olson, S. H., Overvad, K., Patel, A. V., Peeters, P. H., Rajkovic, A., Riboli, E., Risch, H. A., Shu, X. O., Thomas, G., Tobias, G. S., Trichopoulos, D., Van Den Eeden, S. K., Virtamo, J., Wactawski-Wende, J., Wolpin, B. M., Yu, H., Yu, K., Zeleniuch-Jacquotte, A., Chanock, S. J., Hartge, P. & Hoover, R. N. (2009). *Genome-wide association study identifies variants in the ABO locus associated with susceptibility to pancreatic cancer.* Nature Genetics, 41, 986–990.

Asa, S. L. (2011). *Pancreatic endocrine tumors.* Modern Pathology, 24 Suppl 2, S66–77.

Andea, A., Sarkar, F. & Adsay V. N. (2003). *Clinicopathological correlates of pancreatic intraepithelial neoplasia: a comparative analysis of 82 cases with and 152 cases without pancreatic ductal adenocarcinoma.* Modern Pathology, 16, 996–1006.

Antonarakis, E. S., Carducci, M. A., Eisenberger, M. A., Denmeade, S. R., Slovin, S. F., Jelaca-Maxwell, K., Vincent, M. E., Scher, H. I. & Morris, M. J. (2012). *Phase I rapid dose-escalation study of AGS-1C4D4, a human anti-PSCA (prostate stem cell antigen) monoclonal antibody, in patients with castration-resistant prostate cancer: a PCCTC trial.* Cancer Chemotherapy and Pharmacology, 69, 763–771.

Argani, P., Rosty, C., Reiter, R. E., Wilentz, R. E., Murugesan, S. R., Leach, S. D., Ryu, B., Skinner, H. G., Goggins, M., Jaffee, E. M., Yeo, C. J., Cameron, J. L., Kern, S. E. & Hruban, R. H. (2001). *Discovery of new markers of cancer through serial analysis of gene expression: prostate stem cell antigen is overexpressed in pancreatic adenocarcinoma.* Cancer Research, 61, 4320–4324.

Bafna, S., Kaur, S. & Batra, S. K. (2010). *Membrane-bound mucins: the mechanistic basis for alterations in the growth and survival of cancer cells.* Oncogene, 29, 2893–2904.

Bahrenberg, G., Brauers, A., Joost, H. G. & Jakse, G. (2000). *Reduced expression of PSCA, a member of the LY-6 family of cell surface antigens, in bladder, esophagus, and stomach tumors.* Biochemical and Biophysical Research Communications, 275, 783–788.

Bahrenberg, G., Brauers, A., Joost, H. G. & Jakse, G. (2001). *PSCA expression is regulated by phorbol ester and cell adhesion in the bladder carcinoma cell line RT112.* Cancer Letters, 168, 37–43.

Basturk, O., Caoban, I. & Adsay, N. V. (2010). *Pathologic classification and biological behaviour of pancreatic neoplasia..* In Neoptolemos, J. P., Urrutia, R., Abbruzzese, J. L. & Büchler, M. W. (eds.), *Pancreatic cancer* (pp. 39–70). New York: Springer Science+Busines Media.

Biankin, A. V., Waddell, N., Kassahn, K. S., Gingras, M. C., Muthuswamy, L. B., Johns, A. L., Miller, D. K., Wilson, P. J., Patch, A. M., Wu, J., Chang, D. K., Cowley, M. J., Gardiner, B. B., Song, S., Harliwong, I., Idrisoglu, S., Nourse, C., Nourbakhsh, E., Manning, S., Wani, S., Gongora, M., Pajic, M., Scarlett, C. J., Gill, A. J., Pinho, A. V., Rooman, I., Anderson, M., Holmes, O., Leonard, C., Taylor, D., Wood, S., Xu, Q., Nones, K., Fink, J. L., Christ, A., Bruxner, T., Cloonan, N., Kolle, G., Newell, F., Pinese, M., Mead, R. S., Humphris, J. L., Kaplan, W., Jones, M. D., Colvin, E. K., Nagrial, A. M., Humphrey, E. S., Chou, A., Chin, V. T., Chantrill, L. A., Mawson, A., Samra, J. S., Kench, J. G., Lovell, J. A., Daly, R. J., Merrett, N. D., Toon, C., Epari, K., Nguyen, N. Q., Barbour, A., Zeps, N., Kakkar, N., Zhao, F., Wu, Y. Q., Wang, M., Muzny, D. M., Fisher, W. E., Brunicardi, F. C., Hodges, S. E., Reid, J. G., Drummond, J., Chang, K., Han, Y., Lewis, L. R., Dinh, H., Buhay, C. J., Beck, T., Timms, L., Sam, M., Begley, K., Brown, A., Pai, D., Panchal, A., Buchner, N., De Borja, R., Denroche, R. E., Yung, C. K., Serra, S., Onetto, N., Mukhopadhyay, D., Tsao, M. S., Shaw, P. A., Petersen, G. M., Gallinger, S., Hruban, R. H., Maitra, A., Iacobuzio-Donahue, C. A., Schulick, R.

D., Wolfgang, C. L., Morgan, R. A., Lawlor, R. T., Capelli, P., Corbo, V., Scardoni, M., Tortora, G., Tempero, M. A., Mann, K. M., Jenkins, N. A., Perez-Mancera, P. A., Adams, D. J., Largaespada, D. A., Wessels, L. F., Rust, A. G., Stein, L. D., Tuveson, D. A., Copeland, N. G., Musgrove, E. A., Scarpa, A., Eshleman, J. R., Hudson, T. J., Sutherland, R. L., Wheeler, D. A., Pearson, J. V., McPherson, J. D., Gibbs, R. A. & Grimmond, S. M. (2012). Pancreatic cancer genomes reveal aberrations in axon guidance pathway genes. Nature, 491, 399–405.

Botrugno, O. A., Fayard, E., Annicotte, J. S, Haby, C., Brennan, T., Wendling, O., Tanaka, T., Kodama, T., Thomas, W., Auwerx, J. & Schoonjans, K. (2004). Synergy between LRH-1 and beta-catenin induces G1 cyclin-mediated cell proliferation. Molecular Cell, 15, 499–509.

Brune, K. A., Lau, B., Palmisano, E., Canto, M., Goggins, MG., Hruban, R. H. & Klein, A. P. (2010). Importance of age of onset in pancreatic cancer kindreds. Journal of the National Cancer Institute, 102, 119–126.

Cao, D., Ji, H. & Ronnett, B. M. (2005). Expression of mesothelin, fascin, and prostate stem cell antigen in primary ovarian mucinous tumors and their utility in differentiating primary ovarian mucinous tumors from metastatic pancreatic mucinous carcinomas in the ovary. The International Journal of Gynecological Pathology, 24, 67–72.

Cao, H., Le, D. & Yang, L. X. (2013). Current status in chemotherapy for advanced pancreatic adenocarcinoma. Anticancer Research, 33, 1785–1791.

Casey, J. R., Petranka, J. G., Kottra, J., Fleenor, D. E. & Rosse. W. F. (1994). The structure of the urokinase-type plasminogen activator receptor gene. Blood, 84, 1151–1156.

Chapman, E. J., Kelly, G. & Knowles, M. A. (2008). Genes involved in differentiation, stem cell renewal, and tumorigenesis are modulated in telomerase-immortalized human urothelial cells. Molecular Cancer Research, 6, 1154–1168.

Chari, S. T., Leibson, C. L., Rabe, K. G., Timmons, L. J., Ransom, J., de Andrade, M. & Petersen, G. M. (2008). Pancreatic cancer-associated diabetes mellitus: prevalence and temporal association with diagnosis of cancer. Gastroenterology, 134, 95–101.

Chatterjee, S. & Mayor, S. (2001). The GPI-anchor and protein sorting. Cellular and Molecular Life Sciences, 58, 1969–1987.

de Nooij-van Dalen, A. G., van Dongen, G. A., Smeets, S. J., Nieuwenhuis, E. J., Stigter-van Walsum, M., Snow, G. B. & Brakenhoff, R. H. (2003). Characterization of the human Ly-6 antigens, the newly annotated member Ly-6K included, as molecular markers for head-and-neck squamous cell carcinoma. International Journal of Cancer, 103, 768–774.

Dim, D. C., Jiang, F., Qiu, Q., Li, T., Darwin, P., Rodgers, W. H. & Peng H. Q. (2011). The usefulness of S100P, mesothelin, fascin, prostate stem cell antigen, and 14-3-3 sigma in diagnosing pancreatic adenocarcinoma in cytological specimens obtained by endoscopic ultrasound guided fine-needle aspiration. Diagnostic Cytopathology, doi: 10.1002/dc.21684.

Dutruel, C., Bergmann, F., Rooman, I., Zucknick, M., Weichenhan, D., Geiselhart, L., Kaffenberger, T., Rachakonda, P. S., Bauer, A., Giese, N., Hong, C., Xie, H., Costello, J. F., Hoheisel, J., Kumar, R., Rehli, M., Schirmacher, P., Werner, J., Plass, C., Popanda, O. & Schmezer, P. (2013). Early epigenetic downregulation of WNK2 kinase during pancreatic ductal adenocarcinoma development. Oncogene, 2013 Aug 5. doi: 10.1038/onc.2013.312.

Elsamman, E. M., Fukumori, T., Tanimoto, S., Nakanishi, R., Takahashi, M., Toida, K. & Kanayama, H. O. (2006). The expression of prostate stem cell antigen in human clear cell renal cell carcinoma: a quantitative reverse transcriptase-polymerase chain reaction analysis. BJU International, 98, 668–673.

Feldmann, G., Beaty, R., Hruban, R. H. & Maitra, A. (2007). Molecular genetics of pancreatic intraepithelial neoplasia. Journal of Hepato-Biliary-Pancreatic Surgery, 14, 224–232.

Feldmann, G. & Maitra, A. (2010). Molecular pathology of precursor lesions of pancreatic cancer. In Neoptolemos, J.P., Urrutia, R., Abbruzzese, J.L. & Büchler, M.W. (eds.), Pancreatic cancer (pp. 120–141). New York: Springer Science+Busines Media.

Feng, H. C., Tsao, S. W., Ngan, H. Y., Xue, W. C., Kwan, H. S., Siu, M. K., Liao, X. Y., Wong, E. & Cheung, A. N. (2008). Overexpression of prostate stem cell antigen is associated with gestational trophoblastic neoplasia. Histopathology, 52, 167–174.

Franko, J., Feng, W., Yip, L., Genovese, E. & Moser, A. J. (2010). Non-functional neuroendocrine carcinoma of the pancreas: incidence, tumor biology, and outcomes in 2,158 patients. Journal of Gastrointestinal Surgery, 14, 541–548.

Fukushima, N., Sato, N., Prasad, N., Leach, S. D., Hruban, R. H. & Goggins, M. (2004). Characterization of gene expression in mucinous cystic neoplasms of the pancreas using oligonucleotide microarrays. Oncogene, 23, 9042–9051.

Gapstur, S. M., Jacobs, E. J., Deka, A., McCullough, M. L., Patel, A. V. & Thun, M. J. (2011). Association of alcohol intake with pancreatic cancer mortality in never smokers. Archives of Internal Medicine, 171, 444–451.

Geiger, K. D., Hendruschk, S., Rieber, E. P., Morgenroth, A., Weigle, B., Juratli, T., Senner, V., Schackert, G. & Temme, A. (2011). The prostate stem cell antigen represents a novel glioma-associated antigen. Oncology Reports, 26, 13–21.

Ghayouri, M., Boulware, D., Nasir, A., Strosberg, J., Kvols, L. & Coppola, D. (2010). Activation of the serine/threonine protein kinase Akt in enteropancreatic neuroendocrine tumors. Anticancer Research, 30, 5063–5067.

Goggins, M., Hruban, R. H. & Kern, S. E. (2000). BRCA2 is inactivated late in the development of pancreatic intraepithelial neoplasia: evidence and implications. The American Journal of Pathology, 156, 1767–1771.

Grubbs, E. G., Abdel-Wahab, Z., Tyler, D. S. & Pruitt, S. K. (2006). Utilizing quantitative polymerase chain reaction to evaluate prostate stem cell antigen as a tumor marker in pancreatic cancer. Annals of surgical Oncology, 13, 1645–1654.

Gu, Z., Thomas, G., Yamashiro, J., Shintaku, I. P., Dorey, F., Raitano, A., Witte, O. N., Said, J. W., Loda, M. & Reiter, R. E. (2000). Prostate stem cell antigen (PSCA) expression increases with high gleason score, advanced stage and bone metastasis in prostate cancer. Oncogene, 19, 1288–1296.

Gu, Z., Yamashiro, J., Kono, E. & Reiter, R. E. (2005). Anti-prostate stem cell antigen monoclonal antibody 1G8 induces cell death in vitro and inhibits tumor growth in vivo via a Fc-independent mechanism. Cancer Research, 65, 9495–9500.

Harada, T., Chelala, C., Bhakta, V., Chaplin, T., Caulee, K., Baril, P., Young, B. D. & Lemoine, N. R. (2008). Genome-wide DNA copy number analysis in pancreatic cancer using high-density single nucleotide polymorphism arrays. Oncogene, 27, 1951–1960.

Harewood, G. C. & Wiersema, M. J. (2002). Endosonography-guided fine needle aspiration biopsy in the evaluation of pancreatic masses. American Journal of Gastroenterology, 97, 1386–1391.

Hingorani, S. R., Petricoin, E. F., Maitra, A., Rajapakse, V., King, C., Jacobetz, M. A., Ross, S., Conrads, T. P., Veenstra, T. D., Hitt, B. A., Kawaguchi, Y., Johann, D., Liotta, L. A., Crawford, H. C., Putt, M. E., Jacks, T., Wright, C. V., Hruban, R. H., Lowy, A. M. & Tuveson, D. A. (2003). Preinvasive and invasive ductal pancreatic cancer and its early detection in the mouse. Cancer Cell, 4, 437–450.

Hong, S. M., Vincent, A., Kanda, M., Leclerc, J., Omura, N., Borges, M., Klein, A. P., Canto, M. I., Hruban, R. H. & Goggins, M. (2012). Genome-wide somatic copy number alterations in low-grade PanINs and IPMNs from individuals with a family history of pancreatic cancer. Clinical Cancer Research, 18, 4303–4312.

Hruska, M., Keefe, J., Wert, D., Tekinay, A. B., Hulce, J. J., Ibañez-Tallon, I. & Nishi, R. (2009). Prostate stem cell antigen is an endogenous lynx1-like prototoxin that antagonizes alpha7-containing nicotinic receptors and prevents programmed cell death of parasympathetic neurons. Journal of Neuroscience, 29, 14847–14854.

Jain, A., Lam, A., Vivanco, I., Carey, M. F. & Reiter, R. E. (2002). Identification of an androgen-dependent enhancer within the prostate stem cell antigen gene. Molecular Endocrinology, 16, 2323–2337.

Jiao, Y., Shi, C., Edil, B. H., de Wilde, R. F., Klimstra, D. S., Maitra, A., Schulick, R. D., Tang, L. H., Wolfgang, C. L., Choti, M. A., Velculescu, V. E., Diaz, L. A. Jr, Vogelstein, B., Kinzler, K. W., Hruban, R. H. & Papadopoulos, N. (2011). DAXX/ATRX, MEN1, and mTOR pathway genes are frequently altered in pancreatic neuroendocrine tumors. Science, 331, 1199–1203.

Jones, S., Zhang, X., Parsons, D. W., Lin, J. C., Leary, R. J., Angenendt, P., Mankoo, P., Carter, H., Kamiyama, H., Jimeno, A., Hong, S. M., Fu, B., Lin, M. T., Calhoun, E. S., Kamiyama, M., Walter, K., Nikolskaya, T., Nikolsky, Y., Hartigan, J., Smith, D. R., Hidalgo, M., Leach, S. D., Klein, A. P., Jaffee, E. M., Goggins, M., Maitra, A., Iacobuzio-Donahue, C., Eshleman, J. R., Kern, S. E., Hruban, R. H., Karchin, R., Papadopoulos, N., Parmigiani, G., Vogelstein, B., Vel-

culescu, V. E. & Kinzler, K. W. (2008). Core signaling pathways in human pancreatic cancers revealed by global genomic analyses. Science, 321, 1801–1806.

Kawaguchi, T., Sho, M., Tojo, T., Yamato, I., Nomi, T., Hotta, K., Hamada, K., Suzaki, Y., Sugiura, S., Kushibe, K., Nakajima, Y. & Taniguchi, S. (2010). Clinical significance of prostate stem cell antigen expression in non-small cell lung cancer. Japanese Journal of Clinical Oncology, 40, 319–326.

Klimstra, D. S., Hruban, R. H. & Pitman, M. B. (2007). Pancreas. In Mills S. E. (ed.), Histology for pathologists (pp. 723–760). Philadelphia: Lippincot Williams & Wilkins, Wolters Kluwer business.

Korínek, V., Stefanová, I., Angelisová, P., Hilgert, I. & Horejsí, V. (1991). The human leucocyte antigen CD48 (MEM-102) is closely related to the activation marker Blast-1. Immunogenetics, 33, 108–112.

Krausch, M., Raffel, A., Anlauf, M., Schott, M., Willenberg, H., Lehwald, N., Hafner, D., Cupisti, K., Eisenberger, C. F. & Knoefel, W. T. (2011). Loss of PTEN expression in neuroendocrine pancreatic tumors. Hormone and Metabolic Research, 43, 865–871.

Krymskaya, V. P. & Goncharova, E. A. (2009). PI3K/mTORC1 activation in hamartoma syndromes: therapeutic prospects. Cell Cycle, 8, 403–413.

Kufe, D. W. (2009). Mucins in cancer: function, prognosis and therapy. Nature Review Cancer, 9, 874–885.

Klein, A. P., Brune, K. A., Petersen, G. M., Goggins, M., Tersmette, A. C., Offerhaus, G. J., Griffin, C., Cameron, J. L., Yeo, C. J., Kern, S. & Hruban, R. H. (2004). Prospective risk of pancreatic cancer in familial pancreatic cancer kindreds. Cancer Research, 64, 2634–2638.

Li, C., Wu, J. J., Hynes, M., Dosch, J., Sarkar, B., Welling, T. H., Pasca di Magliano, M. & Simeone, D. M. (2011). c-Met is a marker of pancreatic cancer stem cells and therapeutic target. Gastroenterology, 141, 2218–2227.

Liu, H., Shi, J., Anandan, V., Wang, H. L., Diehl, D., Blansfield, J., Gerhard, G. & Lin, F. (2012). Reevaluation and identification of the best immunohistochemical panel (pVHL, Maspin, S100P, IMP-3) for ductal adenocarcinoma of the pancreas. Archives of Pathology & Laboratory Medicine, 36, 601–609.

Low, M. G. & Finean, J. B. (1977). Release of alkaline phosphatase from membranes by a phosphatidylinositol-specific phospholipase C. Biochemical Journal, 167, 281–284.

Low, S. K., Kuchiba, A., Zembutsu, H., Saito, A., Takahashi, A., Kubo, M., Daigo, Y., Kamatani, N., Chiku, S., Totsuka, H., Ohnami, S., Hirose, H., Shimada, K., Okusaka, T., Yoshida, T., Nakamura, Y. & Sakamoto, H. (2010). Genome-wide association study of pancreatic cancer in Japanese population. PLoS One, 5, e11824.

Lukyanchuk, V. V., Friess, H., Kleeff, J., Osinsky, S. P., Ayuni, E., Candinas, D. & Roggo, A. (2003). Detection of circulating tumor cells by cytokeratin 20 and prostate stem cell antigen RT-PCR in blood of patients with gastrointestinal cancers. Anticancer Research, 23, 2711–2716.

Maitra, A., Adsay, N. V., Argani, P., Iacobuzio-Donahue, C., De Marzo, A., Cameron, J. L., Yeo, C. J. & Hruban, R. H. (2003). Multicomporent analysis of the pancreatic adenocarcinoma progression model using a pancreatic intraepithelial neoplasia tissue microarray. Modern Pathology, 16, 902–912.

Marra, E., Uva, P., Viti, V., Simonelli, V., Dogliotti, E., De Rinaldis, E., Lahm, A., La Monica, N., Nicosia, A., Ciliberto, G. & Palombo, F. (2010). Growth delay of human bladder cancer cells by Prostate Stem Cell Antigen downregulation is associated with activation of immune signaling pathways. BMC Cancer, 10, 129.

McCarthy, D. M., Maitra, A., Argani, P., Rader, A. E., Faigel, D. O., Van Heek, N. T., Hruban, R. H. & Wilentz, R. E. (2003). Novel markers of pancreatic adenocarcinoma in fine-needle aspiration: mesothelin and prostate stem cell antigen labeling increases accuracy in cytologically borderline cases. Applied Immunohistochemistry & Molecular Morphology, 11, 238–243.

McKay, J. D., Hung, R. J., Gaborieau, V., Boffetta, P., Chabrier, A., Byrnes, G., Zaridze, D., Mukeria, A., Szczenia-Dabrowska, N., Lissowska, J., Rudnai, P., Fabianova, E., Mates, D., Bencko, V., Foretova, L., Janout, V., McLaughlin, J., Shepherd, F., Montpetit, A., Narod, S., Krokan, H. E., Skorpen, F., Elvestad, M. B., Vatten, L., Njølstad, I., Axelsson, T., Chen, C., Goodman, G., Barnett, M., Loomis, M. M., Lubiñski, J., Matyjasik, J,. Lener, M., Oszutowska, D., Field, J., Liloglou, T., Xinarianos, G., Cassidy, A., Vineis, P., Clavel-Chapelon, F., Palli, D., Tumino, R., Krogh,

V., Panico, S., González, C. A., Ramón Quirós, J., Martínez, C., Navarro, C., Ardanaz, E., Larrañaga, N., Kham, K. T., Key, T., Bueno-de-Mesquita, H. B., Peeters, P. H., Trichopoulou, A., Linseisen, J., Boeing, H., Hallmans, G., Overvad, K., Tjønneland, A., Kumle, M., Riboli, E., Zelenika, D., Boland, A., Delepine, M., Foglio, M., Lechner, D., Matsuda, F., Blanche, H., Gut, I., Heath, S., Lathrop, M. & Brennan, P. (2008). Lung cancer susceptibility locus at 5p15.33. Nature Genetics, 40, 1404–1406.

Moore, M. L., Teitell, M. A., Kim, Y., Watabe, T., Reiter, R. E., Witte, O. N. & Dubey, P. (2008). Deletion of PSCA increases metastasis of TRAMP-induced prostate tumors without altering primary tumor formation. Prostate, 68, 139–151.

Morris, M. J., Eisenberger, M. A., Pili, R., Denmeade, S. R., Rathkopf, D., Slovin, S. F., Farrelly, J., Chudow, J. J., Vincent, M., Scher, H. I. & Carducci, M. A. (2012). A phase I/IIA study of AGS-PSCA for castration-resistant prostate cancer. Annals of Oncology, 23, 2714–2719.

Murphy, S. J., Hart, S. N., Lima, J. F., Kipp, B. R., Klebig, M., Winters, J. L., Szabo, C., Zhang, L., Eckloff, B. W., Petersen, G. M., Scherer, S. E., Gibbs, R. A., McWilliams, R. R., Vasmatzis, G. & Couch, F. J. (2013). Genetic Alterations Associated With Progression From Pancreatic Intraepithelial Neoplasia to Invasive Pancreatic Tumor. Gastroenterology, doi: 10.1053/j.gastro.2013.07.049.

Oliveira-Cunha, M., Byers, R. J. & Siriwardena, A. K. (2011). Poly(A) RT-PCR measurement of diagnostic genes in pancreatic juice in pancreatic cancer. British Journal of Cancer, 104, 514–519.

Ono, H., Hiraoka, N., Lee, Y. S., Woo, S. M., Lee, W. J., Choi, I. J., Saito, A., Yanagihara, K., Kanai, Y., Ohnami, S., Chiwaki, F., Sasaki, H., Sakamoto, H., Yoshida, T. & Saeki, N. (2012a). Prostate stem cell antigen, a presumable organ-dependent tumor suppressor gene, is down-regulated in gallbladder carcinogenesis. Genes Chromosomes and Cancer, 51, 30–41.

Ono, H., Yanagihara, K., Sakamoto, H., Yoshida, T. & Saeki, N. (2012b). Prostate stem cell antigen gene is expressed in islets of pancreas. Anatomy & Cell Biology, 45, 149–154.

Petersen, G. M., de Andrade, M., Goggins, M., Hruban, R. H., Bondy, M., Korczak, J. F., Gallinger, S., Lynch, H. T., Syngal, S., Rabe, K. G., Seminara, D. & Klein, A. P. (2006). Pancreatic cancer genetic epidemiology consortium. Cancer Epidemiology, Biomarkers & Prevention, 15, 704–710.

Petersen, G. M., Amundadottir, L., Fuchs, C. S., Kraft, P., Stolzenberg-Solomon, R. Z., Jacobs, K. B., Arslan, A. A., Bueno-de-Mesquita, H. B., Gallinger, S., Gross, M., Helzlsouer, K., Holly, E. A., Jacobs, E. J., Klein, A. P., LaCroix, A., Li, D., Mandelson M. T., Olson S. H., Risch H. A., Zheng, W., Albanes, D., Bamlet, W. R., Berg, C. D., Boutron-Ruault, M. C., Buring, J. E., Bracci, P. M., Canzian, F., Clipp, S., Cotterchio, M., de Andrade, M., Duell, E. J., Gaziano, J. M., Giovannucci, E. L., Goggins, M., Hallmans, G., Hankinson, S. E., Hassan, M., Howard, B., Hunter, D. J., Hutchinson, A., Jenab, M., Kaaks, R., Kooperberg, C., Krogh, V., Kurtz, R. C., Lynch, S. M., McWilliams, R. R., Mendelsohn, J. B., Michaud, D. S., Parikh, H., Patel, A. V., Peeters, P. H., Rajkovic, A., Riboli, E., Rodriguez, L., Seminara, D., Shu, X. O., Thomas, G., Tjønneland, A., Tobias, G. S., Trichopoulos, D., Van Den Eeden, S. K., Virtamo, J., Wactawski-Wende, J., Wang, Z., Wolpin, B. M., Yu, H., Yu, K., Zeleniuch-Jacquotte, A., Fraumeni, J. F. Jr., Hoover, R. N., Hartge, P. & Chanock, S. J. (2010). A genome-wide association study identifies pancreatic cancer susceptibility loci on chromosomes 13q22.1, 1q32.1 and 5p15.33. Nature Genetics, 42, 224–228.

Pierce, B. L. & Ahsan, H. (2011). Genome-wide "pleiotropy scan" identifies HNF1A region as a novel pancreatic cancer susceptibility locus. Cancer Research, 71, 4352–4358.

Powell, S. K., Cunningham, B. A., Edelman, G. M. & Rodriguez-Boulan, E. (1991). Targeting of transmembrane and GPI-anchored forms of N-CAM to opposite domains of a polarized epithelial cell. Nature, 353, 76–77.

Rafnar, T., Sulem, P., Stacey, S. N., Geller, F., Gudmundsson, J., Sigurdsson, A., Jakobsdottir, M., Helgadottir, H., Thorlacius, S., Aben, K. K., Blöndal, T., Thorgeirsson, T. E., Thorleifsson, G., Kristjansson, K., Thorisdottir, K., Ragnarsson, R., Sigurgeirsson, B., Skuladottir, H., Gudbjartsson, T., Isaksson, H. J., Einarsson, G. V., Benediktsdottir, K. R., Agnarsson, B. A., Olafsson, K., Salvarsdottir, A., Bjarnason, H., Asgeirsdottir, M., Kristinsson, K. T., Matthiasdottir, S., Sveinsdottir, S. G., Polidoro, S., Höiom, V., Botella-Estrada, R., Hemminki, K., Rudnai, P., Bishop, D. T., Campagna, M., Kellen, E., Zeegers, M. P., de Verdier, P., Ferrer, A., Isla, D., Vidal, M. J., Andres, R., Saez, B., Juberias, P., Banzo, J., Navarrete, S., Tres, A., Kan, D., Lindblom, A., Gurzau, E., Koppova, K., de Vegt, F., Schalken, J. A., van der Heijden, H. F., Smit, H. J., Termeer, R. A., Oosterwijk, E., van Hooij, O., Nagore, E., Porru, S., Steineck, G.,

Hansson, J., Buntinx, F., Catalona, W. J., Matullo, G., Vineis, P., Kiltie, A. E., Mayordomo, J. I., Kumar, R., Kiemeney, L. A., Frigge, M. L., Jonsson, T., Saemundsson, H., Barkardottir, R. B., Jonsson, E., Jonsson, S., Olafsson, J. H., Gulcher, J. R., Masson, G., Gudbjartsson, D. F., Kong, A., Thorsteinsdottir, U. & Stefansson, K. (2009). Sequence variants at the TERT-CLPTM1L locus associate with many cancer types. Nature Genetics, 41, 221–227.

Reid, R. A., Bronson, D. D., Young, K. M. & Hemperly, J. J. (1994). Identification and characterization of the human cell adhesion molecule contactin. Brain Research Molecular Brain Research, 21, 1–8.

Reiter, R. E., Gu, Z., Watabe, T., Thomas, G., Szigeti, K., Davis, E., Wahl, M., Nisitani, S., Yamashiro, J., Le Beau, M. M., Loda, M. & Witte, O. N. (1998). Prostate stem cell antigen: a cell surface marker overexpressed in prostate cancer. Proceedings of the National Academy of Sciences of the United States of America, 95, 1735–1740.

Rijnboutt, S., Jansen, G., Posthuma, G., Hynes, J. B., Schornagel, J. H. & Strous, G. J. (1996). Endocytosis of GPI-linked membrane folate receptor-alpha. Journal of Cell Biology, 132, 35–47.

Roberts, W. L. & Rosenberry, T. L. (1985). Identification of covalently attached fatty acids in the hydrophobic membrane-binding domain of human erythrocyte acetylcholinesterase. Biochemical and Biophysical Research Communications, 133, 621–627.

Saeki, N., Ono, H., Sakamoto, H. & Yoshida, T. (2013). Genetic factors related to gastric cancer susceptibility identified using a genome-wide association study. Cancer Science, 104, 1–8.

Sakamoto, H., Yoshimura, K., Saeki, N., Katai, H., Shimoda, T., Matsuno, Y., Saito, D., Sugimura, H., Tanioka, F., Kato, S., Matsukura, N., Matsuda, N., Nakamura, T., Hyodo, I., Nishina, T., Yasui, W., Hirose, H., Hayashi, M., Toshiro, E., Ohnami, S., Sekine, A., Sato, Y., Totsuka, H., Ando, M., Takemura, R., Takahashi, Y., Ohdaira, M., Aoki, K., Honmyo, I., Chiku, S., Aoyagi, K., Sasaki, H., Ohnami, S., Yanagihara, K., Yoon, K. A., Kook, M. C., Lee, Y. S., Park, S. R., Kim, C. G., Choi, I. J., Yoshida, T., Nakamura, Y. & Hirohashi, S. (2008). Genetic variation in PSCA is associated with susceptibility to diffuse-type gastric cancer. Nature Genetics, 40, 730–740.

Sato, N., Maitra, A., Fukushima, N., van Heek, N. T., Matsubayashi, H., Iacobuzio-Donahue, C. A,. Rosty, C. & Goggins, M. (2003). Frequent hypomethylation of multiple genes overexpressed in pancreatic ductal adenocarcinoma. Cancer Research, 63, 4158–4166.

Shete, S., Hosking, F. J., Robertson, L. B., Dobbins, S. E., Sanson, M., Malmer, B., Simon, M., Marie, Y., Boisselier, B., Delattre, J. Y., Hoang-Xuan, K., El Hallani, S., Idbaih, A., Zelenika, D., Andersson, U., Henriksson, R., Bergenheim, A. T., Feychting, M., Lönn, S., Ahlbom, A., Schramm, J., Linnebank, M., Hemminki, K., Kumar, R., Hepworth, S. J., Price, A., Armstrong, G., Liu,Y., Gu, X., Yu, R., Lau, C., Schoemaker, M., Muir, K., Swerdlow, A., Lathrop, M., Bondy, M. & Houlston, R. S. (2009). Genome-wide association study identifies five susceptibility loci for glioma. Nature Genetics, 41, 899–904.

Smith, J. P., Harms, J. F., Matters, G. L., McGovern, C. O., Ruggiero, F. M., Liao, J., Fino, K. K., Ortega, E. E., Gilius, E. L. & Phillips, J. A. 3rd. (2012). A single nucleotide polymorphism of the cholecystokinin-B receptor predicts risk for pancreatic cancer. Cancer Biology & Therapy, 13, 164–174.

Stacey, S. N., Sulem, P., Masson, G., Gudjonsson, S. A., Thorleifsson, G., Jakobsdottir, M., Sigurdsson, A., Gudbjartsson, D. F., Sigurgeirsson, B., Benediktsdottir, K. R., Thorisdottir, K., Ragnarsson, R., Scherer, D., Hemminki, K., Rudnai, P., Gurzau, E., Koppova, K., Botella-Estrada, R., Soriano, V., Juberias, P., Saez, B., Gilaberte, Y., Fuentelsaz, V., Corredera, C., Grasa, M., Höiom, V., Lindblom, A., Bonenkamp, J. J., van Rossum, M. M., Aben, K. K., de Vries, E., Santinami, M., Di Mauro, M. G., Maurichi, A., Wendt, J., Hochleitner, P., Pehamberger, H., Gudmundsson, J., Magnusdottir, D. N., Gretarsdottir, S., Holm, H., Steinthorsdottir, V., Frigge, M. L., Blondal, T., Saemundsdottir, J., Bjarnason, H., Kristjansson, K., Bjornsdottir, G., Okamoto, I., Rivoltini, L., Rodolfo, M., Kiemeney, L. A., Hansson, J., Nagore, E., Mayordomo, J. I., Kumar, R., Karagas, M. R., Nelson, H. H., Gulcher, J. R., Rafnar, T., Thorsteinsdottir, U., Olafsson, J. H., Kong, A. & Stefansson, K. (2009). New common variants affecting susceptibility to basal cell carcinoma. Nature Genetics, 41, 909–914.

Stipp, C. S., Litwack, E. D. & Lander, A. D. (1994). Cerebroglycan: an integral membrane heparan sulfate proteoglycan that is unique to the developing nervous system and expressed specifically during neuronal differentiation. Journal of Cell Biology, 124, 149–960.

Stolzenberg-Solomon, R. Z., Cross, A. J., Silverman, D. T., Schairer, C., Thompson, F. E., Kipnis, V., Subar, A. F., Hollenbeck, A., Schatzkin, A. & Sinha, R. (2007). Meat and meat-mutagen intake and pancreatic cancer risk in the NIH-AARP cohort. Cancer Epidemiology, Biomarkers & Prevention, 16, 2664–2675.

Struyk, A. F., Canoll, P. D., Wolfgang, M. J., Rosen, C. L., D'Eustachio, P. & Salzer, J. L. (1995). Cloning of neurotrimin defines a new subfamily of differentially expressed neural cell adhesion molecules. Journal of Neuroscience, 15, 2141–2156.

Suraneni, M. V., Schneider-Broussard, R., Moore, J. R., Davis, T. C., Maldonado, C. J., Li, H., Newman, R. A., Kusewitt, D., Hu, J., Yang, P. & Tang, D. G. (2010). Transgenic expression of 15-lipoxygenase 2 (15-LOX2) in mouse prostate leads to hyperplasia and cell senescence. Oncogene, 29, 4261–4275.

Tanaka, M., Komatsu, N., Terakawa, N., Yanagimoto, Y., Oka, M., Sasada, T., Mine, T., Gouhara, S., Shichijo, S., Okuda, S. & Itoh, K. (2007). Increased levels of IgG antibodies against peptides of the prostate stem cell antigen in the plasma of pancreatic cancer patients. Oncology Report, 18, 161–166.

Tang, S., Bonaroti, J., Unlu, S., Liang, X., Tang, D., Zeh, H. J. & Lotze, M. T. (2013). Sweating the small stuff: microRNAs and genetic changes define pancreatic cancer. Pancreas, 42, 740–759.

Tanikawa, C., Urabe, Y., Matsuo, K., Kubo, M., Takahashi, A., Ito, H., Tajima, K., Kamatani, N., Nakamura, Y. & Matsuda, K. (2012). A genome-wide association study identifies two susceptibility loci for duodenal ulcer in the Japanese population. Nature Genetics, 44, 430–434,

Tran, C. P., Lin, C., Yamashiro, J. & Reiter, R. E. (2002). Prostate stem cell antigen is a marker of late intermediate prostate epithelial cells. Molecular Cancer Research, 1, 113–121.

Treanor, J. J., Goodman, L., de Sauvage, F., Stone, D. M., Poulsen, K. T., Beck, C. D., Gray, C., Armanini, M. P., Pollock, R. A., Hefti, F., Phillips, H. S., Goddard, A., Moore, M. W., Buj-Bello, A., Davies, A. M., Asai, N., Takahashi, M., Vandlen, R., Henderson, C. E. & Rosenthal, A. (1996). Characterization of a multicomponent receptor for GDNF. Nature, 382, 80–83.

Trikudanathan, G., Philip, A., Dasanu, C. A. & Baker, W. L. (2011). Association between Helicobacter pylori infection and pancreatic cancer. A cumulative meta-analysis. Journal of the Pancreas, 12, 26–31.

Tse, A. G., Barclay, A. N., Watts, A. & Williams, A.F. (1985). A glycophospholipid tail at the carboxyl terminus of the Thy-1 glycoprotein of neurons and thymocytes. Science, 230, 1003–1008.

Vincent, A., Herman, J., Schulick, R., Hruban, R. H. & Goggins, M. (2011). Pancreatic cancer. Lancet, 378, 607–620.

Watabe, T., Lin, M., Ide, H., Donjacour, A. A., Cunha, G. R., Witte, O. N. & Reiter, R. E. (2002). Growth, regeneration, and tumorigenesis of the prostate activates the PSCA promoter. Proceedings of the National Academy of Sciences of the United States of America, 99, 401–406.

Wang, Y., Broderick, P., Webb, E., Wu, X., Vijayakrishnan, J., Matakidou, A., Qureshi, M., Dong, Q., Gu, X., Chen, W. V., Spitz, M. R., Eisen, T., Amos, C.I. & Houlston, R. S. (2008). Common 5p15.33 and 6p21.33 variants influence lung cancer risk. Nature Genetics, 40, 1407–1409.

Wang, X., Liu, Y., Ren, H., Yuan, Z., Li, S., Sheng, J., Zhao, T., Chen, Y., Liu, F., Wang, F., Huang, H. & Hao, J. (2011). Polymorphisms in the hypoxia-inducible factor-1α gene confer susceptibility to pancreatic cancer. Cancer Biology & Therapy, 12, 383–387.

Wente, M. N., Jain, A., Kono, E., Berberat, P. O., Giese, T., Reber, H. A., Friess, H., Büchler, M. W., Reiter, R. E. & Hines, O. J. (2005). Prostate stem cell antigen is a putative target for immunotherapy in pancreatic cancer. Pancreas, 31, 119–125.

Wilentz, R. E., Geradts, J., Maynard, R., Offerhaus, G. J., Kang, M., Goggins, M., Yeo, C. J., Kern, S. E. & Hruban, R. H. (1998). Inactivation of the p16 (INK4A) tumor-suppressor gene in pancreatic duct lesions: loss of intranuclear expression. Cancer Research, 58, 4740–4744.

Wilentz, R. E., Iacobuzio-Donahue, C. A., Argani, P., McCarthy, D. M., Parsons, J. L., Yeo, C. J., Kern, S. E. & Hruban, R. H. (2000). Loss of expression of Dpc4 in pancreatic intraepithelial neoplasia: evidence that DPC4 inactivation occurs late in neoplastic progression. Cancer Research, 60, 2002–2006.

Wolpin, B. M., O'Reilly, E. M., Ko, Y. J., Blaszkowsky, L. S., Rarick, M., Rocha-Lima, C. M., Ritch, P., Chan, E., Spratlin, J., Macarulla, T., McWhirter, E., Pezet, D., Lichinitser, M., Roman, L., Hartford, A., Morrison, K., Jackson, L., Vincent, M., Reyno, L. & Hidalgo, M. (2013). Global, multicenter, randomized, phase II trial of gemcitabine and gemcitabine plus AGS-1C4D4 in patients with previously untreated, metastatic pancreatic cancer. Annals of Oncology, 24, 1792–1801.

Wu, C., Miao, X., Huang, L., Che, X., Jiang, G., Yu, D., Yang, X., Cao, G., Hu, Z., Zhou, Y., Zuo, C., Wang, C., Zhang, X., Zhou, Y., Yu, X., Dai, W., Li, Z., Shen, H., Liu, L., Chen, Y., Zhang, S., Wang, X., Zhai, K., Chang, J., Liu, Y., Sun, M., Cao, W., Gao, J., Ma, Y., Zheng, X., Cheung, S. T., Jia, Y., Xu, J., Tan, W., Zhao, P., Wu, T., Wang, C. & Lin, D. (2011). Genome-wide association study identifies five loci associated with susceptibility to pancreatic cancer in Chinese populations. Nature Genetics, 44, 62–66.

Wu, X., Ye, Y., Kiemeney, L. A., Sulem, P., Rafnar, T., Matullo, G., Seminara, D., Yoshida, T., Saeki, N., Andrew, A. S., Dinney, C. P., Czerniak, B., Zhang, Z. F., Kiltie, A. E., Bishop, D. T., Vineis, P., Porru, S., Buntinx, F., Kellen, E., Zeegers, M. P., Kumar, R., Rudnai, P., Gurzau, E., Koppova, K., Mayordomo, J. I., Sanchez, M., Saez, B., Lindblom, A., de Verdier, P., Steineck, G., Mills, G. B., Schned, A., Guarrera, S., Polidoro, S., Chang, S. C., Lin, J., Chang, D. W., Hale, K. S., Majewski, T., Grossman, H. B., Thorlacius, S., Thorsteinsdottir, U., Aben, K. K., Witjes, J. A., Stefansson, K., Amos, C. I., Karagas, M. R. & Gu, J. (2009). Genetic variation in the prostate stem cell antigen gene PSCA confers susceptibility to urinary bladder cancer. Nature Genetics, 41, 991–995.

Yamamoto, K., Okamoto, A., Isonishi, S., Ochiai, K. & Ohtake, Y. (2001). A novel gene, CRR9, which was up-regulated in CDDP-resistant ovarian tumor cell line, was associated with apoptosis. Biochemal and Biophysical Research Communications, 280, 1148–1154.

Zekri, M., Harb, J., Bernard, S., Poirier, G., Devaux, C. & Meflah, K. (1989). Differences in the release of 5'-nucleotidase and alkaline phosphatase from plasma membrane of several cell types by PI-PLC. Comparative Biochemistry and Physiology. B, Comparative biochemistry, 93, 673–679.

Zhang, Y., Morris, J. P. 4th, Yan, W., Schofield, H. K., Gurney, A., Simeone, D. M., Millar, S. E., Hoey, T., Hebrok, M. & Pasca di Magliano, M. (2013a). Canonical Wnt signaling is required for pancreatic carcinogenesis. Cancer Research, 73, 4909–4922.

Zhang, J., Francois, R., Iyer, R., Seshadri, M., Zajac-Kaye, M. & Hochwald, S. N. (2013b). Current understanding of the molecular biology of pancreatic neuroendocrine tumors. Journal of the National Cancer Institute, 105, 1005–1017.

Zhigang, Z. & Wenlu, S. (2005). Complete androgen ablation suppresses prostate stem cell antigen (PSCA) mRNA expression in human prostate carcinoma. Prostate, 65, 299–305.

Zhou, C.F., Ji, J., Yuan, F., Shi, M., Zhang, J., Liu, B. Y. & Zhu, Z. G. (2011). mTOR activation in well differentiated pancreatic neuroendocrine tumors: a retrospective study on 34 cases. Hepatogastroenterology, 58, 2140–2103.

Zinc, Zinc Transporters and Type 2 Diabetes

Stephen A Myers
Collaborative Research Network
School of Health Sciences
Federation University Australia, Australia

Alex Nield
Collaborative Research Network
School of Health Sciences
Federation University Australia, Australia

1   Introduction

Insulin resistance is an important characteristic of Type 2 Diabetes (T2D) and is commonly associated with obesity, hypertension and cardiovascular disease (Carsten, 2000; Hulver and Lynis, 2004). Insulin resistance reduces insulin-stimulated glucose disposal due to multiple post-receptor intracellular defects in insulin signaling with subsequent reductions in glucose transport, glucose oxidation and incorporation of glucose into glycogen (Abdul-Ghani and DeFronzo, 2010; Peppa *et al.*, 2010). The intracellular post-receptor regulatory effects of insulin include the regulation of the cellular glucose transport system, adaptive changes in gene expression and subsequent biosynthesis and action of the enzymes involved in the preservation of metabolism, and the modulation of genes that contribute to increased pro-mitotic, proliferative and anti-apoptotic activity of cells (Taton *et al.*, 2010). Accordingly, the reduced activity of insulin action in any, or all of these post-receptor regulatory actions is insulin resistance. Given that insulin resistance usually precedes the development of T2D and is a major component of the progressive nature of this disease (Pagel-Langenickel *et al.*, 2010), understanding the pathophysiology of insulin resistance will enable the development of therapeutic strategies to prevent or manage disease progression. Although many theories have been forthcoming, the primary mechanism of insulin resistance remains largely elusive.

In this context, research on T2D has revealed an exciting role for zinc signaling in this disease. Ionic zinc has insulin "mimetic" activity where it is involved in insulin receptor signal transduction and insulin storage, secretion and distribution (Fukada *et al.*, 2011). In peripheral tissue such as fat and muscle, zinc ions facilitate insulin-induced glucose transport and glycaemic control through the regulation of essential pathways involved in glucose homeostasis (Jansen *et al.*, 2009). However there is insufficient information on how the concentration of free ionic zinc in cells is controlled. The proteins that transport zinc presumably facilitate cell signaling processes that contribute to glycaemic control in peripheral tissue through the modulation of ionic zinc concentrations in the cytosol. For example, aberrant subcellular partitioning or signaling of zinc could contribute to altered insulin responsiveness (Mocchegiani *et al.*, 2008) and therefore facilitate insulin resistance. However, how zinc transporter proteins effectively facilitate zinc flux and contribute to cellular metabolism is not clear.

Accordingly, this review will discuss the zinc transporter gene family and what is currently known regarding their various roles in cellular signaling in disease processes with a particular focus on T2D. It is envisaged that understanding the potential relevance of dysfunctional ionic zinc partitioning in diseases such as T2D will created opportunities for translating basic research into clinically important applications. Therefore, knowing the specific molecular targets of ionic zinc in cellular signaling in the context of insulin resistance and T2D will provide opportunities to develop novel therapeutic approaches to prevent disease progression or treat this disease.

2   Type 2 Diabetes Mellitus

Type 2 Diabetes (T2D) is a progressive and chronic metabolic disease that is rapidly increasing in prevalence worldwide. In 2030, it is predicted that adults diagnosed with this disorder will rise from the current count of 246 million to 552 million (Pal and McCarthy, 2013). Patients with T2D are predisposed to a number of microvascular and macrovascular complications and therefore have a significant increase in mortality and morbidity (Shin *et al.*, 2012). Consequently, T2D is an important global public health problem due to the considerable cost of appropriate disease control and management of chronic complications (Shin *et al.*, 2012). For example, diabetes cost the global economy nearly US $50 billion in 2010 and that figure is expected to increase to US $745 billion in 2030 (Bloom *et al.*, 2011).

Lifestyle factors that lead to obesity, in particular poor nutrition and reduced physical activity, contribute to the development of T2D. In this context, for the prevention of factors leading to T2D, it is vital that blood glucose levels are maintained within a normal range (i.e. fasting blood glucose of less than 100 mg/dL and a 2 hour postprandial blood glucose of less than 140 mg/dL are usually considered normal) (Nyenwe *et al.*, 2011). Medical nutrition therapy and exercise programs are the basis for managing T2D, however the majority of patients with this disease also require pharmacotherapy to manage this disorder successfully (Kourtoglou, 2011).

T2D results when the endocrine pancreas fails to meet increasing metabolic demands and compensate for peripheral tissue insulin resistance (Osto *et al.*, 2013) and usually develops in patients with pancreatic β-cell dysfunction in the presence of insulin resistance in peripheral tissue such as liver, fat and muscle (Lin and Sun, 2010). Insulin resistance is described as a reduced and/or delayed response to insulin in peripheral tissue and is generally associated with dysfunctional insulin signaling rather than the production of insulin (Lin and Sun, 2010). Even in the absence of T2D, insulin resistance is often associated with hypertension, obesity, polycystic ovarian syndrome, dyslipidemia and atherosclerosis (Saltiel and Pessin, 2002). In T2D, the majority of patients will eventually require the administration of insulin, either alone or in combination with other antidiabetic agents to control their diabetes (Kourtoglou, 2011).

Recently there has been a growing interest in the role of zinc signaling in T2D based on the fact that reduced levels of serum zinc have been observed in patients with diabetes (Basaki *et al.*, 2012; Jansen *et al.*, 2009; Jansen *et al.*, 2012; Zhao *et al.*, 2011) and zinc supplementation in several animal models of T2D and human patients showed improved glycaemic control (Adachi *et al.*, 2006; Jansen *et al.*, 2009; Jayawardena *et al.*, 2012; Liu *et al.*, 2011a; Pathak *et al.*, 2011; Wang *et al.*, 2012). The clinical relevance of zinc in T2D is further emphasized by recent developments in our understanding of dysregulation of zinc partitioning in this disease (Mocchegiani *et al.*, 2008). T2D is characterized by defects in both insulin secretion and insulin sensitivity, of which zinc is particularly important based on its role in insulin receptor signal transduction (Haase *et al.*, 2005a, 2005b), and insulin storage and secretion (Figlewicz *et al.*, 1984; Vardatsikos *et al.*, 2013).

3   Zinc

Zinc is one of the most important trace elements in nature where it is indispensable for the growth and development of microorganisms, plants and animals (Chasapis *et al.*, 2011). In the human body there is approximately 2-4 g of total zinc making it the most abundant trace metal in tissue next to iron (approximately 4 g which is localized primarily in blood). Zinc is found in relatively high abundance with the highest concentration of zinc is found in the prostate (84-211 μg/g), while the pancreas contains 140 μg/g; muscle has approximately 51 μg/g of zinc while in plasma approximately 14-16 μM of zinc can be measured, which contributes to the mobile zinc pool that is required for cellular distribution (Jansen *et al.*, 2009). At the cellular level, approximately 30-40% of total cellular zinc is found in the nucleus, approximately 50% in the cytosol and its organelles, and the remainder in the plasma membrane (Vallee *et al.*, 1993). Zinc found in these compartments is essentially bound to macromolecules including zinc proteins/enzymes, lipids, and DNA/RNA (Chasapis *et al.*, 2011; Maret, 2011a, 2011b). In fact, research of the human genome has established that approximately 10% of the proteome consists of potential zinc-binding proteins (Andreini *et al.*, 2006). Accordingly, the compartmentalization, availability, transport and re-distribution of zinc must be tightly controlled in order to maintain cellular zinc homeostasis. Thus, the mechanisms dedicated to controlling these processes is principally achieved by the metallothioneins [for a comprehensive review see (Maret, 2011a), and references therein], and a family of transmembrane zinc transporter proteins (Kambe, 2011; Myers *et al.*, 2012).

Zinc ions are widely used as a cofactor for numerous proteins, and in addition to their structural and catalytic role, zinc facilitates information transfer and cellular control (Maret, 2011a, 2011b). In fact, zinc is critical for the function of over 300 enzymes including members of all classes. These include the oxidoreductases, transferases, hydrolases, lyases, isomerases and ligases, and are examples of all the six enzymes classes established by the International Union of Biochemistry (Vallee and Falchuk, 1993). Zinc is also involved in a number of cellular processes including extracellular signal recognition; second messenger activity; protein phosphorylation and dephosphorylation, and the regulation of transcription factors (Beyersmann and Haase, 2001).

Zinc has insulin-mimetic and anti-diabetic effects in cells and animal models of type 1 and T2D. The molecular mechanisms responsible for the insulin-mimetic effects of zinc include the activation of several key signaling molecules of the insulin signaling pathway such as the extracellular signal-regulated kinase 1/2 (ERK1/2) and phosphatidylinositol 3-kinase (PI3-K)/protein kinase B/Akt (PKB/Akt) pathways (Vardatsikos *et al.*, 2013). Moreover, disturbances of zinc homeostasis are associated with several disease states including diabetes, liver cirrhosis (Bode *et al.*, 1988), cancer (Dufner-Beattie *et al.*, 2004) and impaired function of the immune system (Haase *et al.*, 2006). However, the molecular mechanisms responsible for alterations in cellular zinc status that lead to dysfunctional signaling and disease are unknown.

3.1   Zinc and health: brief historical perspectives

The importance of zinc in biological systems was first described in 1869 where it was shown to be essential for the growth of *Aspergillus niger,* the common bread mold (Raulin, 1869). Subsequently, zinc was found to be vital for the growth of plants (Sommer *et al.*, 1926) and rats (Todd *et al.*, 1934). In 1955 it was identified that parakeratosis in swine was due a deficiency in zinc (Tucker and Salmon, 1955) and the addition of zinc to food rations with established cases of this disease produced immediate and rapid weight gain and essentially eliminated the skin lesions (Lewis *et al.*, 1956). Moreover, chickens with a severe deficiency in zinc were slow growing, had abnormal respiration, poor calcification of bone, and evidence of parakeratosis (O'Dell *et al.*, 1958). Although by 1960 several experiments reported the essentiality of zinc in several animal models; due to its abundance, zinc deficiency and subsequent clinical manifestations in humans was considered unlikely (Prasad, 2012).

The idea that zinc was essential for humans was first discovered in 1958 where symptoms of severe anemia, growth retardation, hypogonadism, heptosplenomegaly, skin abnormalities and mental lethargy and geophagia (clay eating) in men from Iran were attributed to zinc deficiency (Prasad *et al.*, 1961). Subsequently, many other studies have identified the importance of dietary zinc in humans (Alves *et al.*, 2012; Atasoy and Ulusoy, 2012; Bribiescas, 2003; Coble *et al.*, 1971; Hambidge *et al.*, 1972; Makonnen *et al.*, 2003; Ronaghy *et al.*, 1969; Sandstead *et al.*, 1967), and the recognition that zinc deficiency is potentially a widespread problem in both developing and developed countries (Ackland *et al.*, 2006). Although zinc deficiency has compound effects on human health, perturbations in cellular ionic zinc status can lead to several chronic diseases including cancer, cardiovascular disease, Alzheimer's disease and diabetes (Bosomworth *et al.*, 2013; Devirgiliis *et al.*, 2007, Mocchegiani *et al.*, 2008).

4   Zinc Transporters

Zinc transporters belong to a family of transmembrane proteins that control zinc transport across cellular membranes and contribute to the uptake, distribution and compartmentalization of this metal ion (Myers *et al.*, 2012) (Figure 1). The zinc transporters[1] belong to two major gene families: the ZnT proteins (solute-linked carrier 30, SLC30) and the ZIP (Zrt/Irt-like, solute-linked carrier 39, SLC39) (Kambe, 2011; Liuzzi *et al.*, 2004). Among these, in mammals there are ten members of the zinc efflux (SLC30/ZnT; Znt1-10) transporters proteins that transport zinc out of the cell or into subcellular compartments in the presence of high cytoplasmic zinc, and fourteen members of the zinc influx (SLC39/ZIP; ZIP1-14) proteins that transport zinc into the cell or out of subcellular compartments when cytosolic zinc is low or depleted (Figure 1) (Gaither and Eide, 2001).

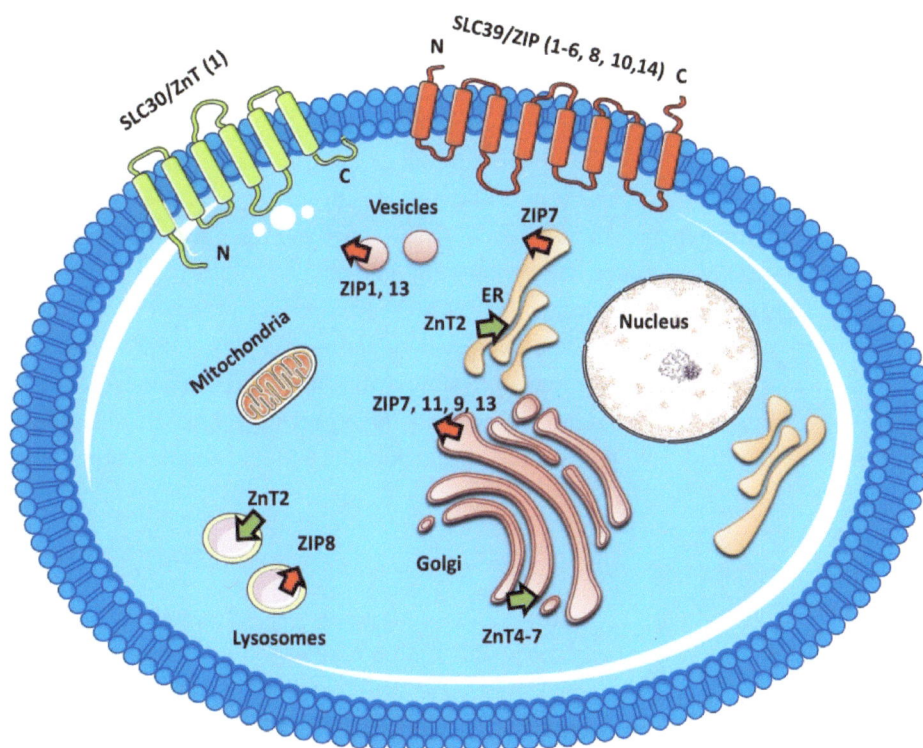

Figure 1: Cellular localization of the ZIP and ZnT zinc transporters. Green arrows depict the ZnTs while red arrows show the ZIP family. The position of the arrows indicates the direction of zinc flux. Note: Golgi (Golgi apparatus) and ER (endoplasmic reticulum). Figure was produced using Servier Medical Art, http://www.servier.com/.

---

[1] The alias terminology ZIP and ZnT (SLC39 and SLC30, respectively) will be used throughout for consistency.

5.1   The SLC39/ZIP family

The first member of the ZIP family of transporters to be identified was in *Saccharomyces cerevisiae* based on a similarity to that of Irt1p, an Fe(II) transporter from *Arabidopsis thaliana* (Eide *et al.*, 1996; Zhao *et al.*, 1996). The *ZRT1* gene was found to encode a zinc transporter protein with a high affinity for zinc and moreover, this transporter was induced at the transcriptional level in zinc-depleted conditions (Zhao *et al.*, 1996). Furthermore, a mutation in this gene eliminated the high-affinity uptake of zinc and inhibited growth on zinc-limiting media suggesting that ZRT1 is necessary for growth in zinc-limiting conditions. Since the discovery of ZRT1, fourteen gene members have been identified in mammals designated *SLC39A1-SLC39A14,* (Table 1) encoding for the proteins ZIP1-14, respectively (Jeong and Eide, 2013). Most ZIP transporters have a predicted 8 transmembrane domain (TMD) with the N- and C-termini localized extra-cytoplasmically (Figure 1). A long loop region that often contains a histidine-rich region is localized between TMD III and TMD IV (Jeong and Eide, 2013) where it is thought to be involved in binding metal ions. Indeed, studies in PC-3 prostate cancer cells identified that mutation of one or both histidine residues in the loop region (H_{158} and H_{160}) of ZIP1 resulted in a decrease in zinc accumulation in PC-3 cells (Milon *et al.*, 2006). More recently, a loop region located between TM II and III of the IRT1 transporter from *Arabidopsis thaliana* was shown to have unique zinc-binding features where imidazoles from two histidines (His-96 and His-116), a cysteine thiolate (Cys-109) and one of a glutamic acid carboxyl group was responsible for the formation of the zinc-IRT1 complex, and thus the transport of zinc ions (Potocki *et al.*, 2013). These data are supported by earlier studies in the zinc-binding protein ZnuA from *Escherichia coli* where bound zinc was coordinated by three histidine residues (His-78, His-161 and His-225) and one glutamate residue (Glu-77) (Li *et al.*, 2007).

The ZIP transporters are expressed in a range of tissue types and their proteins are localized to distinct subcellular compartments. In addition to regulation by intracellular and extracellular zinc concentrations, many of these transporters are also regulated by hormones and cytokines (Table 1) (Lichten and Cousins, 2009). Such diverse regulation, tissue expression patterns and subcellular localization of these transporters provides some insight into their many physiological roles. Moreover, the ZIP transporters are implicated in a number of pathophysiological processes including prostate, breast and pancreatic cancer, carotid artery disease, acrodermatitis enteropathica, schizophrenia, Ehlers-Danlos syndrome, and asthma (Table 1).

5.2   The SLC30/ZnT family

The mammalian SLC30 zinc transporters belong to a large family of cation diffusion facilitators (CDF/ZnT) and include zinc transporter members with similar topology from bacteria, fungi, nematodes, insects, plants and mammals (Huang and Tepaamorndech, 2013). Members of this family are predicted to have six transmembrane (TM) domains and a histidine-rich loop between TMD IV and TMD V with the N- and C-termini on the cytoplasmic side of the membrane (Palmiter and Huang, 2004) (Figure 1). At present, there is little information available on the structure of the ZnTs, however, one CDF bacterial homologs, Yiip from *Escherichia coli* has been characterized functionally and has 25-30% sequence similarity to their mammalian counterparts (Lu and Fu, 2007). The Yiip protein is a homodimer consisting of two 32.9-kDa integral membrane proteins composed of six TMD (Wei *et al.*, 2004) and a tetrahedral zinc-binding site that is essential for transport (Lu and Fu, 2007).

Gene/protein	Tissue expression and cellular localization	Regulation of ZIP transporters	Disease/pathology association
Slc39a1/ZIP1	Ubiquitously expressed, plasma membrane	[↑] Prolactin and testosterone (LNCaP and PC3 prostate cancer cells)[b]	Prostate cancer
Slc39a2/ZIP2	Blood, prostate, plasma membrane	Unknown	Carotid artery disease
Slc39a3/ZIP3	Mammary gland, prostate, plasma membrane, intracellular compartments	[↑] Prolactin (mammary gland)[c]	Pancreatic cancer[l]
Slc39a4/ZIP4	Small intestine, stomach, colon, kidney, brain, plasma membrane, apical membranes	[↓] Zinc deficiency (embryonic visceral yolk sack isolated from pregnant mice)[d]	Pancreatic cancer, acrodermatitis enteropathica (AE)
Slc39a5/ZIP5	Pancreas, kidney, liver, spleen, colon, stomach, plasma membrane, basolateral membranes	Unknown	Unknown
Slc39a6/ZIP6	Ubiquitously expressed, plasma membrane	[↑] Estrogen, [↓] Tamoxifen and fulvestrant (MCF-7 breast cancer cells)[e], [↑] glucose (pancreatic mouse islets)[f]	Breast cancer; cervical cancer[m]
Slc39a7/ZIP7	Ubiquitously expressed, Golgi apparatus, endoplasmic reticulum	[↑] Estrogen (MCF-7 breast cancer cells)[e], [↑] glucose (pancreatic mouse islets)[f]	Breast cancer
Slc39a8/ZIP8	Ubiquitously expressed, vesicles	[↑] TNF-α (monocytes[g], human lung epithelial cells, hLECs)[h]	Inflammation
Slc39a9/ZIP9	Ubiquitously expressed, trans-Golgi network	Unknown	Unknown
Slc39a10/ZIP10	Ubiquitously expressed, plasma membrane	[↑] Thyroid hormone (rat intestines and kidney)[i]	Breast cancer
Slc39a11/ZIP11	Mammary gland, testes[a], stomach[a], small and large intestine[a], Golgi apparatus	[↑] Zinc (spleen and liver in gavage-fed mice)[a]	Unknown
Slc39a12/ZIP12	Retina, brain, testis, lung	Unknown	Schizophrenia, neuronal differentiation[n]
Slc39a13/ZIP13	Ubiquitously ex-pressed, Golgi apparatus	Unknown	Ehlers-Danlos syndrome
Slc39a14/ZIP14	Ubiquitously ex-pressed, plasma membrane	[↑] Estrogen, [↓] tamoxifen and fulvestrant (MCF-7 breast cancer cells)[e]; [↑] IL-6 (mouse liver parenchymal cells[j], adipose tissue and muscle)[k]	Asthma, inflammmation[k]

Table Source: modified from Myers et al. 2012 and references herein. Regulation of zinc transporters: [↑] Upregulation; [↓] Down regulation, [a] Yu et al., 2013; [b] Costello et al., 1999; [c] Kelleher et al., 2011; [d] Dufner-Beattie et al., 2004; [e] Taylor et al., 2007; [f] Bellomo et al., 2011; [g] Begum et al., 2002; [h] Besecker et al., 2008; [i] Pawan et al., 2007; [j] Liuzzi et al., 2005; [k] Beker et al., 2012; [l] Costello et al., 2012; [m] Zhao et al., 2007; [n] Chowanadisai et al., 2013.

Table 1: SlC39/ZIP transporters: tissue expression and cellular localization, regulation and disease/pathology association.

The first mammalian ZnT transporter (ZnT1) was isolated from a rat kidney cDNA library where it was shown to facilitate zinc resistance to zinc toxicity in the zinc-sensitive baby hamster kidney (BHK) cell line (Palmiter and Findley, 1995). Since the discovery of ZnT1, ten members of the mammalian SLC30 family have been identified and designated *SLC30A1-SLC30A10* and encoding for the proteins ZnT1-10, respectively (Table 2) (Huang and Tepaamorndech, 2013). Similar to the ZIP family members, the ZnTs are expressed in a wide-range of tissues; have specific subcellular localizations and are implicated in a number of pathophysiological disease states (Table 2). Equally, they are also regulated by intracellular and extracellular zinc status, hormones and cytokines and other molecules (Table 2).

6   Zinc, Zinc Transporters and Cell Signaling

Zinc transporters typically act as zinc sensors and respond to cellular zinc availability to maintain intracellular zinc homeostasis. Cellular homeostasis of zinc is complex and there are a number of significant and comprehensive reviews on these processes (Jeong and Eide, 2013; Kambe, 2011; Liuzzi and Cousins, 2004; Myers *et al.*, 2012, and references therein). Therefore, this section aims to briefly present a number of important processes by which zinc and zinc transporters maintain cellular homeostasis. A particular focus will be made to highlight the role of these transporters in cellular signaling. Zinc mimics the action of hormones, growth factors and cytokines and given the large number of zinc transporters that are dedicated to controlling zinc homeostasis (Table 1 and Table 2); it is not surprising that this ion is quickly taking precedence as a leading signaling molecule analogous to calcium. In this context, the processes of cellular zinc signaling have been designated into two main mechanisms of action; these are 1) early zinc signaling (EZS), and 2) late zinc signaling (LZS).

6.1   Early and late zinc signaling

EZS is a transcriptional-independent mechanism that involves a rapid intracellular change in levels of free zinc ions that occurs in minutes due to an extracellular stimulus (Fukada *et al.*, 2011). This mechanism was first reported in bone marrow-derived mast cells (BMMCs) where treatment of these cells with the high affinity IgE receptor (FcεRI) resulted in a rapid increase (within minutes) in intracellular free zinc from the perinuclear region that includes the endoplasmic reticulum (ER) (Yamasaki *et al.*, 2007). This zinc 'wave' as defined by these authors was also observed under conditions in which either the extracellular zinc influx or the exocytosis of zinc-rich granules, was blocked. LZS is also triggered by an extracellular signal but involves transcriptional-dependent changes in expression of proteins implicated in zinc homeostasis such as storage proteins or transporters (Yamasaki *et al.*, 2007). In LZS the intracellular zinc concentrations are usually altered over several hours following an external stimulus (Fukada *et al.*, 2011). Since zinc has an important role in maintaining cellular function, and dysregulation or altered partitioning of intracellular zinc causes disease in humans and animal models (Foster and Samman, 2010; Fukada *et al.*, 2011; Haase and Maret, 2005a; Jansen *et al.*, 2012; Pfaffl and Windisch, 2003; Prasad, 1991), understanding the proteins that transport zinc into and out of cells and subcellular organelles (the ZnTs and ZIPs) will be important in identifying novel therapeutic opportunities.

Gene/protein	Tissue expression and cellular localization	Regulation of ZnT transporters	Disease/pathology association
Slc30a1/ZnT1	Ubiquitously expressed, plasma membrane	[↑] Zinc (intestine, liver and kidney[e], pancreatic cancer cells[f], HeLa cells[g], [↑] nitric oxide (rat cerebral cortex)[h], [↓] Cadmium (mouse decidua, yolk sac, and embryo)[i]	Alzheimer's disease, heart disease, pancreatic cancer
Slc30a2/ZnT2	Pancreas, kidney, testis, epithelial cells, small intestine, prostate, vesicles, lysosomes	[↑] Zinc (intestine, liver and kidney)[e], [↑] Nitric oxide (rat cerebral cortex)[h], [↑] Prolactin (human mammary epithelial cells)[j]; [↑] neurotrophic factors (retinal pigment epithelium cell lines)[k]	Low zinc milk concentrations
Slc30a3/ZnT3	Brain, testis, vascular smooth muscle cells[a]; adipose tissue[b], synaptic vesicles	[↓] angiotensin (vascular smooth muscle)[a], [↑] High glucose (INS-1E cells)[b]; [↓] Chronic metabolic acidosis (rat duodenal epithelial cells)[j]; [↑] Synthetic androgen R1881 (AIDL prostate cancer cells)[l]	Alzheimer's disease
Slc30a4/ZnT4	Mammary gland, brain, small intestine, placenta, blood, epithelial cells, intracellular compartments	[↑] Nitric oxide (rat cerebral cortex)[h]	Lethal Zn-deficient milk production, Alzheimer's disease, asthma
Slc30a5/ZnT5	Ubiquitously expressed, secretory vesicles, Golgi apparatus	[↑] Low glucose (INS-1E cells)[b], [↑] TPEN (HeLa cells)[g], [↓] High dietary zinc (human ileal mucosa and Caco-2 cells)[m]	Osteopenia
Slc30a6/ZnT6	Small intestine, liver, brain, adipose tissue, secretory vesicles, Golgi apparatus	Unknown	Alzheimer's disease
Slc30a7/ZnT7	Retina, small intestine, liver, blood, epithelial cells, spleen, secretory vesicles, Golgi apparatus	[↑] TPEN (HeLa cells)[g]	Prostate cancer
Slc30a8/ZnT8	Pancreatic β-cells, retina[c], secretory vesicles	[↑] Exendin-4 (pancreas in db/db mice)[n], [↓] High glucose (INS-1E cells)[b]	Type 1 and 2 diabetes mellitus, retinopathy
Slc30a9/ZnT9	Ubiquitously expressed, cytoplasm, nucleus	Unknown	
Slc30a10/ZnT10	Liver, brain, small intestine[d], Golgi apparatus	[↓] Angiotensin (vascular smooth muscle)[a]	Parkinson's disease, dystonia, liver disease, Alzheimer's disease

Table Source: modified from Myers et al. 2012 and references herein. Regulation of zinc transporters: [↑] Upregulation; [↓] Down regulation, [a] Patrushev et al., 2012; [b] Smidt and Rungby., 2012; [c] Deniro and Al-Mohanna., 2012; [d] Bosomworth et al., 2012; [e] Liuzzi et al., 2001; [f] Jayaraman et al., 2011; [g] Devergnas et al., 2004; [h] Aguilar-Alonso et al., 2008; [i] Fernandez et al., 2007; [j] Wongdee et al., 2009; [k] Leung et al., 2008; [l] Iguchi et al., 2004; [m] Cragg et al., 2005 [n] Liu et al., 2011b.

Table 2: SlC30/ZnT transporters: tissue expression, cellular localization and regulation, and disease association.

6.2 Zinc and cellular signaling

The role of zinc and its function as a signaling mediator is well established and the literature is replete with many important findings (see, Fukada *et al.*, 2011, and references therein). Early studies suggesting that zinc ions could function as a signaling molecule were identified in rat adipocytes where it was shown that zinc stimulated lipogenesis that was independent, and additive to that of insulin (Coulston and Dandona, 1980). Similarly, rat adipocytes treated with zinc for 30 minutes stimulated cAMP phospodiesterase and the translocation of the glucose transporter to the plasma membrane that was not dependent on insulin receptor stimulated kinase activity (Ezaki, 1989). Zinc was also shown to induce EGF receptor phosphorylation and subsequent EGF signaling cascade in human airway bronchial cells (Wu *et al.*, 1999).

Since these early studies implicating zinc as a cellular signaling molecule, there is increasing evidence that this ion is implicated in extracellular signal recognition (Yamasaki *et al.*, 2007), second messenger metabolism (Zhao *et al.*, 2011), protein kinase activity (Tang and Shay, 2001), protein phosphorylation (Pandey *et al.*, 2010; Yoshikawa *et al.*, 2004) and the modulation of transcription factors (Rutherford and Bird, 2004). These studies highlight zinc's dynamic role as a cellular second messenger in the control of cellular systems that are associated with insulin signaling and glucose homeostasis (Hwang *et al.*, 2011; Mocchegiani *et al.*, 2008; Yamasaki *et al.*, 2007).

In this context, the mechanisms of zinc and its insulin-mimetic activity have been delineated in glucose (Ilouz *et al.*, 2002; May and Contoreggi, 1982; Moniz *et al.*, 2011; Simon and Taylor, 2001; Tang and Shay, 2001; Wijesekara *et al.*, 2009; Yoshikawa *et al.*, 2004) and lipid (Coulston and Dandona, 1980; Yoshikawa *et al.*, 2004) metabolism. For example, zinc mediates control of glucose homeostasis through the inhibition of protein tyrosine phosphatases (PTPs) which are an important class of enzymes involved in the removal of phosphate groups (Haase and Maret, 2003, 2005a; Wilson *et al.*, 2012; Yamasaki *et al.*, 2007). Thus, in the context of the insulin receptor (IR), the inhibition of protein tyrosine phosphatases by zinc facilitates an increase in the net phosphorylation of the IR and activates its signaling cascade (Haase and Maret, 2003, 2005a). For example, the elevated expression and activity of PTP1B (a negative regulator of insulin and leptin signaling pathways) in the liver of hyperglycemic insulin receptor substrate 2 (IRS2$^{-/-}$) mice facilitated the association of the IR with PTP1B and impaired IR/IRS1-mediated insulin signaling (González-Rodríguez *et al.*, 2010). Similarly, zinc inhibition of PTP1B augments tyrosine phosphorylation of the IGF-1 receptor and the insulin receptor substrate 1 in C6 rat glioma cells (Haase and Maret, 2003) and mice lacking PTP1B are lean and have increased insulin sensitivity (Xue *et al.*, 2007).

Thus, the zinc-mediated effect on cellular homeostasis is numerous and includes the stimulation of glucose uptake and lipogenesis in adipocytes (Tang and Shay, 2001), tyrosine phosphorylation of the insulin/IGF-1 receptor and insulin receptor substrate-1 (Haase and Maret., 2003, 2005a; Pandey *et al.*, 2010), activation of epidermal growth factor receptor (Pandey *et al.*, 2010; Taylor *et al.*, 2008), inhibition of protein tyrosine phosphatase (PTP) (Haase and Maret, 2005a; Mocchegiani *et al.*, 2008) and subsequent activation of mitogen-activated protein kinases (MAPKs) including extracellular-signal-regulated kinases 1 and 2 (ERK1/2), c-Jun N-terminal kinase (JNK) and p38 (Hogstrand *et al.*, 2009) and an increase in glycogen synthesis through the inhibition of glycogen synthase kinase-3 (Ilouz *et al.*, 2002).

6.3   Zinc transporters in cellular signaling

The fundamental and diverse role of zinc transporters in maintaining zinc flux in cells defines the critical importance of zinc ions in cellular homeostasis. Although zinc has an important role in mediating cell signaling; the transporters responsible for zinc modulation in cells and their involvement in cell signaling are less defined. Accordingly, specific findings that contribute to the emerging notion that zinc transporters that control zinc flux, and thus cell signaling, will be briefly discussed.

6.3.1   ZnTs and ZIPs in cellular signaling

The processes of cellular signaling are complex and extremely critical for cellular function in normal health and disease states. Although there are numerous examples in the literature of proteins implicated in cellular signal transduction, knowledge regarding the role of zinc transporters in these processes is limited. However, recent research is starting to unravel the mechanisms by which zinc transporters can contribute to cellular homeostasis through their contribution to the transport of the mobile zinc pool in the cytosol that contributes to cellular regulatory events. As mentioned, studies on the mechanisms of zinc transporters and subsequent zinc signaling in cellular processes are limited. However, given the well-known role of these proteins in transporting zinc into and out of cells and subcellular organelles, we can extrapolate the importance of zinc transporters and zinc flux in facilitating cell signaling from studies that have overexpressed or reduced the expression of these proteins in cell and animal models.

Studies in the cervical cancer cell line (HeLa) found that a reduction in the expression of ZIP6 limited growth and the prevention of the *in vitro* migration and matrigel invasion capacity of cancer cells. This process was via a reduction in the levels of p44/42 MAPK and phospho-p44/42 MAPK, and subsequent Snail and Slug (two important transcription factors implicated in epithelial-to-mesenchymal transition (EMT)) signaling (Zhao *et al.*, 2007). These data suggest that ZIP6 expression is required for HeLa cell invasion and metastasis. In support of these studies, the overexpression of ZIP6 in human androgen-refractory prostate cancer cells (ARCaP) facilitated an EMT by upregulating the matrix metalloproteinase (MMP) 2 and MMP 9 which resulted in the shedding of heparin binding-EGF and subsequent epidermal growth factor receptor (EGFR) phosphorylation and downstream ERK signaling (Lue *et al.*, 2011). These studies established a link between ZIP6 expression and EGFR-ERK signaling in facilitating EMT and prostate cancer migration, invasion and metastasis.

In other cancer-related studies, the reduction of ZIP7 by small-interfering RNA (siRNA) in tamoxifen-resistant (TamR) MCF-7 cells was responsible for the inactivation of epithelial growth factor receptor/IGF-1 receptor/Src signaling by reducing the availability of intracellular zinc levels (Taylor *et al.*, 2008). It was suggested by these authors that the effective removal of ZIP7 may provide a mechanism to inhibit zinc-induced activation of growth factor receptors and thus provide an opportunity to target tumor growth and development. In fact, ZIP7 has been identified as a key zinc transporter implicated in the "zinc wave" and is suggested to be a "*gatekeeper*" of cytosolic zinc release from the ER (Taylor *et al.*, 2012). Recent evidence in TamR MCF-7 breast cancer cells suggests that ZIP7 is phosphorylated by casein kinase 2 and is associated with the regulated 'gated' release of zinc from intracellular stores leading to the activation of tyrosine kinases and the phosphorylation of AKT and extracellular signalling kinases 1 and 2 (Taylor *et al.*, 2012).

In other studies, intracellular zinc has been shown to regulate signaling pathways in T cell and lymphocytes however it is not clear how this signaling occurs. Accordingly, it was observed in ZIP9 deficient chicken DT40, B lymphocyte cells that Akt and Erk phosphorylation was reduced and resulted in an increase in PTPase activity (Taniguchi *et al.*, 2013). Furthermore, overexpression of human ZIP9 in the chicken ZIP9 knockout DT40 cells restored Akt and Erk phosphorylation while PTPase activity was decreased in response to zinc treatment. These data suggest that ZIP9 increases cytosolic zinc and activation of cell signaling by inhibition of PTPases in these cells (Taniguchi *et al.*, 2013).

In metabolic studies, glucose stimulation of pancreatic insuinoma RIN5mf cells that had an overexpression of ZnT7, resulted in an increase in insulin secretion (Huang *et al.*, 2010). This was also associated with an increase in insulin biosynthesis and a subsequent increase in cellular insulin content and suggested that ZnT7 plays an important role in insulin expression. Similarly, ZnT7 null mice were more susceptible to diet-induced glucose intolerance and insulin resistance and this was associated with a reduction in the expression of the insulin receptor (IR), IR substrate 1, IR substrate 2 and Akt mRNA in primary skeletal myotubes (Huang *et al.*, 2012). In other studies on ZnT7, the overexpression of this transporter in mouse osteoblasts MC3T3-E1 cells facilitated cytoprotection from H_2O_2 oxidative stress-induced apoptosis via the activation PI3K/Akt and MAPK/ERK pathways (Liang *et al.*, 2013).

ZnT3, ZnT5 and ZnT8 gene expression is differentially regulated by glucose in INS-1E cells and a ZnT3 'knock down' decreased insulin gene expression and secretion and resulted in hyperglycemia in streptozotocin-treated ZnT3 null mice (Smidt *et al.*, 2009). Similarly, elevated glucose concentrations increased free cytosolic zinc in mouse pancreatic islets and were associated with an increase in the mRNA expression of ZIP6-8 (Bellomo *et al.*, 2011). These authors suggested that glucose induces cytosolic zinc leading to the processing and storage of insulin and associated increase in the ZIP importers.

Fasting gluconeogenesis is impaired in the livers of ZIP14 knockout mice which is attributable to dysregulation of G-protein coupled receptor (GPCR) signaling (Hojyo *et al.*, 2011). The reduction in signaling is due to reduced levels of basal cAMP as a consequence of increased phosphodiesterase (PDE) activity and suggests that ZIP14 plays a role in facilitating GPCR-mediated cAMP-CREB activity by reducing basal PDE in the liver (Hojyo *et al.*, 2011). Moreover, ZIP14 null mice have greater body fat, hypoglycemia and increase levels of insulin that was concomitant with increased liver glucose and increase insulin receptor, PI3K and Akt phosphorylation (Beker *et al.*, 2012).

Recently we have identified that the reduction in ZIP7 by siRNA in mouse skeletal muscle C2C12 cells is associated with the downregulation of several genes implicated in glucose metabolism including the IR, IR-substrate 1, IR-substrate 2, Glut4 and glycogen branching enzyme (Gbe) (Myers *et al.* 2013). This was concomitant with a reduction in glycogen synthesis and pAKT and suggests that ZIP7 controls glycogen synthesis in these cells via pAKT and Glut4 signaling.

Given that the zinc transporters are involved in the cellular regulation of signal transduction pathways in a number of biological systems, and specifically, their ability to modulate pathways involved in glucose and lipid metabolism, suggests that these transporters will have significance in disease states associated with insulin resistance and type 2 diabetes. Although several studies in cell and animal models have provided some insight into the mechanisms of zinc transporters in the context of metabolic processes associated with insulin signaling and insulin resistance, their role in type 2 diabetes remains vague.

7   Zinc, Zinc Transporters and Type 2 Diabetes

Type 2 diabetes (T2D) is a complex disorder characterized by insulin resistance and impaired glucose homeostasis. Recently, intensive research has aimed to elucidate the role that dysfunctional zinc signaling plays in this disease. Moreover, given that the global incidence of T2D is escalating at an alarming rate

(Zimmet, 2002), there is considerable interest in understanding the molecular mechanisms of zinc transport and zinc action on cellular pathways associated with glucose metabolism. Although dietary zinc supplements given to animal models of diabetes and human diabetic patients has shown some benefits in improving glycaemic control (Hwang *et al.*, 2011; Jansen *et al.*, 2009; Jayawardena *et al.*, 2012; Simon and Taylor, 2001; Song *et al.*, 2001), there are also contradictory outcomes in human studies on zinc supplementation to treat diabetes (see, Miao *et al.*, 2013, for a comprehensive review and references therein), and is beyond the scope of this review. While these studies on zinc supplementation as an adjunct therapy to treat diabetes are ongoing, the transporters implicated in controlling zinc flux in cells and their role in diabetes is limited.

7.1 ZnT8 and diabetes

Zinc has an integral role in the processing, storage, secretion and action of insulin in response to changes in elevated glucose concentrations (Mocchegiani *et al.*, 2008; Wijesekara *et al.*, 2009). Zinc is required for the storage of insulin in the secretory granules of the pancreas as an inactive Zn^{2+}-insulin hexamer. When released into blood serum, a change in pH drives dissociation of the hexamer into a monomer which is the physiologically active form of insulin (Xu *et al.*, 2011). To date, the most well-studied zinc transporter in diabetes is ZnT8. This transporter is almost exclusively expressed in the β-cells of the pancreas where it plays a crucial role in transporting zinc into insulin secretory vesicles and therefore is critical for the synthesis, storage and action of insulin (for comprehensive reviews, see Chimienti *et al.*, 2005; Kawasaki., 2012; Mocchegiani *et al.*, 2008 and references therein).

It has been shown in pancreatic INS-1 cells that overexpression of ZnT8 facilitated glucose-stimulated insulin secretion (Chimienti *et al.*, 2006) while reduced expression of this transporter in these cells resulted in a reduction in insulin content and secretion in response to a hyperglycaemic stimulus (Fu *et al.*, 2009). Moreover, mice with a target-specific ZnT8 knockout in pancreatic β-cells show compromised glucose tolerance (Wijesekara *et al.*, 2010) while global ZnT8 null mice showed abnormalities in diet-dependent glucose tolerance, insulin secretion (Nicolson *et al.*, 2009; Pound *et al.*, 2009) and body weight (Hardy *et al.*, 2012; Nicolson *et al.*, 2009). An association of ZnT8 with diabetes risk in humans emerged when a non-synonymous single nucleotide polymorphism (SNP) (rs13266634 C>T) which changes an arginine (R) to tryptophan (W) at amino acid position 325 was identified as a susceptibility locus of T2D in genome-wide association studies in European patients (Kommoju and Reddy, 2011; Saxena *et al.*, 2007; Sladek *et al.*, 2007; Xu *et al.*, 2012). The rs13266634 SNP disrupts a protein kinase A and protein kinase C recognition motif that alters the function of this transporter (Kawasaki, 2012). Accordingly, defects in ZnT8 protein structure will affect the accumulation of zinc ions in the secretory granule where insulin is matured and stored as hexamers bound to zinc ions (Nicolson *et al.*, 2009). In this context, the risk allele of ZnT8 was found to be associated with impaired conversion of proinsulin to insulin in human patients (Kirchhoff *et al.*, 2008).

It is well-established that type 1 diabetes (T1D) is associated with autoimmune-mechanisms (type 1A) and both genetic and environmental factors affect the disease onset and progression (Kawasaki, 2012). T1D is characterized by the selective destruction of the β-cells of the pancreas resulting in significant insulin deficiency and subsequent hyperglycemia. Circulating autoantibodies targeting pancreatic β-cell proteins are currently the most reliable biomarkers in the early stage of T1D and therefore provides utility for therapeutic intervention. To date, the four major humoral autoantigens in T1D are [pro]-insulin, glutamic acid decarboxylase (GAD65), insulinoma-associated antigen 2 (IA-2) and ZnT8 (Wenzlau and Hutton, 2013).

The discovery of ZnT8 as the fourth humoral autoantigen involved microarray gene expression profiling of human and rodent pancreas and islet cells that were subsequently screened with new-onset T1D and prediabetic sera (Wenzlau *et al.*, 2007). These studies identified that ZnT8 is a diabetes-associated autoantigen where autoantibodies were found in 60-80% of new onset cases of T1D (Wenzlau *et al.*, 2007). Recent genome-wide association studies revealed that the above mentioned SNP rs13266634 is a key determinant of humoral autoreactivity to ZnT8 (Wenzlau *et al.*, 2008; Kawasaki *et al.*, 2008). Moreover, autoantibodies that recognize ZnT8R, ZnT8W, or both at the polymorphic site are common in newly diagnosed T1D patients (Skarstrand *et al.*, 2013). However, it is not clear on the importance of ZnT8 epitope-specific autoantibodies and β-cell destruction in T1D. Nevertheless, because ZnT8 plays a critical role in insulin biology, and has recently emerged as a genetic marker for diabetes, it represents an attractive candidate for therapy for the treatment of diabetes and other disorders related to pancreatic pathology.

7.2   Other zinc transporters and type 2 diabetes

A recent study investigated the effect of zinc and α-linolenic acid (ALA) supplementation on circulating concentrations of inflammatory markers and zinc transporter gene expression in peripheral blood mononuclear cells (PBMCs) of forty-three postmenopausal women with T2D (Foster *et al.*, 2013). These studies identified that zinc and ALA supplementation had no effect on inflammatory markers, however, circulating base levels of the inflammatory cytokine IL-6 could predict the expression levels of mRNA for ZnT5, ZnT7, ZIP1, ZIP7 and ZIP10 in such that each unit increase in IL-6 produced an 8%-15% increase in zinc transporter gene expression (Foster *et al.*, 2013). These authors suggest that IL-6 increases the expression of this group of zinc transporters to facilitate the redistribution of zinc into PBMC organelles as part of a coordinated inflammatory response.

Apart from research in animal models and cell culture systems (see 6.2 Zinc and cellular signaling and 6.3 Zinc transporters in cellular signaling) there is little additional information available on the role of other members of the zinc transporter family in human type 2 diabetes.

8   Zinc, Zinc transporters and therapeutic utility

The relevance of intracellular zinc signaling for normal physiology and for the pathogenesis of several disease states including T2D has recently been highlighted. Although zinc supplementation in zinc-deficient T2D patients might be appropriate treatment in genetically susceptible individuals, the potential mechanisms that lead to dysfunctional intracellular zinc signaling and altered zinc subcellular distribution, rather than zinc deficiency will require the development innovative drugs that target zinc transporters for example. Moreover, several issues regarding zinc supplementation for T2D patients requires intensive investigation as this type for treatment may not have the maximal benefit required to improve glycaemic control. Although zinc in general is less toxic, excessive zinc intake may have undesirable effects such as the elevation of HbA1c and high blood pressure (Miao *et al.*, 2013).

While zinc has insulin-mimetic actions and is implicated in cellular signaling events, its application in the clinical setting in lowering blood glucose in patients with T2D is complicated by the fact that absorption rates are low and high doses and long-term supplementation are required. In this context, several zinc complexes have been developed to overcome these complexities (see Miao *et al.*, 2013 for a comprehensive review). Zinc complexes with nicotinamide, maltol, amino acids, picolinic acid, picolinamide, and their derivatives have high insulin-mimetic activities *in vitro* and *in vivo* studies, however it was found that these complexes were only effective in lowering blood glucose in T2D subjects by giving daily injections (Yoshikawa *et al.*, 2003). For example, daily intraperitoneal injections of a zinc complex with maltol (Zn(ma)$_2$) normalized blood glucose levels in KKA^y mice with T2D (Yoshikawa *et al.*, 2001).

In the context of a clinical application for zinc complexes, it is desirable to identify therapies that can be administered orally. Accordingly, many studies have aimed to synthesis novel zinc complexes that have insulin-mimetic activities that can be administered orally. For example, the daily oral administration of the zinc complex Zn(II)-thioallixin-*N*-methyl (Zn(tanm)$_2$) over four weeks significantly improved hyperglycemia, glucose intolerance, insulin resistance, hyperleptinemia, obesity and hypertension in KKA^y mice (Adachi *et al.*, 2006). Similarly, the development and synthesis of a novel of zinc complex [Di(1-oxy-2-pyridinethiolato)Zn] displayed superior insulin-mimetic and anti-diabetic activity compared to ZnCl$_2$ or the clinically administered pioglitazone in KKA^y diabetic rats (Yoshikawa *et al.*, 2011). Moreover, this complex was shown to have high gastrointestinal absorption when compared to ZnCl$_2$ alone. Although zinc complexes have been shown to have beneficial effects in animal models of T2D, their utility and efficacy in human diabetes is not known. Accordingly, opportunities for translating zinc-complex therapies in animal models of diabetes into clinically relevant applications will require intensive investigation into the properties of these zinc complexes, their absorption rates, tissue distribution, toxicity, insulin-mimetic activity and efficacy in ameliorating blood glucose levels in human T2D.

Given our current understanding on the role of zinc as a critical modulator of cellular signaling and homeostasis, and the fact that the storage, compartmentalization and cellular distribution of zinc is tightly regulated by zinc transporters, it is reasonable that dysregulation of zinc flux will play an important role in disease processes. Moreover, the processes of zinc-related cellular dysfunction are predominately due to alternations in the proteins that control zinc flux and homeostasis rather than an issue of zinc deficiency or accumulation. Accordingly, drugs that target zinc transporters may provide utility to correct or improve dysfunctional zinc homeostasis and could therefore be more efficient than zinc supplementation. Although zinc is implicated in cellular signaling events, several questions remain to be resolved: For example, what extracellular stimulus regulates the expression of the zinc transporters? Are the zinc transporters differentially regulated in a tissue or cell-specific manner? How does each specific zinc transporter regulate cellular signaling pathways? Moreover, genetic studies such as the targeted, tissue-specific disruption of these transporters in animal models will assist in determining the function of these proteins.

9   Summary

- Zinc is an essential trace element that is indispensable for the growth and development of organisms.
- The ZIP and ZnT zinc transporter family are involved in regulating the intracellular availability of zinc in cells to maintain homeostasis.
- Zinc is an insulin-mimetic involved in cellular signaling events.
- Dysfunction zinc signaling is implicated in a number of disease states including liver cirrhosis, cancer, impaired immune function and diabetes.
- A single nucleotide polymorphism in the zinc transporter, ZnT8 is associated with greater risk for the development of T2D.

- Zinc supplementation in T2D patients with zinc deficiency has shown to be beneficial in some cases but not all.
- Novel zinc complexes for lowering blood glucose in animal models of T2D are promising but will require extensive clinical trials to determine their efficacy in humans.
- Drugs that target altered zinc transporter activity or dysfunctional zinc signaling may provide utility to understand aberrant zinc homeostasis in diseases such as T2D.

10   Conclusion

Zinc is an essential trace element that is implicated in a numerous normal and patho-physiological cellular functions. The emerging role of zinc as an insulin mimetic and the ubiquitous nature of this ion in maintaining cellular function suggests that abnormal cellular partitioning and levels of zinc will have biological and clinical effects. Although our current understandings on the role of zinc transporters in type 2 diabetes is limited, it is clear from studies on ZnT8 that this family of transporters has utility for the development of novel diabetic therapies. While ZnT8 plays a significant role in insulin biology and therefore represents an attractive target for diabetes therapy, the other members of the zinc transporter family in diabetes are less defined. However, we can speculate from the information presented in this review that the other transporters are involved in processes that facilitate insulin signaling and glycaemic control and therefore could offer exciting new targets that are amendable to therapeutic intervention in the treatment of diseases associated with insulin resistance and type 2 diabetes.

References

Abdul-Ghani, M.A., & DeFronzo, R. A. (2010). Pathogenesis of Insulin Resistance in Skeletal Muscle. Journal of Biomedicine and Biotechnology, doi:10.115/2010/476279.

Ackland, M. L., & Michalczyk, A. (2006). Zinc deficiency and its inherited disorders-a review. Genes & Nutrition, 1, 41-50.

Adachi, Y., Yoshida, J., Kodera, Y., Kiss, T., Jakusch, T., Enyedy, E. A., Yoshikawa, Y., & Sakurai, H. (2006). Oral administration of a zinc complex improves type 2 diabetes and metabolic syndromes. Biochemical and Biophysical Research Communications, 351, 165-170.

Aguilar-Alonso, P., Martinez-Fong, D., Pazos-Salazar, N. G., Brambila, E., Gonzalez-Barrios, J. A., Mejorada, A., Flores, G., Millan-Perezpena, L., Rubio, H., & Leon-Chavez, B. A. (2008). The increase in zinc levels and upregulation of zinc transporters are mediated by nitric oxide in the cerebral cortex after transient ischemia in the rat. Brain Research, 1200, 89-98.

Alves, C. X., Vale, S. H., Dantas, M. M., Maia, A. A., Franca, M. C., Marchini, J. S., Leite, L. D., & Brandao-Neto, J. (2012). Positive effects of zinc supplementation on growth, GH, IGF1, and IGFBP3 in eutrophic children. Journal of Pediatric Endocrinology and Metabolism, 25, 881-887.

Andreini, C., L. Banci, I. Bertini and A. Rosato (2006). Counting the zinc-proteins encoded in the human genome. Journal of Proteome Research, 5, 196-201.

Atasoy, H. B., & Ulusoy, Z. I. (2012). The relationship between zinc deficiency and children's oral health. Pediatric Dentistry, 34, 383-386.

Basaki, M., Saeb, M., Nazifi, S., & Shamsaei, H. A. (2012). Zinc, Copper, Iron, and Chromium Concentrations in Young Patients with Type 2 Diabetes Mellitus. Biological Trace Element Research, 148, 161-164.

Begum, N. A., Kobayashi, M., Moriwaki, Y., Matsumoto, M., Toyoshima, K., & Seya, T. (2002). Mycobacterium bovis BCG cell wall and lipopolysaccharide induce a novel gene, BIGM103, encoding a 7-TM protein: identification of a new protein family having Zn-transporter and Zn-metalloprotease signatures. Genomics, 80, 630-645.

Beker Aydemir, T., Chang, S. M., Guthrie, G. J., Maki, A. B., Ryu, M. S., Karabiyik, A., & Cousins, R. J. (2012). Zinc transporter ZIP14 functions in hepatic zinc, iron and glucose homeostasis during the innate immune response (endotoxemia). PLoS One, 7, e48679.

Bellomo, E. A., Meur, G., & Rutter, G. A. (2011). Glucose Regulates Free Cytosolic Zn^{2+} Concentration, Slc39 (ZiP), and Metallothionein Gene Expression in Primary Pancreatic Islet β-Cells. Journal of Biological Chemistry, 286, 25778-25789.

Besecker, B., Bao, S., Bohacova, B., Papp, A., Sadee, W., & Knoell, D. L. (2008). The human zinc transporter SLC39A8 (Zip8) is critical in zinc-mediated cytoprotection in lung epithelia. American Journal of Physiology - Lung Cellular and Molecular Physiology, 294, L1127-L1136.

Beyersmann, D., & Haase, H. (2001). Functions of zinc in signaling, proliferation and differentiation of mammalian cells. BioMetals, 14:331-341.

Bloom, D. E., Cafiero, E. T., Jane-Llopis, E., Abrahams-Gessel, S., Bloom, L. R., Fathima, S., Feigl, A. B., Gaziano, T., Mowafi, M., Pandya, A., Prettner, K., Rosenberg, L., Seligman, B., Stein, A. Z., & Weinstein, C. (2011). The Global Economic Burden of Noncommunicable Diseases. Geneva: World Economic Forum, Geneva Switzerland. www.weforum.org/EconomicsOfNCD

Bode, J. C., Hanisch, P., Henning, H., Koenig, W., Richter, F. W., & Bode, C. (1988). Hepatic zinc content in patients with various stages of alcoholic liver disease and in patients with chronic active and chronic persistent hepatitis. Hepatology, 8:1605-1609.

Bosomworth, H. J., Adlard, P. A., Ford, D., & Valentine, R. A. (2013). Altered Expression of ZnT10 in Alzheimer's Disease Brain. PLoS One, 8, e65475.

Bosomworth, H. J., Thornton, J. K., Coneyworth, L. J., Ford, D., & Valentine, R. A. (2012). Efflux function, tissue-specific expression and intracellular trafficking of the Zn transporter ZnT10 indicate roles in adult Zn homeostasis. Metallomics, 4, 771-779.

Bribiescas, R. G. (2003). Effects of oral zinc supplementation on serum leptin levels in Ache males of eastern Paraguay. American Journal of Human Biology, 15, 681-687.

Carsten, S-P. (2000). Signalling aspects of insulin resistance in skeletal muscle: mechanisms induced by lipid oversupply. Cellular Signalling, 12, 583-594.

Chasapis, C., Loutsidou, A., Spiliopoulou, C., & Stefanidou, M. (2011). Zinc and human health: an update. Archives of Toxicology, 86, 1-14.

Chimienti, F., Devergnas, S., Pattou, F., Schuit, F., Garcia-Cuenca, R., Vandewalle, B., Kerr-Conte, J., Van L., Leentje, G., Didier, F. A., & Seve, M. (2006). In vivo expression and functional characterization of the zinc transporter ZnT8 in glucose-induced insulin secretion. Journal of Cell Science, 119, 4199-4206.

Chimienti, F., Favier, A., & Seve, M. (2005). ZnT-8, A Pancreatic Beta-Cell-Specific Zinc Transporter. BioMetals, 18, 313-317.

Chowanadisai, W., Graham, D. M., Keen, C. L., Rucker, R. B., & Messerli, M. A. (2013). Neurulation and neurite extension require the zinc transporter ZIP12 (slc39a12). Proceedings of the National Academy of Sciences, 110, 9903-9908.

Coble, Y. D., Jr., Bardin, C. W., Ross, G. T., & Darby, W. T. (1971). Studies of endocrine function in boys with retarded growth, delayed sexual maturation and zinc deficiency. The Journal of Clinical Endocrinology & Metabolism, 32, 361-367.

Costello, L. C., Zou, J., Desouki, M. M., & Franklin, R. B. (2012). Evidence for changes in RREB-1, ZIP3, and Zinc in the early development of pancreatic adenocarcinoma. Journal of Gastrointestinal Cancer, 43, 570-578.

Costello, L. C., Liu, Y., Zou, J., & Franklin, R. B. (1999). *Evidence for a Zinc Uptake Transporter in Human Prostate Cancer Cells Which Is Regulated by Prolactin and Testosterone. Journal of Biological Chemistry, 274, 17499-17504.*

Coulston, L., & Dandona, P. (1980). *Insulin-like Effect of Zinc on Adipocytes. Diabetes, 29, 665-667.*

Cragg, R. A., Philips, S. R., Piper, J. M., Varma, J. S., Campbell, F. C., Mathers, J. C & Ford, D. (2005). *Homeostatic regulation of zinc transporters in the human small intestine by dietary zinc supplementation. Gut, 54, 469-478.*

Deniro, M., & Al-Mohanna, F. A. (2012). *Zinc transporter 8 (ZnT8) expression is reduced by ischemic insults: a potential therapeutic target to prevent ischemic retinopathy. PLoS One, 7, e50360.*

Devergnas, S., Chimienti, F., Naud, N., Pennequin, A., Coquerel, Y., Chantegrel, J., Favier, A., & Seve, M. (2004). *Differential regulation of zinc efflux transporters ZnT-1, ZnT-5 and ZnT-7 gene expression by zinc levels: a real-time RT–PCR study. Biochemical Pharmacology, 68, 699-709.*

Devirgiliis, C., P. D. Zalewski, G. Perozzi and C. Murgia (2007). *Zinc fluxes and zinc transporter genes in chronic diseases. Mutation Research, 622, 84-93.*

Dufner-Beattie, J., Kuo, Y. M., Gitschier, J., & Andrews, G. K. (2004). *The Adaptive Response to Dietary Zinc in Mice Involves the Differential Cellular Localization and Zinc Regulation of the Zinc Transporters ZIP4 and ZIP5. Journal of Biological Chemistry, 279, 49082-49090.*

Eide, D., Broderius, M., Fett, J., & Guerinot, M. L. (1996). *A novel iron-regulated metal transporter from plants identified by functional expression in yeast. Proceedings of the National Academy of Sciences, 93, 5624-5628.*

Ezaki, O. (1989). *IIb group metal ions (Zn2+, Cd2+, Hg2+) stimulate glucose transport activity by post-insulin receptor kinase mechanism in rat adipocytes. Journal of Biological Chemistry, 264, 16118-16122.*

Fernandez, E. L., Dencker, L, & Tallkvist, J. (2007). *Expression of ZnT-1 (Slc30a1) and MT-1 (Mt1) in the conceptus of cadmium treated mice. Reproductive Toxicology, 24, 353-358.*

Figlewicz, D. P., Forhan, S. E., Hodgson, A. T., & Grodsky, G. M. (1984). *^{65}Zinc and endogenous zinc content and distribution in islets in relationship to insulin content. Endocrinology, 115, 877-881.*

Foster, M., Petocz, P., & Samman, S. (2013). *Inflammation markers predict zinc transporter gene expression in women with type 2 diabetes mellitus. The Journal of Nutritional Biochemistry, 24, 1655-1661.*

Foster, M., & Samman, S. (2010). *Zinc and redox signaling: perturbations associated with cardiovascular disease and diabetes mellitus. Antioxidants & redox signaling, 13, 1549-1573.*

Fu, Y., Tian, W., Pratt, E. B., Dirling, L. B., Shyng, S. L., Meshul, C. K., & Cohen, D. M. (2009). *Down-Regulation of ZnT8 Expression in INS-1 Rat Pancreatic Beta Cells Reduces Insulin Content and Glucose-Inducible Insulin Secretion. PLoS One, 4, e5679.*

Fukada, T., Yamasaki, S., Nishida, K., Murakami, M., & Hirano, T. (2011). *Zinc homeostasis and signaling in health and diseases. Journal of Biological Inorganic Chemistry, 16, 1123-1134.*

Gaither, L. A. & Eide, D (2001). *Eukaryotic zinc transporters and their regulation. BioMetals, 14, 251-270.*

González-Rodríguez, Á., Gutierrez, J. A. M., Sanz-González, S., Ros, M., Burks, D. J., & Valverde, Á. M. (2010). *Inhibition of PTP1B Restores IRS1-Mediated Hepatic Insulin Signaling in IRS2-Deficient Mice. Diabetes, 59, 588-599.*

Haase, H., & Maret, W. (2003). *Intracellular zinc fluctuations modulate protein tyrosine phosphatase activity in insulin/insulin-like growth factor-1 signaling. Experimental Cell Research, 291, 289-298.*

Haase, H., & Maret, W. (2005a). *Fluctuations of cellular, available zinc modulate insulin signaling via inhibition of protein tyrosine phosphatases. Journal of Trace Elements in Medicine and Biology, 19, 37-42.*

Haase, H., & Maret, W. (2005b). *Protein Tyrosine Phosphatases as Targets of the Combined Insulinomimetic Effects of Zinc and Oxidants. BioMetals, 18, 333-338.*

Haase, H., Mocchegiani, E., & Rink, L. (2006). *Correlation between zinc status and immune function in the elderly. Biogerontology, 7:412-428.*

Hambidge, K. M., Hambidge, C., Jacobs, M., & Baum, J. D. (1972). Low levels of zinc in hair, anorexia, poor growth, and hypogeusia in children. Pediatric Research, 6, 868-874.

Hardy, A. B., Wijesekara, N., Genkin, I., Prentice, K. J., Bhattacharjee, A., Kong, D., Chimienti, F., & Wheeler, M. B. (2012). Effects of high-fat diet feeding on Znt8-null mice: differences between beta-cell and global knockout of Znt8. American Journal of Physiology: Endocrinology and Metabolism, 302, E1084-1096.

Hogstrand, C., Kille, P., Nicholson, R. I., & Taylor, K. M. (2009). Zinc transporters and cancer: a potential role for ZIP7 as a hub for tyrosine kinase activation. Trends in Molecular Medicine, 15, 101-111.

Hojyo, S., Fukada, T., Shimoda, S., Ohashi, W., Bin, B-H., Koseki, H., & Hirano, T. (2011). The Zinc Transporter SLC39A14/ZIP14 Controls G-Protein Coupled Receptor-Mediated Signaling Required for Systemic Growth. PLoS One, 6, e18059.

Huang, L., Kirschke, C. P., Lay, Y. E., Levy, L. B., Lamirande, D. E., & Zhang, P. H. (2012). Znt7-null mice are more susceptible to diet-induced glucose intolerance and insulin resistance. Journal of Biological Chemistry. 287:33883-33896.

Huang, L., & Tepaamorndech, S. (2013). The SLC30 family of zinc transporters – A review of current understanding of their biological and pathophysiological roles. Molecular Aspects of Medicine, 34, 548-560.

Huang, L., Yan, M., & Kirschke, C. P. (2010). Over-expression of ZnT7 increases insulin synthesis and secretion in pancreatic β-cells by promoting insulin gene transcription. Experimental Cell Research, 316, 2630-2643.

Hulver, M. W., & Lynis D, G. (2004). The molecular mechanism linking muscle fat accumulation to insulin resistance. Proceedings of the Nutrition Society, 63, 375-380.

Hwang, I., Yoon, T., Kim, C., Cho, B., Lee, S., & Song, M. K. (2011). Different roles of zinc plus arachidonic acid on insulin sensitivity between high fructose- and high fat-fed rats. Life Sciences, 88, 278-284.

Iguchi, K., Otsuka, T., Usui, S., Ishii, K., Onishi, T., Sugimura, Y., & Hirano, K. (2004). Zinc and metallothionein levels and expression of zinc transporters in androgen-independent subline of LNCaP cells. Journal of Andrology, 25, 154-161.

Ilouz, R., Kaidanovich, O., Gurwitz, D., & Eldar-Finkelman, H. (2002). Inhibition of glycogen synthase kinase-3β by bivalent zinc ions: insight into the insulin-mimetic action of zinc. Biochemical and Biophysical Research Communications, 295, 102-106.

Jansen, J., Karges, W., & Rink, L. (2009). Zinc and diabetes — clinical links and molecular mechanisms. Journal of Nutritional Biochemistry, 20, 399-417.

Jansen, J., Rosenkranz, E., Overbeck, S., Warmuth, S., Mocchegiani, E., Giacconi, R., Weiskirchen, R., Karges, W., & Rink, L. (2012). Disturbed zinc homeostasis in diabetic patients by in vitro and in vivo analysis of insulinomimetic activity of zinc. The Journal of Nutritional Biochemistry, 23, 1458-1466.

Jayaraman, A. K., & Jayaraman, S. (2011). Increased level of exogenous zinc induces cytotoxicity and up-regulates the expression of the ZnT-1 zinc transporter gene in pancreatic cancer cells. The Journal of Nutritional Biochemistry, 22, 79-88.

Jayawardena, R., Ranasinghe, P., Galappatthy, P., Malkanthi, R. L. D. K., Constantine, G. R., & Katulanda, P. (2012). Effects of zinc supplementation on diabetes mellitus: a systematic review and meta-analysis. Diabetology & Metabolic Syndrome, 4, 13.

Jeong, J., & Eide, D. J. (2013). The SLC39 family of zinc transporters. Molecular Aspects of Medicine, 34, 612-619.

Kambe, T. (2011). An Overview of a Wide Range of Functions of ZnT and Zip Zinc Transporters in the Secretory Pathway. Bioscience Biotechnology and Biochemistry, 75, 1036-1043.

Kawasaki, E. (2012). ZnT8 and type 1 diabetes [Review]. Endocrine Journal, advpub, 1203050683-1203050683.

Kelleher, S. L., McCormick, N. H., Velasquez, V., & Lopez, V. (2011). Zinc in Specialized Secretory Tissues: Roles in the Pancreas, Prostate, and Mammary Gland. Advances in Nutrition: An International Review Journal, 2, 101-111.

Kirchhoff, K., Machicao, F., Haupt, A., Schafer, S. A., Tschritter, O., Staiger, H., Stefan, N., Haring, H-U., & Fritsche, A. (2008). Polymorphisms in the TCF7L2, CDKAL1 and SLC30A8 genes are associated with impaired proinsulin conversion. Diabetologia, 51:597-601.

Kommoju, U. J., & Reddy, B. M. (2011). Genetic etiology of type 2 diabetes mellitus: a review. International Journal of Diabetes in Developing Countries, 31, 51-64.

Kourtoglou, G. I. (2011). Insulin therapy and exercise. Diabetes Research and Clinical Practice, 93, Supplement 1, S73-S77.

Leung, K. W., Liu, M., Xu, X., Seiler, M. J., Barnstable, C. J., & Tombran-Tink, J. (2008). Expression of ZnT and ZIP zinc transporters in the human RPE and their regulation by neurotrophic factors. Investigative Ophthalmology and Visual Science, 49, 1221-1231.

Lewis, P. K. Jr., Hoekstra, W. G., Grummer, R. H., & Philips, P. H. (1956). The Effect of Certain Nutritional Factors including Calcium, Phosphorus and Zinc on Parakeratosis in Swine. Journal of Animal Science, 15, 741-751.

Li, H, & Jogl, G. (2007). Crystal Structure of the Zinc-binding Transport Protein ZnuA from Escherichia coli Reveals an Unexpected Variation in Metal Coordination. Journal of Molecular Biology, 368, 1358-1366.

Liang, D., Xiang, L., Yang, M., Zhang, X., Guo, B., Chen, Y., Yang, L., & Cao, J. (2013). ZnT7 can protect MC3T3-E1 cells from oxidative stress-induced apoptosis via PI3K/Akt and MAPK/ERK signaling pathways. Cellular Signalling, 25, 1126-1135.

Lichten, L. A., & Cousins, R. J. (2009). Mammalian Zinc Transporters: Nutritional and Physiologic Regulation. Annual Review of Nutrition, 29, 153-176.

Lin, Y., & Sun, Z. (2010). Current views on type 2 diabetes. Journal of Endocrinology, 204, 1-11.

Liu, B. Y., Jiang, Y. Z., Lu, Z. Y., Li, S. F., Lu, D. B., & Chen, B. (2011b). Down-regulation of zinc transporter 8 in the pancreas of db/db mice is rescued by Exendin-4 administration. Molecular Medicine Reports, 4, 47-52.

Liu, J., Bao, W., Jiang, M., Zhang, Y., Zhang, X., & Liu, L. (2011a). Chromium, Selenium, and Zinc Multimineral Enriched Yeast Supplementation Ameliorates Diabetes Symptom in Streptozotocin-Induced Mice. Biological Trace Element Research, 1-10.

Liuzzi, J. P., Blanchard, R. K., & Cousins, R. J. (2001). Differential Regulation of Zinc Transporter 1, 2, and 4 mRNA Expression by Dietary Zinc in Rats. The Journal of Nutrition, 131, 46-52.

Liuzzi, J. P., & Cousins, R. J. (2004). Mammalian Zinc Transporters. Annual Review of Nutrition, 24, 151-172.

Liuzzi, J. P., Lichten, L. A., Rivera, S., Blanchard, R. K., Aydemir, T. B., Knutson, M. D., Ganz, T., & Cousins, R. J. (2005). Interleukin-6 regulates the zinc transporter Zip14 in liver and contributes to the hypozincemia of the acute-phase response. Proceedings of the National Academy of Sciences, 102, 6843-6848.

Lu, M., & Fu, D. (2007). Structure of the Zinc Transporter YiiP. Science, 317, 1746-1748.

Lue, H. W., Yang, X., Wang, R., Qian, W., Xu, R. Z. H., Lyles, R., Osunkoya, A. O., Zhou, B. P., Vessella, R. L., Zayzafoon, M., Liu, Z-R., Zhau, H. E., & Chung, L. W. K. (2011). LIV-1 Promotes Prostate Cancer Epithelial-to-Mesenchymal Transition and Metastasis through HB-EGF Shedding and EGFR-Mediated ERK Signaling. PLoS One, 6, e27720.

Makonnen, B., Venter, A., & Joubert, G. (2003). A randomized controlled study of the impact of dietary zinc supplementation in the management of children with protein-energy malnutrition in Lesotho. II: Special investigations. Journal of Tropical Pediatrics, 49, 353-360.

Maret, W. (2011a). Metals on the move: zinc ions in cellular regulation and in the coordination dynamics of zinc proteins. BioMetals, 24, 411-418.

Maret, W. (2011b). New perspectives of zinc coordination environments in proteins. Journal of Inorganic Biochemistry, 111, 110-116.

May, J. M., & Contoreggi, C. S. (1982). The mechanism of the insulin-like effects of ionic zinc. Journal of Biological Chemistry, 257, 4362-4368.

Miao, X., Sun, W., Fu, Y., Miao, L., & Cai, Lu. (2013). Zinc homeostasis in the metabolic syndrome and diabetes. Frontiers of Medicine, 7, 31-52.

Milon, B., Wu, Q., Zou, J., Costello, L. C., & Renty, F. B. (2006). Histidine residues in the region between transmembrane domains III and IV of hZip1 are required for zinc transport across the plasma membrane in PC-3 cells. Biochimica et Biophysica Acta (BBA) - Biomembranes, 1758, 1696-1701.

Mocchegiani, E., Giacconi, R., & Malavolta, M. (2008). Zinc signalling and subcellular distribution: emerging targets in type 2 diabetes. Trends in Molecular Medicine, 14, 419-428.

Moniz, T., Amorim, M. J., Ferreira, R., Nunes, A., Silva, A., Queirós, C., Leite, A., Gameiro, P., Sarmento, B., Remião, F., Yoshikawa, Y., Sakurai, H., & Rangel, M. (2011). Investigation of the insulin-like properties of zinc(II) complexes of 3-hydroxy-4-pyridinones: Identification of a compound with glucose lowering effect in STZ-induced type I diabetic animals. Journal of Inorganic Biochemistry, 105, 1675-1682.

Myers, S. A., Nield, A., Chew, G. S., & Myers, M. A. (2013) The Zinc Transporter, Slc39a7 (Zip7) Is Implicated in Glycaemic Control in Skeletal Muscle Cells. PLoS ONE, 8:e79316.

Myers, S. A., Nield, A., & Myers, M. (2012). Zinc Transporters, Mecahnisms of Action and Therapeutic Utility: Implications for Type 2 Diabetes Mellitus. Journal of Nutrition and Metabolism, doi:10.1155/2012/173712).

Nicolson, T. J., Bellomo, E. A., Wijesekara, N., Loder, M. K., Baldwin, J. M., Gyulkhandanyan, A. V., Koshkin, V., Tarasov, A. I., Carzaniga, R., Kronenberger, K., Taneja, T. K., da Silva Xavier, G., Libert, S., Froguel, P., Scharfmann, R., Stetsyuk, V., Ravassard, P., Parker, H., Gribble, F. M., Reimann, F., Sladek, R., Hughes, S. J., Johnson, P. R.V., Masseboeuf, M., Burcelin, R., Baldwin, S. A., Liu, M., Lara-Lemus, R., Arvan, P., Schuit, F. C., Wheeler, M. B., Chimienti, F., & Rutter, G. A. (2009). Insulin Storage and Glucose Homeostasis in Mice Null for the Granule Zinc Transporter ZnT8 and Studies of the Type 2 Diabetes–Associated Variants. Diabetes, 58, 2070-2083.

Nyenwe, E. A., Jerkins, T. W., Umpierrez, G. E., & Kitabchi, A. E. (2011). Management of type 2 diabetes: evolving strategies for the treatment of patients with type 2 diabetes. Metabolism, 60, 1-23.

O'Dell, B. L., Newberne, P. M., & Savage, J. E. (1958). Significance of dietary zinc for the growing chicken. The Journal of Nutrition, 65, 503-518.

Osto, M., Zini, E., Reusch, C. E., & Lutz, T. A. (2013). Diabetes from humans to cats. General and Comparative Endocrinology, 182, 48-53.

Pagel-Langenickel, I., Bao, J., Pang, L., & Sack, M. N. (2010). The Role of Mitochondria in the Pathophysiology of Skeletal Muscle Insulin Resistance. Endocrine Reviews, 31, 25-51.

Pal, A., & McCarthy, M. I. (2013). The genetics of type 2 diabetes and its clinical relevance. Clinical Genetics, 83, 297-306.

Palmiter, R. D, & Findley, S. D. (1995). Cloning and functional characterization of a mammalian zinc transporter that confers resistance to zinc. EMBO J., 14, 639-649.

Palmiter, R. D, & Huang, L. (2004). Efflux and compartmentalization of zinc by members of the SLC30 family of solute carriers. Pflugers Archiv., 447, 744-751.

Pawan, K., Sharma, N., Kumar, S., Radha, K. R., Prasad, R. (2007). Upregulation of Slc39a10 gene expression in response to thyroid hormones in intestine and kidney. Biochimica et Biophysica Acta (1769), 117–123.

Pandey, N., Vardatsikos, G., Mehdi, M., & Srivastava, A. (2010). Cell-type-specific roles of IGF-1R and EGFR in mediating Zn^{2+}-induced ERK1/2 and PKB phosphorylation. Journal of Biological Inorganic Chemistry, 15, 399-407.

Pathak, A., Sharma, V., Kumar, S., & Dhawan, D. (2011). Supplementation of zinc mitigates the altered uptake and turnover of ^{65}Zn in liver and whole body of diabetic rats. BioMetals, 24, 1027-1034.

Patrushev, N., Seidel-Rogol, B., & Salazar, G. (2012). Angiotensin II requires zinc and downregulation of the zinc transporters ZnT3 and ZnT10 to induce senescence of vascular smooth muscle cells. PLoS One, 7, e33211.

Peppa, M., Koliaki, C., Nikolopoulos, P., & Raptis, S. A. (2010). Skeletal Muscle Insulin Resistance in Endocrine Disease. Journal of Biomedicine and Biotechnology, 10.1155/2010/527850.

Pfaffl, M. W., & Windisch, W. (2003). Influence of zinc deficiency on the mRNA expression of zinc transporters in adult rats. Journal of Trace Elements in Medicine and Biology, 17, 97-106.

Potocki, S., Valensin, D., Camponeschi, F., & Kozlowski, H. (2013). The extracellular loop of IRT1 ZIP protein - the chosen one for zinc? Journal of Inorganic Biochemistry. doi: 10.1016/j.jinorgbio.2013.05.003

Pound, L. D., Sarkar, S. A., Benninger, R. K. P., Wang, Y. D., Suwanichkul, A., Shadoan, M. K., Printz, R. L., Oeser, J. K., Lee, C. E., Piston, D. W., McGuinness, O. P., Hutton, J. C., Powell, D. R., & O'Brien, R. M. (2009). Deletion of the mouse Slc30a8 gene encoding zinc transporter-8 results in impaired insulin secretion. Biochemical Journal, 421, 371-376.

Prasad, A. (1991). Discovery of human zinc deficiency and studies in an experimental human model. The American Journal of Clinical Nutrition, 53, 403-412.

Prasad, A. S., Halsted, J. A., & Nadimi, M. (1961). Syndrome of iron deficiency anemia, hepatosplenomegaly, hypogonadism, dwarfism and geophagia. American Journal of Medicine, 31, 532-546.

Prasad, A. S. (2012). Discovery of human zinc deficiency: 50 years later. Journal of Trace Elements in Medicine and Biology, 26, 66-69.

Raulin, J. (1869). Etudes clinique sur la vegetation. Annales des Scienceas Naturelle: Botanique, 11, 93-299.

Rink, L. (2011). Zinc in Human Health. Amsterdam, Netherlands: IOS Press BV, pp.577.

Ronaghy, H., Fox, M. R., Garnsm, Israel, H., Harp, A., Moe, P. G., & Halsted, J. A. (1969). Controlled zinc supplementation for malnourished school boys: a pilot experiment. American Journal of Clinical Nutrition, 22, 1279-1289.

Rutherford, J. C., & Bird, A. J. (2004). Metal-Responsive Transcription Factors That Regulate Iron, Zinc, and Copper Homeostasis in Eukaryotic Cells. Eukaryotic Cell, 3, 1-13.

Rutter, G. A. (2010). Think zinc: New roles for zinc in the control of insulin secretion. Islets, 2, 49-50.

Saltiel, A. R., & Pessin, J. E. (2002). Insulin signaling pathways in time and space. Trends in Cell Biology, 12, 65-71.

Sandstead, H. H., Prasad, A. S., Schulert, A. R., Farid, Z., Miale, A., Jr., Bassilly, S., & Darby, W. J. (1967). Human zinc deficiency, endocrine manifestations and response to treatment. American Journal of Clinical Nutrition, 20, 422-442.

Saxena, R., Voight, B. F., Lyssenko, V., Burtt, N. P., de Bakker, P. I. W., Chen, H., Roix, J. J., Kathiresan, S., Hirschhorn, J. N., Daly, M. J., Hughes, T. E., Groop, L., Altshuler, D., Almgren, P., Florez, J. C., Meyer, J., Ardlie, K., Bengtsson B. K., Isomaa, B., Lettre, G., Lindblad, U., Lyon, H. N., Melander, O., Newton-Cheh, C., Nilsson, P., Orho-Melander, M., Råstam, L., Speliotes, E. K., Taskinen, M-R., Tuomi, T., Guiducci, C., Berglund, A., Carlson, J., Gianniny, L., Hackett, R., Hall, L., Holmkvist, J., Laurila, E., Sjögren, M., Sterner, M., Surti, A., Svensson, M., Svensson, M., Tewhey, R., Blumenstiel, B., Parkin, M., DeFelice, M., Barry, R., Brodeur, W., Camarata, J., Chia, N., Fava, M., Gibbons, J., Handsaker, B., Healy, C., Nguyen, K., Gates, C., Sougnez, C., Gage, D., Nizzari, M., Gabriel, S. B., Chirn, G-W., Ma, Q., Parikh, H., Richardson, D., Ricke, D., & Purcell, S. (2007). Genome-Wide Association Analysis Identifies Loci for Type 2 Diabetes and Triglyceride Levels. Science, 316, 1331-1336.

Skarstrand, H., Lernmark, A & Vaziri-Sani, F. (2013). Antigenicity and Epitope Specificity of ZnT8 Autoantibodies in Type 1 Diabetes. Scandinavian Journal of Immunology, 77:21-29.

Shin, J. A., Lee, J. H., Kim, H. S., Choi, Y. H., Cho, J. H., & Yoon, K. H. (2012). Prevention of diabetes: a strategic approach for individual patients. Diabetes/Metabolism Research and Reviews, 28, 79-84.

Simon, S. F., & Taylor, C. G. (2001). Dietary Zinc Supplementation Attenuates Hyperglycemia in db/db Mice. Experimental Biology and Medicine, 226, 43-51.

Sladek, R., Rocheleau, G., Rung, J., Dina, C., Shen, L., Serre, D., Boutin, P., Vincent, D., Belisle, A., Hadjadj, S., Balkau, B., Heude, B., Charpentier, G., Hudson, T. J., Montpetit, A., Pshezhetsky, Al. V., Prentki, M., Posner, B. I., Balding, D. J., Meyre, D., Polychronakos, C., & Froguel, P. (2007). A genome-wide association study identifies novel risk loci for type 2 diabetes. Nature, 445, 881-885.

Smidt, K., & Rungby, J. (2012). ZnT3: a zinc transporter active in several organs. Biometals, 25,1-8.

Smidt, K., Jessen, N., Petersen, A. B., Larsen, A., Magnusson, N., Jeppesen, J. B., Stoltenberg, M., Culvenor, J. G., Tsatsanis, A., Brock, B., Schmitz, O., Wogensen, L., Bush, A. I., & Rungby, J. (2009). SLC30A3 Responds to Glucose- and Zinc Variations in beta-Cells and Is Critical for Insulin Production and In Vivo Glucose-Metabolism During beta-Cell Stress. PLoS One, 4, e568410.

Sommer, A. L., & Lipman, C. B. (1926). Evidence on the indispensable nature of zinc and boron for higher green plants. Plant Physiology, 1, 231-249.

Song, M. K., Rosenthal, M. J., Hong, S., Harris, D. M., Hwang, I., Yip, I., Golub, M. S., Ament, M. E., & Go, V. L. W. (2001). Synergistic antidiabetic activities of zinc, cyclo (His-Pro), and arachidonic acid. Metabolism, 50, 53-59.

Tang, X. H., & Shay, N. F. (2001). Zinc Has an Insulin-Like Effect on Glucose Transport Mediated by Phosphoinositol-3-Kinase and Akt in 3T3-L1 Fibroblasts and Adipocytes. The Journal of Nutrition, 131, 1414-1420.

Taniguchi, M., Fukunaka, A., Hagihara, M., Watanabe, K., Kamino, S., Kambe, T., Enomoto, S., & Hiromura, M. (2013). Essential role of the zinc transporter ZIP9/SLC39A9 in regulating the activations of Akt and Erk in B-cell receptor signaling pathway in DT40 cells. PLoS One, 8, e58022.

Taton, J., Piatkiewicz, P., & Czech, A. (2010). Molecular physiology of cellular glucose transport - a potential area for clinical studies in diabetes mellitus. Endokrynologia Polska, 61, 303-310.

Taylor, K. M., Morgan, H. E., Smart, K., Zahari, N. M., Pumford, S., Ellis, I. O., Robertson, J. F., & Nicholson, R. I. (2007). The emerging role of the LIV-1 subfamily of zinc transporters in breast cancer. Molecular Medicine, 13, 396-406.

Taylor, K. M., Hiscox, S., Nicholson, R. I., Hogstrand, C., & Kille, P. (2012). Protein Kinase CK2 Triggers Cytosolic Zinc Signaling Pathways by Phosphorylation of Zinc Channel ZIP7. Science Signaling, 5, ra11.

Taylor, K. M., Vichova, P., Jordan, N., Hiscox, S., Hendley, R., & Nicholson, R. I. (2008). ZIP7-Mediated Intracellular Zinc Transport Contributes to Aberrant Growth Factor Signaling in Antihormone-Resistant Breast Cancer Cells. Endocrinology, 149, 4912-4920.

Todd, W. R., Elvehjem, C. A., & Hart, E. B. (1934). Zinc in the nutrition of the rat. The American Journal of Physiology, 107, 146-156.

Tucker, H. F, & Salmon, W. D. (1955). Parakertosis or zinc deficiency disease in pig. Proceedings of the Society for Experimental Biology and Medicine, 88, 613-616.

Vallee, B. L., & Falchuk, K. H. (1993). The biochemical basis of zinc physiology. Physiological Reviews, 73, 79-118.

Vardatsikos, G., Pandey, N. R., & Srivastava, A. K. (2013). Insulino-mimetic and anti-diabetic effects of zinc. Journal of Inorganic Biochemistry, 120, 8-17.

Wang, X., Li, H., Fan, Z., & Liu, Y. (2012). Effect of zinc supplementation on type 2 diabetes parameters and liver metallothionein expressions in Wistar rats. Journal of Physiology and Biochemistry, 68, 1-10.

Wei, Y., Li, H., & Fu, D. (2004). Oligomeric State of the Escherichia coli Metal Transporter YiiP. Journal of Biological Chemistry, 279, 39251-39259.

Wenzlau, J. M & Hutton, J. C. (2013). Novel Diabetes Autoantibodies and Prediction of Type 1 Diabetes. Current Diabetes Reports, 13, 608-615.

Wenzlau, J. M., Juhl, K., Yu, L., Moua, O., Sarkar, S. A., Gottlieb, P., Rewers, M., Eisenbarth, G. S., Jensen, J., Davidson, H. W., & Hutton, J. C. (2007). The cation efflux transporter ZnT8 (Slc30A8) is a major autoantigen in human type 1 diabetes. Proceedings of the National Academy of Sciences, 104, 17040-17045.

Wenzlau, J. M., Liu, Y., Yu, L., Moua, O., Fowler, K. T., Rangasamy, S., Walters, J., Eisenbarth, G. S., Davidson, H. W., & Hutton, J. C. (2008). A common non-synonymous single nucleotide polymorphism in the SLC30A8 gene determines ZnT3 autoantibody specificity in type 1 diabetes. Diabetes, 57:2693-2697.

Wijesekara, N., Chimienti, F., & Wheeler, M. B. (2009). Zinc, a regulator of islet function and glucose homeostasis. Diabetes, Obesity and Metabolism, 11, 202-214.

Wijesekara, N., Dai, F. F., Hardy, A. B., Giglou, P. R., Bhattacharjee, A., Koshkin, V., Chimienti, F., Gaisano, H. Y., Rutter, G. A., & Wheeler, M. B. (2010). Beta cell-specific Znt8 deletion in mice causes marked defects in insulin processing, crystallisation and secretion. Diabetologia, 53, 1656-1668.

Wilson, M., Hogstrand, C., & Maret, W. (2012). Picomolar Concentrations of Free Zinc(II) Ions Regulate Receptor Protein-tyrosine Phosphatase β Activity. Journal of Biological Chemistry, 287, 9322-9326.

Wongdee, K., Teerapornpuntakit, J., Riengrojpitak, S., Krishnamra, N., & Charoenphandhu, N. (2009). Gene expression profile of duodenal epithelial cells in response to chronic metabolic acidosis. Molecular Cell Biochemistry, 321, 173-188.

Wu, W., Graves, L. M., Jaspers, I., Devlin, R. B., Reed, W., & Samet, J. M. (1999). Activation of the EGF receptor signaling pathway in human airway epithelial cells exposed to metals. American Journal of Physiology, 277(5 Pt 1), L924-931.

Xu, J., Wang, J., & Chen, B. (2012). SLC30A8 (ZnT8) variations and type 2 diabetes in the Chinese Han population. Genetics and Molecular Research, 11, 1592-1598.

Xu, Y., Yan, Y., Seeman, D., Sun, L., & Dubin, P. L. (2011). Multimerization and Aggregation of Native-State Insulin: Effect of Zinc. Langmuir. doi: 10.1021/la202902a

Xue, B., Kim, Y. B., Lee, A., Toschi, E., Bonner-Weir, S., Kahn, C. R., Neel, B. G., & Kahn, B. B. (2007). Protein-tyrosine Phosphatase 1B Deficiency Reduces Insulin Resistance and the Diabetic Phenotype in Mice with Polygenic Insulin Resistance. Journal of Biological Chemistry, 282, 23829-23840.

Yamasaki, S., Sakata-Sogawa, K., Hasegawa, A., Suzuki, T., Kabu, K., Sato, E., Kurosaki, T., Yamashita, S., Tokunaga, M., Nishida, K., & Hirano, T. (2007). Zinc is a novel intracellular second messenger. The Journal of Cell Biology, 177, 637-645.

Yoshikawa, Y., Murayama, A., Adachi, Y., Sakurai, H., & Yasui, H. (2011). Challenge of studies on the development of new Zn complexes (Zn(opt)$_2$) to treat diabetes mellitus. Metallomics, 3:686-692.

Yoshikawa, Y., Ueda, E., Miyake, H., Sakurai, H., & Kojima, Y. (2001). Insulinomimetic bis(maltolato)zinc(II) Complex: Blood Glucose Normalizing Effect in KK-A^y Mice with Type 2 Diabetes Mellitus. Biochemical and Biophysical Research Communications, 281, 1190-1193.

Yoshikawa, Y., Ueda, E., Sakurai, H., & Kojima, Y. (2003). Anti-diabetes Effect of Zn(II)/Carnitine Complex by Oral Administration. Chemical and Pharmaceutical Bulletin, 51:230-231. 281:1190-1193.

Yoshikawa, Y., Ueda, E., Kojima, Y., & Sakurai, H. (2004). The action mechanism of zinc(II) complexes with insulinomimetic activity in rat adipocytes. Life Sciences, 75, 741-751.

Yu, Y., Wu, A., Zhang, Z., Yan, G., Zhang, F., Zhang, L., Shen, X., Hu, R., Zhang, Y., Zhang, K., & Wang, F. (2013). Characterization of the GufA subfamily member SLC39A11/Zip11 as a zinc transporter. Journal of Nutritional Biochemistry. doi: 10.1016/j.jnutbio.2013.02.010

Zhao, H., & Eide, D. (1996). The yeast ZRT1 gene encodes the zinc transporter protein of a high-affinity uptake system induced by zinc limitation. Proceedings of the National Academy of Sciences, 93, 2454-2458.

Zhao, L., Chen, W., Taylor, K. M., Cai, B., & Li, X. (2007). LIV-1 suppression inhibits HeLa cell invasion by targeting ERK1/2-Snail/Slug pathway. Biochemical and Biophysical Research Communications, 363, 82-88.

Zhao, Y., Tan, Y., Dai, J., Wang, B., Li, B., Guo, L., Cui, J., Wang, G., Li, W., & Cai, L. (2011). Zinc deficiency exacerbates diabetic down-regulation of Akt expression and function in the testis: essential roles of PTEN, PTP1B and TRB3. The Journal of Nutritional Biochemistry, 23, 1018-1026.

Zimmet, P. (2002). Review: Epidemiology of diabetes — its history in the last 50 years. The British Journal of Diabetes & Vascular Disease, 2, 435-439.

Stress and Thyroid Disease

Atsushi Fukao
Ibaraki City Public Health Medical Center, Japan

Junta Takamatsu
Takamatsu Thyroid Clinic, Japan

Akira Miyauchi
Kuma Hospital, Japan

Toshiaki Hanafusa
Department of Internal Medicine (I)
Osaka Medical College, Japan

1   Introduction

Graves' disease (GD) is one of the most frequently seen thyroid disorders characterized by hyperthyroidism, goiter and extrathyroidal manifestations such as exophthalmos. Various genetic factors and environmental factors affect pathogenesis of GD (Akamizu, 1997). In particular, the role of emotional stress including psychosocial strain, trauma and stressful life events has been the subject of considerable debate since Caleb Parry (1825) who first described the syndrome of hyperfunction of the thyroid gland attributed the disorder in his young female patient to the fear she had experienced when thrown out of her wheelchair when coming down a hill, fast. Graves, Basedow and others reported similar debates. There are many reports on the association between stress and the onset of GD or thyrotoxicosis. However, most early reports were anecdotal and various epidemiologically problems. Recently, many epidemiologically improved study have demonstrated that GD patients had more stress than controls subjects prior to the onset of hyperthyroidism and stress had an unfavorable effect on the prognosis of GD. If stress affect the prognosis of GD, psychosomatic therapeutic approaches may improve the disease.

This review described the role of psychosocial factors including personality traits as well as stresses on the etiology of thyroid diseases for physicians to be able to utilize in the clinical setting. Our recent studies in GD were also included in this paper. Because there are some studies about the relationships between stress and other thyroid diseases including Hashimoto's thyroiditis, Plummer' disease and benign thyroid nodule, we introduced these reports.

2   Stress and GD

2.1   Emotional Stresses on the Onset of GD

To this day, many research efforts are still directed at exploring the possible role of stress on the onset of GD. These early reports were followed by epidemiological observations of an increase of GD or thyrotoxicosis during major wars, a condition named "Kriegbasedow". Indeed, the incidence of GD significantly increased in Scandinavian countries during WW II (1939-1945) and returned to normal rates after the war (Gorman, 1990). Bram (1936) found that 2842 patients in 3343 GD patients (85%) had experienced trauma before disease had occurred. But this study and other early studies (Lids & Whitehorn, 1949; Mandelbrote & Wittkower, 1955; Hadden & McDevitt, 1974) were uncontrolled and more recent authors have used unstandardized research instruments or inadequate epidemiological method, small size, improper controls, poor differential diagnosis within thyrotoxicosis.

Winsa *et al* (1991) has reported the first large population-based case-control study demonstrating a relationship between stress and GD. 208 (95%) of 219 eligible patients with newly diagnosed GD and 372 (80%) of all selected matched controls answered an identical mailed questionnaire about marital status, occupation, drinking and smoking habits, physical activity, familial occurrence of thyroid disease, life events, social support and personality. Compared with controls, GD patients claimed to have had more negative life events in 12 months preceding the diagnosis, and negative life-event scores were also significantly higher (odds ratio 6.3, 95% confidence interval 2.7-14.7, for the category with the highest negative score). When results were adjusted for possible confounding factors in multivariate analysis, risk estimates were almost unchanged. After this report, many case control studies were reported. Sonino *et al* (1993) reported by structured interview that 70 GD patients had reported significantly more life events compared to 70 controls. They also have had more independent events on thyrotoxicosis that had an objective negative impact according to an independent rater, unaware whether the events had occurred in patients or controls. Kun (1995) reported by questionnaires that 95 GD patients had reported more daily hassles as well as negative life events compared to 95 controls. Radosaljevic et al (1996) reported by structured interview that 100 GD patients had reported more independent life events and potentially dependent life events on illness compared to 100 controls. Yoshiuchi et al (1998) reported by questionnaires that 182 female GD patients had reported more life events compared to 228 controls but daily hassles were not significant different. Matos-Santos et al (2001) reported by structured interview that 31 GD patients had reported more stressful life events compared to 30 toxic nodular goiter (Plummer's disease) patients and 31 controls, and no significant differences were found between toxic nodular goiter patients and controls. Paunkovic et al (1998) also reported that the incidence of GD significantly increased in eastern Serbia during the civil war from 1992 to 1995, and the incidents of Plummer's disease did not increase for the same period. These retrospective data suggest the positive relationship between stress and the onset of GD.

Conversely, some authors obtained contradictory findings. Gray and Hoffenberg (1985) found no association between stressful life events in 50 thyrotoxic patients by structured interview. However, this study have some methodological problems that the date of onset of symptoms was uncertain, thyrotoxic patients include GD and toxic nodule and 50 control subjects were not healthy subjects but non toxic goiter. Chiovato et al (1998) could not find past or present GD patients in 87 patients with panic disorder encompassing a total of 478 patient-years of exposure to recent endogenous stress unrelated to life events. Martin-du Pan (1998) evaluated the role of major stress and pregnancy in triggering autoimmune thyroid disease in 98 GD patients and 97 patients with benign thyroid nodules. There were no significant differences of stress factors between two groups, and generally the role of stress in triggering GD seemed weak and dubious compared to the role of pregnancy and the postpartum period. Effraimidis et al (2011) reported a prospective cohort study on the association between stress and the onset of autoimmune thyroid disease (AITD) in 521 euthyroid women who were 1st or 2nd degree relatives of AITD patients. They could not find that stress factors (stressful life events, daily hassles and negative feeling) involved in the onset of GD including development of TPOAb and hyperthyroidism.

Some criticisms of case-control studies were proposed (Chiovato & Pinchera, 1996; Mizokami, et al, 2004). There are some general methodological problems and limitations in studies dealing stress, especially preceding retrospective studies based on the assessment of life events preceding thyrotoxicosis or the diagnosis of GD. Firstly, the main scientific problem is the difficulty in defining "stress" and objectively quantifying individual stressors. Second, the recall bias cannot be avoided in retrospective studies. GD patients may be more prone to recall stressful life events than healthy controls. Third, it is impossible to date the onset of GD precisely. Thus stressful life events may occur after the onset of GD. Some studies investigated life events in the 12 months before diagnosis, rather than before the first symptoms or signs. However, some events could have occurred between the onset and diagnosis. Finally, thyrotoxicosis itself can cause psychological disturbance and behavioral changes such as anxiety and depression, which may have an effect on life events. So, some stressful life events may be the consequence rather than the trigger for disease development. Though each above-mentioned study was planned with various devices, some problems remained. So the role of stress on the onset of GD is still controversial.

2.2   Emotional Stresses on the Clinical Course of GD

2.2.1   Previous Studies

On the other hand, there are case reports in which emotional stress induced an exacerbation and relapse of hyperthyroidism. Ferguson-Rayport (1956) reported that the course of thyrotoxicosis in 20 patients during antithyroid drug (ATD) treatment had seemed to be related to the patient's ability to cope with life stress psychologically, especially when confronted with loss or bereavement. If successful solutions were found, the illness subsided; if not, the exacerbation progressed. Voth *et al* (1970) reported that among 239 women the hyperfunctioning regions on thyroid scintiscans had appeared to wax and wine in a direct relationship with life stress followed for 12 years, and some women developed clinical thyrotoxicosis during conditions of severe or prolonged life strain. Yoshiuchi *et al* (1998) investigated the association between the short term outocome of 230 newly diagnosed GD patients, assessed 12 months after the ATD therapy, and stressful life events. They reported that daily hassles at 6 months after beginning therapy were associated with continued hyperthyroid state 12 months later in female patients.

It seems that a therapeutic approach to the patients' psychology such as stress management is effective in improving the prognosis of hyperthyroidism. Indeed, there is a brief interisting report (Benvenga, 1996) in which administration of minor tranquilizer (bromazepam) together with ATD increased the remission rate of hyperthyroidism.

2.2.2   Our Studies on Psychiatric Abnormality and Stress

We (2003) have determined three psychological tests including the Minnesota Multiphasic Personality Inventory (MMPI) for personality traits, the Natsume's Stress Inventory for stressful life events and the Hayashi's Daily Life Stress Inventory for daily life stress in 69 GD patients who had been a euthyroid state after ATD medication for more than two years and 32 healthy subjects (Table 1). When the patients were divided according to prognosis (41 with relapse and 28 with remission), depressive personality traits including hypochondriasis, depression and psychasthenia were significantly more common in the relapsed GD group than those of the remitted group and control group (Table 2). The scores of dally hassles were also significantly greater in the relapsed GD group than in the remitted GD group and control group (Figure1). In the GD patients, stress scores of life events correlated significantly with serumTSH receptor antibody (TRAb) activity ($r = 0.424$, $P < 0.001$) and thyrold volume ($r = 0.480$, $P < 0.001$) (Table 3). The scale scores of depression and psychasthenia showed a positive correlation with scores of dally hassles ($r = 0.535$, $P < 0.001$; $r = 0.580$, $P < 0.001$, respectively), while an inverse correlation with scores of daily uplifts ($r = -0.0373$, $P < 0.05$; $r = -0.322$, $P < 0.05$,respectively) (Table 3).

We (2011) also determined the MMPI for personality traits, the Natsume's Stress Inventory, and the Hayashi's Daily Life Stress Inventory before and during ATD treatment in 64 untreated GD patients. In the untreated thyrotoxic state, depressive personality (T-scores of hypochondriasis, depression or psychasthenia greater than 60 points in MMPI) were found for 44 patients (69%) (Figure 2). For 15 (23%) (group C) of these patients, the scores decreased to the normal range after treatment. However, depressive personality persisted after treatment in the remaining 29 patients (46%) (group A). Normal scores before treatment were found for 20 patients (31%), and the scores were persistently normal for 15 patients (23%) (group D). The remaining 5 patients (8%) (group B) had higher depressive personality after treatment. Such depressive personality was not associated with the severity of hyperthyroidism before treat-

Groups	No. of Subjects	Male / Female	Age (years)	Duration of Therapy (years)	Serum concentration			Thyroid Volume (ml)	MCPA (percent positive) (%)	TGPA (percent positive) (%)
					FT$_4$ (pmol/l)	TSH (mU/l)	TRAb (%)			
Relapsed Graves' disease	41	3/38	39.3±14.6	3.1±0.9 (2.0–5.0)	16.86±4.63	0.76±1.21[*+]	24.9±21.9[#§]	43.8±22.8[#§]	93[**]	29[**]
Remitted Graves' disease	28	1/27	43.4±12.4	2.9±1.0 (2.0–4.7)	16.86±3.60	1.86±2.07	3.8±3.9[¶]	24.4±6.2[¶]	89[**]	39[**]
Controls	32	1/31	36.7±12.6	--	16.22±3.22	1.57±1.23	0.7±2.3	10.2±2.5	0	0

[*] $P < 0.05$, *vs.* controls by Fisher's PLSD test.
[+] $P < 0.05$, *vs.* remitted Graves' disease byFisher's PLSD test.
[#] $P < 0.001$, *vs.* controls by Mann-Whitney's test.
[§] $P < 0.001$, *vs.* remitted Grave's disease by Mann-Whitney's test.
[¶] $P < 0.05$, *vs.* controls by by Mann-Whitney's test.
[**] $P < 0.001$, *vs.* controls by χ^2 test for independence.

Table1: Clinical profiles and thyroid function tests in two groups of GD patients on ATD and normal controls. The data are shown as mean±SD.

Groups	Hypochondriasis	Depression	Conversion Hysteria	Psychopathic deviation	Masculity / Feminity	Paranoia	Psychasthenia	Schizophrenia	Hypomaria	Social Introversion
Relapsed Graves' disease	53.7±10.7[*#]	57.8±13/7[*#]	55.6±9.7[+]	55.0±12.4[+]	50.3±8.9	54.4±12.5[#]	57.5±15.3[*#]	53.6±14.9[+]	49.0±10.2	53.9±10.8
Remitted Graves' disease	48.2±8.6	50.0±9.9	51.6±8.1	51.0±8.0	50.4±9.7	48.1±10.1	50.3±10.9	49.4±9.7	47.3±9.9	51.4±8.5
Controls	46.2±7.9	46.6±8.1	49.5±9.0	48.6±8.6	48.3±6.6	52.6±6.5	46.8±8.6	46.5±7.8	48.1±10.5	48.9±10.0

[*] $P < 0.001$, vs. controls by Fisher's PSD test.
[+] $P < 0.05$, vs. controls by Fisher's PLSD test.
[#] $P < 0.05$, vs. remitted Graves disease by Fisher's PLSD test.

Table2: Comparison of clinical scales of MMPI among the three groups of subjects. The data are shown as mean±SD of T-scores in MMPI. T-scores express the psychiatric tendency by each clinical scale.

	Frequency of life events	Stress scores of life events	Daily hassles score	Daly uplifts score	MMPI depression	MMPI psychastenia	Serum TRAb activity	Thyroid volume	Serum FT$_4$ concentration
Frequency of life events	-	0.933**	0.189	0.173	0.150	0.013	0.396**	0.419*	-0.059
Stress scores of life events		-	0.225	0.194	0.103	0.031	0.424**	0.480*	-0.077
Daily hassles score			-	0.193	0.535**	0.580**	0.009	0.083	-0.083
Daly uplifts score				-	-0.373*	-0.322*	0.054	0.144	-0.088
MMPI depression					-	0.784**	0.063	0.293	0.042
MMPI psychastenia						-	-0.032	-0.162	-0.086
Serum TRAb activity							-	0.527**	0.012
Thyroid volume								-	0.121
Serum FT$_4$ concentration									-

Significant difference: $^{*}P < 0.05$; $^{**}P < 0.001$.

Table 3: Correlation between psychological factors and thyroid-related parameters in 69 GD patients.

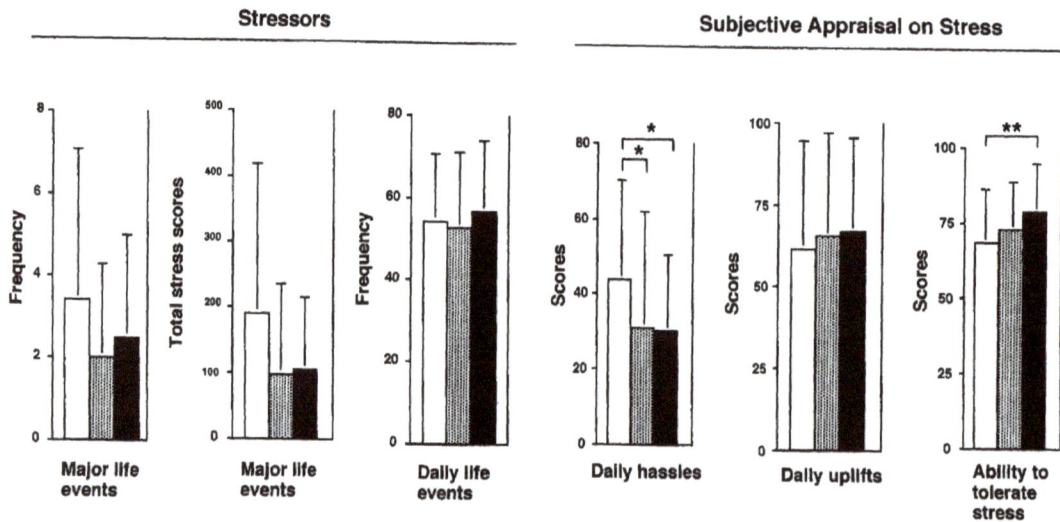

Figure 1: Stressors and subjective appraisal on stress in the three groups of subjects. The data from each group are shown as mean ± SD. Significant differences ($P < 0.05$) between groups are represented by asterisks. Relapsed Graves' disease; Remitted Graves' disease; Controls, $^{*}P < 0.05$ by Mann-Whiney's test. $^{**}P < 0.05$ by Fisher's PLSD test.

Total 64 patients

Depressive personality
before treatment
of thyrotoxic state

(+)
44(69%)

(-)
20(31%)

Depressive personality   (+)
during treatment   29(46%)
of euthyroid state   A

(-)
15(23%)
C

(+)
5(8%)
B

(-)
15(23%)
D

Depression   Non-depression

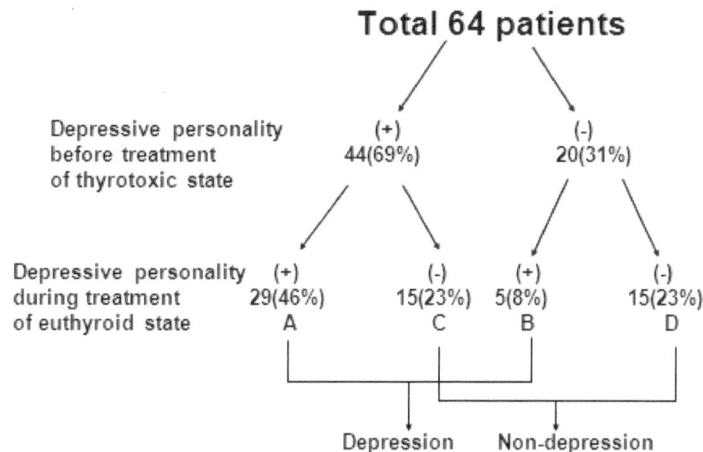

Figure 2: Changes of the depressive personality of Graves' disease patients before and during treatment. Depressive personality show the patients whose T-scores of hypochondriasis, depression or psychasthenia are greater than 60 points in MMPI. GroupA : depressive personality was present before and persisted after treatment.GroupB: depressive personality scores became higher after treatment. GroupC: depressive personality was present before treatment and decreased to within the normal range after treatment GroupD: depressive personality did not appear either before or after treatment.

ment (Figure 3). Thirty four patients with depressive personality even in the euthyroid state (group A and B) had significantly ($P < 0.05$) lower daily uplifts than the remaining 30 patients without depressive personality (group C and D) (Figure 4). Serum TRAb activity at three years after treatment was significantly ($P < 0.05$) greater in the depression group (23 cases) than in the non- depression group (25 cases) (Figure 5). The remission rate at four years after treatment was significantly ($P < 0.05$) lower in the depression group than in the non- depression group (22% vs 52%).

These findings suggest that in ATD treated GD patients, depressive personality during treatment when patients are euthyroid reflects the effect of emotional stresses rather than thyrotoxicosis and that it aggravates hyperthyroidism. So antidepressant may improve the prognosis of GD patients with depression. Indeed, the authors have experienced three cases of first remission after long term ATD treatment together with antidepressants (paroxetine) in GD patients with depression (Fukao, 2010).

2.2.3   Our Studies on Ego States, Depression and Alexithymia

We (2000a) determined three types of questionnaires in 61 ATD-treated GD patients for more than two years (37 with relapse and 24 with remission) and 21 healthy subjects to examine which patterns to cope with patients' feeling and thinking relate to either prognosis of hyperthyroidism or accompanied psychiatric symptoms. The Toronto Alexithymia Scale-20 (TAS-20) including factor 1 (difficulty of identifying feeling), factor 2 (difficulty of describing feeling) and factor 3 (externally oriented thinking) was used for assessment of alexithymic personality relating to psychosomatic disorder. The Tokyo University Egogram (TEG) including terms of critical parent (CP), nuturing parent (NP), adult (A), free child (FC) and adapted child (AC) was used for assessment of ego state. Self-rating Depression Scale (SDS) was also used for assessment of depression.

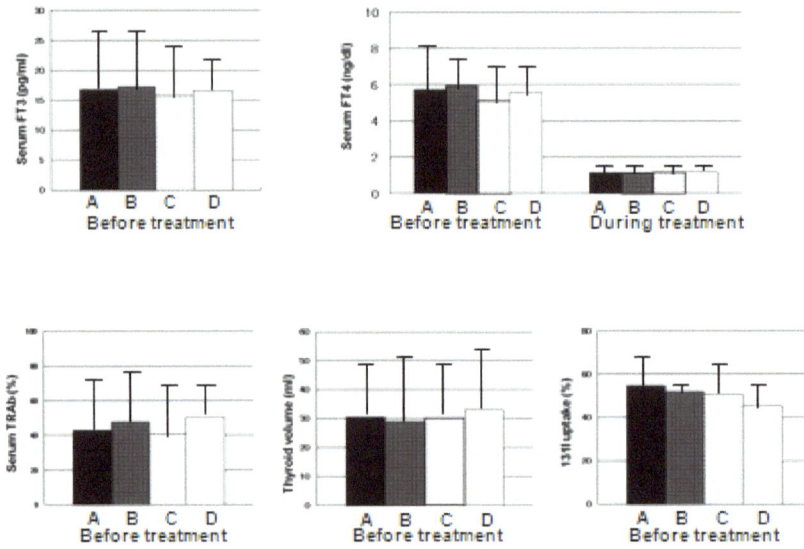

Figure 3: Comparisons of thyroid functions and severity of hyperthyroidism among four groups. The data from each group are shown as mean + SD. Group A (29) : depressive personality was present before and persisted after treatment. Group B (5): depressive personality scores became higher after treatment. Group C (15): depressive personality was present before treatment and decreased to within the normal range after treatment Group D (15): depressive personality did not appear either before or after treatment. There were no significant differences in any parameters among the four groups by ANOVA.

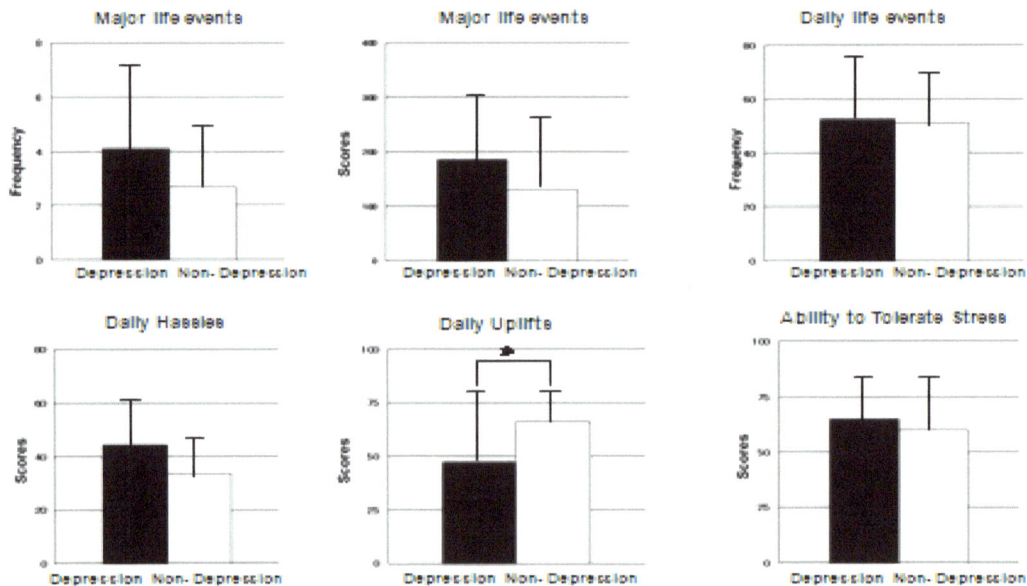

Figure 4: Comparisons of emotional stresses between the depression and non- depression groups. The closed bar express the depression group (34), even in the euthyroid state (group A and B) and open bar express the remaining non- depression group (30) without depressive personality (group C and D). The data from each group are shown as mean+SD. Significant difference : $^{*}P < 0.005$ by Mann-Whitney's test.

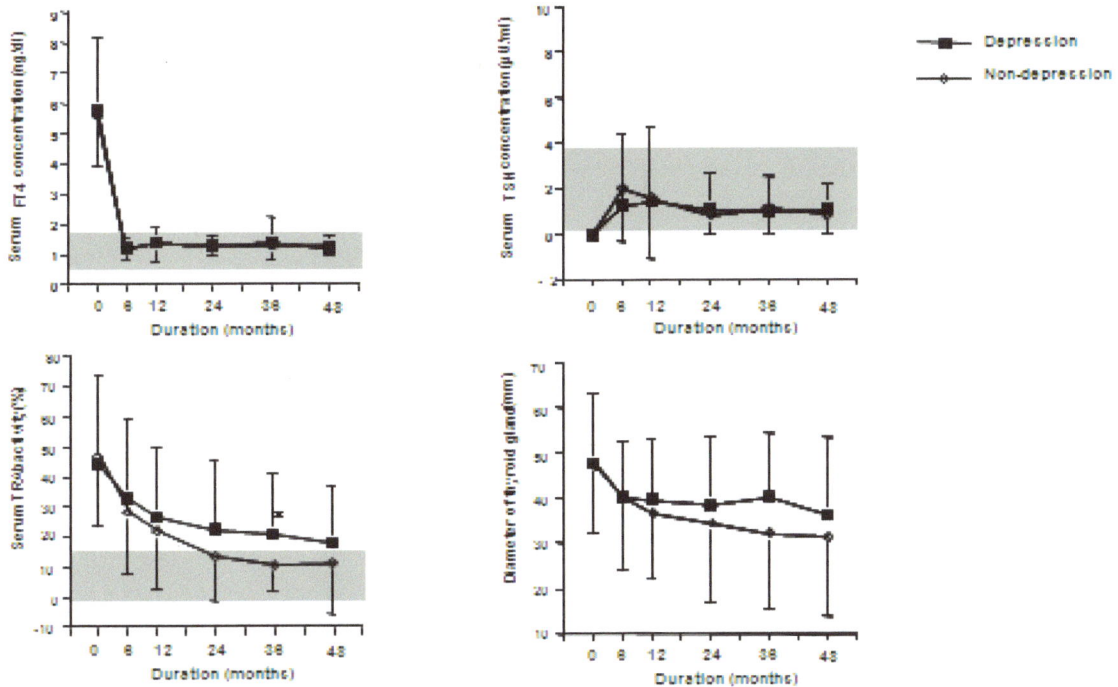

Figure 5: Comparison of the prognosis of hyperthyroidism between the depression and non - depression groups. The data from each group are shown as mean±SD. The gray zone expresses the normal ranges. Significant difference : *$P < 0.05$ by Student t-test. Remission rate: depressive group 22% (5/23) vs non-depressive group 52% (13/25) ($P < 0.05$ by chi-square test).

In TAS-20, total scores, scores of factor 1 and factor 2 were significantly ($P < 0.05$) greater in the relapsed GD group than in the remitted GD group. In TEG, scores of A scale, showing ability of rational consideration, and FC scale, showing ability of describing feeling, were significantly ($P < 0.05$) greater in the remitted GD group than in the relapsed GD group. Scores of AC scale, showing tendency of suppressing feelings, were significantly ($P < 0.05$) lower in the remitted GD group than in the relapsed GD group. Scores of SDS were significantly ($P < 0.001$) greater in the relapsed GD group than in the remitted GD group. In total patients, total scores of TAS-20, scores of factor 1, factor 2, AC scale and SDS significantly ($P < 0.001$) correlated each other. On the other hand, scores of A and FC scales significantly ($P < 0.05$) correlated with total scores of TAS-20, factor 2 and SDS negatively. The results suggest that difficulty of identifying and describing feeling relate to both aggravation of hyperthyroidism and depressive state. Conversely, the ability of describing feeling and rational consideration relate to the good prognosis of hyperthyroidism.

Then, we (2002) carried out a prospective study to confirm the relationship between ego states of GD patients evaluated by TEG and prognosis of hyperthyroidism. Seventy three GD patients were divided into two groups; high A group (44 patients) whose A at euthyroid state after ATD treatment were greater than 50 percentile and low A group (29 patients) whose A were lower than 50 percentile. The relationships between ego states of these groups and prognosis of disease at three years were investigated. Additionally, similar relationships were investigated in another two groups; FC predominant group (40 patients) who's FC was greater than AC and AC predominant group (33 patients) who's AC were greater than FC conversely. Age, sex, rates of smoking, serum FT4, FT3 concentrations, serum TBII (TRAb), TSAb activities, 131I-uptake, goiter size before treatment were not significant different between each groups (Table 4). Serum FT4 and TSH concentrations were not significant different between high A group and low A group during treatment (Figure 6). But serum TBII activity and diameter of thyroid were significantly ($P < 0.05\sim0.001$) higher in low A group than in high A group and remission rate at three years were significantly ($P < 0.01$) lower in low A group than in high A group (10% vs 41%). Remission rate at three years were also significantly ($P < 0.05$) lower in AC predominant group than in FC predominant group (18% vs 40%) (Figure 7).

	Number (male / famale)	Age (years old)	Rate of smoking	Serum thyroid concentration		Serum TSH receptor antibody activity		[123]I – uptake (%)	Thyroid volume (ml)
				FT$_4$ (ng/dl)	FT$_3$ (pg/ml)	TBII (%)	TSAb (%)		
High A group	44 (7/37)	39.7 ±14.3	10/44 (23%)	5.08 ±1.98	16.37 ±7.05	45.8 ±22.8	352.1 ±536.1	48.8 ±11.3	30.0 ±22.9
Low A group	29 (4/25)	34.6 ±13.2	9/29 (31%)	5.29 ±1.63	16.04 ±6.46	48.7 ±24.4	528.9 ±638.0	52.5 ±6.07	28.6 ±14.1

	Number (male / famale)	Age (years old)	Rate of smoking	Serum thyroid concentration		Serum TSH receptor antibody activity		[123]I – uptake (%)	Thyroid volume (ml)
				FT$_4$ (ng/dl)	FT$_3$ (pg/ml)	TBII (%)	TSAb (%)		
FC predominant group	40 (7/33)	37.6 ±13.5	10/40 (25%)	5.17 ±1.93	16.81 ±6.97	47.0 ±22.5	278.4 ±210.8	49.1 ±11.6	28.2 ±16.0
AC predominant group	33 (4/29)	37.8 ±14.9	9/33 (27%)	5.15 ±17.6	15.44 ±6.58	46.7 ±24.6	592.1 ±806.7	51.1 ±7.00	30.8 ±23.8

Table 4: Comparison of pretreatment clinical profiles and thyroid function tests between each groups of GD patients.

These results confirm that ability of rational consideration and expressing feeling of ATD treated GD patients are important to get early remission. It can be concluded that psychotherapies for patients to think rationally, to express feeling and to cope with the stress in the positive manner may be useful in improving the disease prognosis. Indeed, the authors had two cases of patients with successful outcome by conventional medication and psychotherapy (Fukao, 2000b). Recently, Tanaka *et al* (Tanaka, 2013) reported that the remission rate of ATD treated GD patients was significantly higher in the patients group with longer (over than 31 times) psychotherapy than in the patients group with shorter (less than 5 times) psychotherapy.

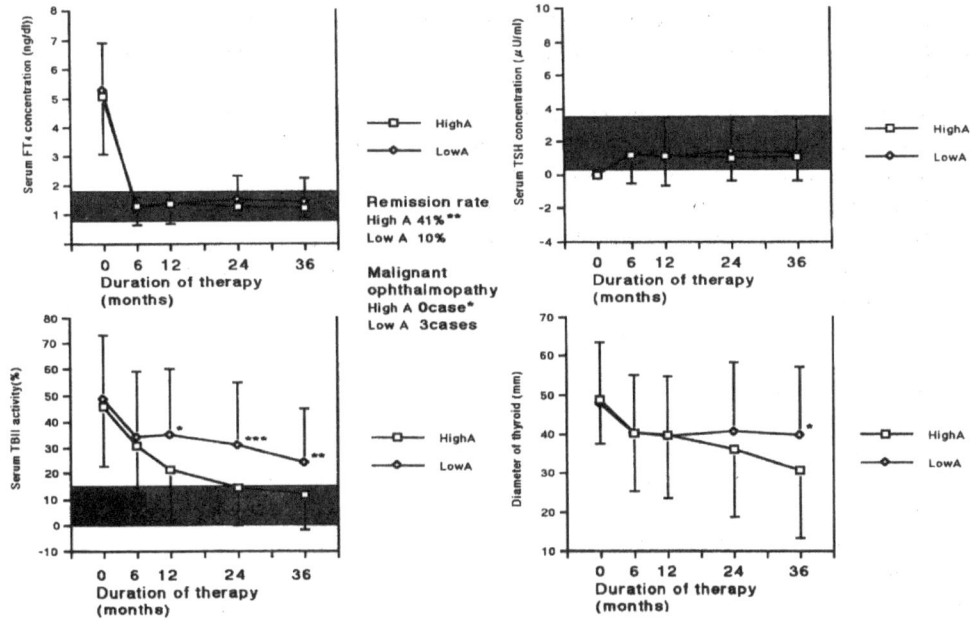

Figure 6: Comparison of prognosis of hyperthyroidism between highA group and low A group.The data from each group are shown as mean±SD. The gray zone express the normal ranges. Significant difference : $^*P < 0.05$; $^{**}P < 0.01$; $^{***}P < 0.001$.

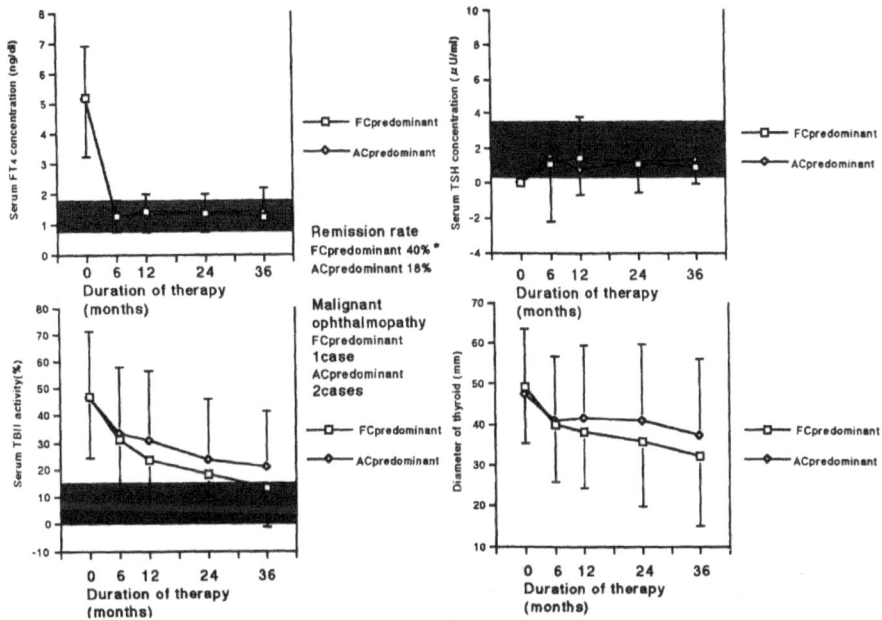

Figure 7: Comparison of prognosis of hyperthyroidism between the FC predominant group and the AC predominant group. The data from each group are shown as mean±SD. The gray zone expresses the normal ranges. Significant difference : $^*P < 0.05$

3   Stress and Hashimoto's Thyroiditis

In contrast to GD, there are few studies on the relationships between stress and Hashimoto's thyroiditis (HT). Two case-control studies (Martin-du Pan, 1998; Oretti *et al*, 2003) evaluated the role of stressful life events in HT or postpartum thyroiditis. They concluded that stress was not a trigger in either condition. Because the onset and clinical course of HT are often insidious and the diagnosis may be delayed until the patients develop overt hypothyroidism, it is difficult to assess the role of stress on the onset and clinical course of disease. A population study (Strieder, 2005) also did not find a relationship between stress and the presence of anti-TPOAb. Effraimidis *et al* (2011) reported a prospective cohort study on the association between stress and the onset of AITD in 521 euthyroid women who were 1st or 2nd degree relatives of AITD patients. They could not find that stress involved in the development of TPOAb and hypohyroidism.

On the other hand, painless thyroiditis often occurs after cure from Cushing's syndrome or discontinuation of glucocorticoid therapy. These situations are similar to the situations after activation of hypothalamic-pituitary-adrenal axis by stress. So that future studies about the role of stress in HT or autoimmune thyroiditis are needed.

4   Stress and Thyroid Nodule

There are also few studies about the relationships between stress and thyroid nodule. All studies were determined stress as control groups in benign thyroid nodule or toxic nodular goiter compared to GD patients. Gray and Hoffenberg (1985) found no association between stressful life events and 50 thyrotoxic patients and 50 non toxic goiters. Martin-du Pan (1998) evaluated the role of major stress in 98 GD patients and 97 patients with benign thyroid nodules. There were no significant differences of stress factors between two groups. Matos-Santos *et al* (2001) reported that 31 GD patients had reported more stressful life events compared to 30 toxic nodular goiter patients and 31 controls, and no significant differences were found between toxic nodular goiter patients and controls. Paunkovic *et al* (1998) also reported that the incidence of GD significantly increased in eastern Serbia during the civil war from 1992 to 1995, and the incidents of Plummer's disease did not increase for the same period. These data suggest that stress is not associated with the etiology of thyroid nodule.

5   Stress and Thyroid Autoimmunity

Mechanism of effects of stress on the pathogenesis of GD is still controversial. Volpe (1991) proposed that a defect of antigen-specific suppressor T-lymphocytes is partially responsible for the initiation of GD. Stress may cause a generalized suppressor T-lymphocytes defect and TRAb may be produced as a result of a specific defect in immunologic surveillance though the relationships are still not established. Some reports (Paschke *et al*, 1990; Harsch *et al*, 1992) that GD patients with depression and anxiety exhibit abnormal peripheral helper/suppressor T-lymphocyte ratios support this hypothesis. GD is generally considered to be a Th2-predominat disease. Both endogenous glucocorticoids and catecholamines at concentrations observed during periods of stress cause a selective suppression of Th1 response and a shift toward Th2-mediated immunity (Elenkov & Chrousos, 1999; Elenkov *et al*, 2000). This Th2 shift may affect the onset or course of GD (Chrousos & Gold, 1992). On the other hand, HT is generally considered to be a Th1-predominat disease. OS chickens, which are an animal model of autoimmune thyroiditis is influenced by a reduced glucocorticoid tonus and painless thyroiditis often occur after cure from Cushing's syndrome or discontinuation of glucocorticoid therapy (Ader *et al*, 1995; Chrousos, 1995). These situations have been associated with increased susceptibility to Th1-mediated immune disorders. This might also include the period that follows cessation of chronic stress or a rebound reaction upon relief of various stressors. Tsatoulis (2006) proposed hypothesis shown in Figure 8. Genetic and environmental factors may induce an aberrant immune response against thyroid autoantigens and render an individual susceptible to develop thyroid autoimmunity. If an individual is under stress, the stress hormones will influence the antigen-presenting cell (APC) to steer the balance toward Th2-type activity. Effector Th2 cells and type 2 cytokines will induce antigen-specific B lymphocytes to produce TRAb. Under these circumstances, the clinical outcome is GD. Conversely, if a susceptible individual is recovering from stress response or the immune suppressive effect of pregnancy, a rebound reaction may create the potential for APCs to activate the Th1-mediated pathway, leading to cellular immunity and destruction of thyroid follicular cells. The likely outcome then will be autoimmune or postpartum thyroiditis respetively. Further researches are needed to confirm the relationship between stress and thyroid autoimmunity.

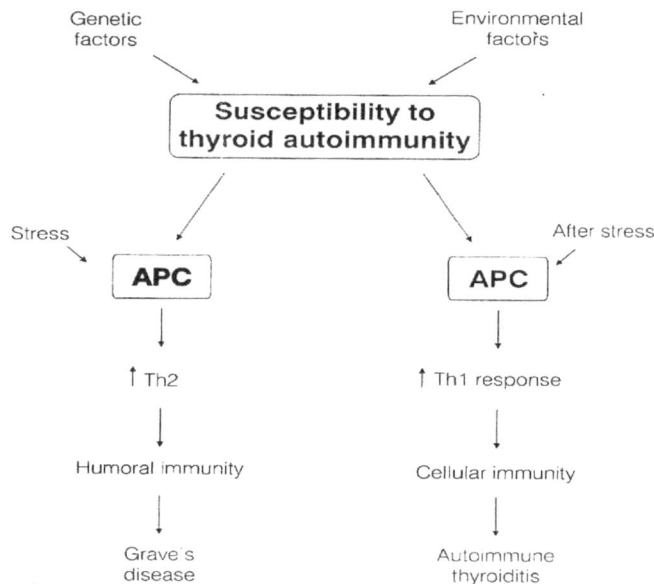

Figure 8: Role of stress in the clinical expression of AITD by Tsatsoulis

6   Conclusion

Although there are many epidemiological and clinical reports on the relationship between stress and the onset of GD, it is still controversial. However, stress affects the prognosis of GD certainly. If further study sample would be enough large, the problems could be solved. Psychosomatic therapeutic approaches including antipsychiatric drugs and/or psychotherapy appear to be useful for improving the prognosis of hyperthyroidism. Stress may influence immune system both directly and indirectly through the activation of the neural and endocrine systems. Further researches are needed to confirm the relationship between stress and thyroid diseases.

References

Akamizu, T., Mori, T. & Nakao, K. (1997). Pathogenesis of Graves' disease: Molecular analysis of anti-thyrotropin receptor antibodies. Endocrine Journal, 44, 633-646.

Ader, R., Cohen, N. & Felten, D. (1995). Psychoneuroimmunology: interaction between the nervous system and the immune system. Lancet, 345, 99-103.

Benvenga, S.(1996). Benzodiazepine and remission of Graves' disease. Thyroid. 6, 659-660.

Bram, I. (1936). Psychiatric trauma in aetiology of Graves' disease. Am J Psychiatr,92, 1077-1094.

Chiovato, L. & Pinchera, A. (1996) . Stressful life events and Graves' disease. Eur J Endocrinol 134, 680-682.

Chiovato, L., Marino, M., & Perugi, G.(1998). Chronic recurrent stress due to panic disorder dose not precipitate Graves' disease. J Endocrinol Invest , 21, 758-764.

Chrousos, G.P. & Gold, P.W. (1992). The concepts of stress and stress system disorders. Overview of physical and behavioral homeostasis. JAMA, 267, 1244-1252.

Chrousos, G.P. (1995). The hypothalamic-pituitary-adrenal axis and immune-mediated inflammation. N Engl J Med, 332, 1351-1362.

Effraimidis, G., Tijssen, J.G.P., Brosschot, J.F. et al. (2012). Involvement of stress in the pathogenesis of autoimmune thyroid disease : a prospective study. Psychoneuroendocrinology, doi;10.1016/j.psyneuen.2011.12.009.

Elenkov, I.J. & Chrousos, G.P.(1999). Stress, cytokine patterns and susceptibility to disease. Bailliere's Clin Endocrinol Metab, 13, 583-595.

Elenkov, I.J., Wilder, R.L., Chrousos, G.P. et al. (2000). The sympathetic nerve –An integrative interface between two supersystems: The brain and immune system. Pharmacol Rev, 52, 595-638.

Ferguson-Rayport, S.M. (1956). The relation of emotional factors to recurrence of thyrotoxicosis. Can Med Assoc, 15,993-1000.

Fukao, A., Takamatsu, J., Matsuo, T. et al. (2000a). Relation of psychological factors to prognosis of Graves' disease : ability of description of feeling and rational consideration (Abstr).Endocr J, 47 Suppl.

Fukao, A., Kurokawa, N., Hosoi, K. et al. (2000b). Successful treatment by psychosomatic medicine in patients with hyperthyroidism due to Graves' disease : report of two cases. Psychosom Med, (Shinryo Naika, written in Japanese), 4, 219-224.

Fukao, A. & Takamatsu, J. (2002).The role of psychological factors on the onset and clinical course of hyperthyroid Graves' disease. Recent Res. Devel. Endocrinol, 3, 369-376.

Fukao A., Takamatsu J., Murakami Y. et al. (2003). The relationship of psychological factors to the prognosis of hyperthyroidism in antithyroid drug-treated patients with Graves' disease. Clin Endocrinol (Oxf), 58, 550-555.

Fukao, A., Takamatsu, J., Tsujimoto, N. et al. (2010). Three Cases of Graves' Disease Patients with Depression Successfully Treated by Antidepressant (Abstr). Endocrine J, 57, suppl.2 s459.

Fukao, A., Takamatsu, J., Kubota, S. et al. (2011). The Thyroid Function of Graves' Disease Patients is Aggravated by Depressive Personality during Antithyroid Drug Treatment.. Bio Psycho Social Med, doi:10.1186/1751-0759-5-9.

Gorman, C.A. (1990). A critical review of the role of stress in hyperthyroidism In The Thyroid Gland, Environment and Autoimmunity. Drexhage H.A., de Vijlder J.T.M. & Wiersinga W.M., Eds. Elsevier Science Publishers. Amsterdam (pp.191-200).

Gray, J. & Hoffenberg, R. (1985). Thyrotoxicosis and stress. Quart J Med, New series, 54, 153-160 .

Hadden, D.R. & McDevitt, D.G. (1974). Environmental stress and thyrotoxicosis. Lancet, 7, 578-578.

Harsch, I., Paschke, R. & Usadel, K.H. (1992). The possible ethiological role of psychological disturbances in Graves' disease. AMA, 19 suppl 1, 62-65.

Kun, A.W.C. (1995) . Life events, daily stresses and coping in patients with Graves' disease. Clin Endocrinol (Oxf), 42:303-308.

Lidz, T. & Whitehorn, J.C. (1949). Psychiatric problems in a thyroid clinic. J Am Psychiat Assoc, 139, 698-701.

Mandelbrote, B.M. & Wittkower, E.D. (1955). Emotional factors in Graves' disease. Psychosom Med,, 17, 109-123.

Matos-Santos, A., Nobre,E.L., Costa, J.G..E. et al. (2001). Relationship between the number and impact of stressful life events and the onset of Graves' disease and toxic nodular goiter. Clin Endocrinol (Oxf), 55, 15-19.

Martin-du Pan, R.C. (1998). Triggering role of stress and pregnancy in the occurrence of 98cases of Graves' disease compared to 95cases of Hashimoto thyroiditis and 97cases of thyroid nodules. Ann Endocrinol (Paris), 59, 107-112.

Mizokami, T., Wu Li, A., El-Kassi, S. et al. (2004). Stress and thyroid autoimmunity . Thyroid, 14, 1047-1055.

Oretti, R.G., Harris, J.H., Parkers, A.B. et al. (2003). Is there an association between life events, postnatal depression and thyroid dysfunction in thyroid antibody positive women? Int J Soc Psychiatry, 49, 70-76.

Parry, C.H. (1825). Collections from the unpublished writings of the late C.H. Parry. Vol.2.London: Underwoods.

Paschke, R., Harsch, I., Schlote, B. et al. (1990). Sequential psychological testing during the course of autoimmune hyper-thyroidism. Klin Wochensc, 68, 942-950.

Paunkovic, N., Paunkovic, J., Palvovic, O. et al. (1998). The significant increase in incidence of Graves' disease increased in eastern Serbia during the civil war in the former Yugoslavia (1992 to 1995). Thyroid, 8, 37-41.

Radosaljevic, V.R., Jankovic, S.M., Marinkovic, J.M. (1996). Stressful life events in the pathogenesis of Graves' disease. Eur J Endocrinol (Oxf), 134, 699-701.

Sonino, N., Girelli, M.E., Boscaro, M. et al. (1993). Life events in the pathogenesis of Graves' disease. A controlled study. Acta Endocrinol, 128, 293-296.

Strieder, T.G.A., Prummel, M.F., Tijssen, J.G.P. et al. (2005). Stress is not associated with thyroid peroxidase autoanti-bodies in euthyroid women. Brain Behav Immun, 19, 203-206.

Tanaka, M., Kanayama, Y., Kawai, T. et al. (2013) On the features of psychotherapy with Graves' disease: from the experiences in a thyroid hospital. Japanese J Psychosom Int Med (written in Japanese), 17,174-179.

Tsatoulis, A. (2006). The role of stress in the clinical expression of thyroid autoimmunity. Ann NY Acad Sci, 1088, 382-395.

Volpe, R. (1991). Graves' disease: pathogenesis. In Werner and Ingbar's The Thyroid, 6th ed, edited by Braverman LE and Utiger RD. Lippincott- Williams & Wilkins. Philadelphia (pp.648-657).

Voth, H.M., Holzman, P.S., Katz, J.B. et al. (1970). Thyroid "hot spots":their relationship to life stress. Psychosom Med, 32, 561-568.

Winsa, B., Adami, H.O., Bergstrom, R. et al. (1991). Stressful life events and Graves' disease. Lancet, 338, 1475-1479.

Yoshiuchi, K., Kumano, H., Nomura, S. et al. (1998). Stressful life events and smoking were associated with Graves' disease in women, but not in men. Psychosom Med, 60:182-185.

Yoshiuchi, K, Kumano, H, Nomura, S. et al. (1998). Psychosocial factors influencing the short term outocome of antithy-roid drug therapy in Graves' disease. Psychosom Med, 60, 592-596.

Current and Future Clinical Applications of Ghrelin

Carine De Vriese
Laboratory of Pharmaceutics and Biopharmaceutics
Université Libre de Bruxelles, Belgium

Jason Perret
Laboratory of Pathophysiological and Nutritional Biochemistry
Université Libre de Bruxelles, Belgium

Christine Delporte
Laboratory of Pathophysiological and Nutritional Biochemistry
Université Libre de Bruxelles, Belgium

1 Introduction

1.1 Ghrelin Synthesis and Tissue Distribution

Ghrelin is a unique 28 amino acids peptide containing an *n*-acylation on the serine in position 3 (Kojima *et al.*, 1999). Ghrelin is the natural ligand of the growth hormone secretagogue receptor (GHS-R1a) stimulating growth hormone secretion (Kojima *et al.*, 1999). However, ghrelin is now recognized as a pleiotropic hormone, that can also induce food intake and weight gain (Cummings *et al.*, 2001; Tshöp *et al.*, 2001; Wren *et al.*, 2001), and promotes gastric emptying (Trudel *et al.*, 2002). Ghrelin is predominantly synthesized and secreted in the blood stream by a discrete subset of endocrine stomach mucosal cells coined P/D1 cells (Sakata *et al.*, 2002) in human and X/A like in rat (Date *et al.*, 2000a; Rindi *et al.*, 2002; Stengel *et al.*, 2010). However, immunoreactive ghrelin is also present in duodenum, jejunum, ileum and colon (Date *et al.*, 2000a; Hosoda *et al.*, 2000; Sakata *et al.*, 2002), and in endocrine (Date *et al.*, 2002; Kageyama *et al.*, 2005; Volante *et al.*, 2002; Prado *et al.*, 2004; Wierup *et al.*, 2002; Wierup & Sundler, 2005) and exocrine (Lai *et al.*, 2007) pancreas. Furthermore, ghrelin is expressed in the central nervous system in arcuate nucleus of the hypothalamus involved in the regulation of food intake (Kojima *et al.*, 1999; Lu *et al.*, 2002) and the pituitary (Korbonits *et al.*, 2001). Finally, ghrelin is expressed in other organs such as kidneys, adrenal glands, lung, liver, gallbladder, thyroid, breast, ovary, prostate, testis, skeletal muscle, myocardium and skin (Ghelardoni *et al.*, 2006; Gnanapavan *et al.*, 2002).

The presence of the acyl group is crucial for ghrelin's activity, as non-octanoylated ghrelin neither virgulbinds nor activates GHS-R1a (Kojima *et al.*, 1999). It is to be noted that there is a growing body of evidence showing that non-acylated ghrelin possesses biological effects, though its mechanism of action remains elusive to date (Baragli *et al.* 2011; Satou and Sagimoto, 2012; De Vriese *et al.*, 2005). Ghrelin acylation is catalyzed during the processing of the peptide by ghrelin *O*-acyltransferase (GOAT), a member of the membrane-bound *O*-acyltransferase family (Gutierrez *et al.*, 2008; Yang *et al.*, 2008). GOAT is coexpressed with acyl ghrelin in ghrelin-expressing tissues (Sakata *et al.*, 2009). GOAT displays a preference for hexanoyl-CoA over octanoyl-CoA as an acyl donor (Ohgusu *et al.*, 2009; Ohgusu *et al.*, 2012). Fasting and satiation could modulate the activity of GOAT as ghrelin levels rise before meals (Cummings *et al.*, 2001; Cummings *et al.*, 2006) and decrease with food intake (Tschöp *et al.*, 2001). Moreover, long term fasting inhibits ghrelin acylation but not total ghrelin secretion, whereas feeding suppresses both acyl and des-acyl ghrelin (Liu *et al.*, 2008). However, the modulation of GOAT mRNA levels by fasting and feeding remain unclear (Gonzalez *et al.*, 2008; Kirchner *et al.*, 2009). Dietary lipids are critical for the activation of GOAT, and consequently ghrelin acylation. Indeed, GOAT knock out mice submitted to a diet containing 10% medium chain triglyceride exhibited lower body weight that can be explained by lower fat mass compared to wild-type mice. Furthermore, large amounts of acyl ghrelin are produced in GOAT transgenic mice only fed with a medium-chain triglycerides supplementation (Kirchner *et al.*, 2009). An essential function of ghrelin could be the maintenance of viability during periods of famine. This hypothesis is supported by the fact that wild-type and GOAT knock out mice submitted to 60% calorie-restricted diet displayed 30% and 75% body weight loss, respectively (Zhao *et al.*, 2010). Plasma GOAT levels depend on metabolic status and are correlated with body mass index. Indeed, low plasma GOAT levels are measured in anorexic patients, while high plasma GOAT levels are detected in obese patients (Goebel-Stengel *et al.*, 2013). Besides, GOAT activity is required for hedonic feeding behavior (Davis *et al.*, 2012).

1.2   Family of Ghrelin Peptides

Since the initial discovery of ghrelin, a family of ghrelin peptides has been identified. This family can be subdivided into two groups based on peptide length (28 or 27 amino acids) or into four groups based on the absence of presence, and the nature, of the acyl group present on Ser3 (non-acylated, octanoylated, decanoylated, decenoylated). Both in stomach and plasma, the major form is octanoylated ghrelin 1-28, but decanoyled ghrelin 1-28, decenoyled ghrelin 1-28, octanoyled ghrelin 1-27 and decanoyled ghrelin 1-27 are also present (Hosoda *et al.*, 2003). Medium-chain fatty acids and medium-chain triacylglycerides ingestion increases ghrelin acylation (Nishi *et al.*, 2005). The variant acylated forms of ghrelin present lower binding affinity than the canonical octanoylated form of ghrelin for GHS-R1a, while non-acylated ghrelin does not bind to GHS-R1a (Hosoda *et al.*, 2003). As non-acylated ghrelin does have established effects, the existence of another high affinity receptor for non-acylated ghrelin is a possibility to be explored.

1.3   Circulating Ghrelin

In human plasma, non-acylated ghrelin accounts for more that 90% of ghrelin immunoreactivity (Shanado *et al.*, 2004). The predominance of non-acylated ghrelin in the bloodstream could results from the shorter half-life of ghrelin compared to des-acyl ghrelin (Akamizu *et al.*, 2005) and ghrelin deacylation by butyrylcholinesterase and other esterase(s), such as platelet-activating factor acetylhydrolase (De Vriese *et al.*, 2004; Hosoda *et al.*, 2004; De Vriese *et al.*, 2007a). The obese phenotype of butyrylcholinesterase knockout mice could not be explained by increased ghrelin, caloric intake, or decreased exercise, suggesting a role of the enzyme in fat catabolism (Li *et al.*, 2008). In rat stomach, ghrelin is deacylated by lysophospholipase I (Shanado *et al.*, 2004; Satou *et al.*, 2010) and degraded by N-terminal proteolysis (Shanado *et al.*, 2004; De Vriese *et al.*, 2004). In rat plasma, carboxylesterase induces ghrelin desoctanoylation (De Vriese *et al.*, 2004). The possible ghrelin deacylation by human paraoxonase (Beaumont *et al.*, 2003) remains controversial (De Vriese *et al.*, 2004). Plasma ghrelin degradation therefore contributes to the difficulty to accurately assess acylated ghrelin levels and consequently its physiological and pathophysiological roles. While circulating des-acyl ghrelin is mostly present as a free peptide, the vast majority of acyl ghrelin is bound to larger molecules and in particular to lipoproteins (Beaumont *et al.*, 2003; De Vriese *et al.*, 2007a; Holmes *et al.*, 2009). The acyl group is required for ghrelin interaction with triglyceride-rich lipoproteins and low-density lipoprotein but not high-density lipoproteins and very high-density lipoproteins. Besides, N- and C-terminal parts of ghrelin interact with high-density lipoproteins and very high-density lipoproteins. These data support the transport of acylated ghrelin by triglyceride-rich lipoproteins and of both ghrelin and des-acyl ghrelin by high-density lipoproteins and very high-density lipoproteins (De Vriese *et al.*, 2007a). Modifications of lipoprotein levels in certain pathophysiological conditions, such as obesity, may affect ghrelin transport as well as free ghrelin levels.

1.4   Ghrelin Receptors

Two spliced variants of GHS-R have been identified: GHS-R1a coupled to G protein and phospholipase C activation and GHS-R1b that can not couple to those effectors (McKee *et al.*, 1997; Smith *et al.*, 1996). GHS-R1b is suggested to be pharmacologically inactive as it does not bind ghrelin and non-acylated ghrelin (Howard *et al.*, 1996). However, GHS-R1b oligomerization with GHS-R1a modulates cell surface expression and signal transduction of GHS-R1a (Chan & Cheng, 2004; Chow *et al.*, 2012). GHS-R1a can form heterodimers with other G-protein coupled receptors such as melanocortin 3 receptor, serotonin 2C receptor and dopamine 1 receptor (Schellekens *et al.*, 2013). The formation of these heterodimers leads to attenuated ghrelin signalling (Schellekens *et al.*, 2013; Rediger *et al.*, 2011).

1.5   Physiological Actions of Ghrelin

Physiological functions of ghrelin, have expanded considerably since its discovery and now includes not only growth hormone secretion (Date *et al.*, 2000b; Hataya *et al.*, 2001; Malagon *et al.*, 2003, Takaya *et al.*, 2000), but also food intake stimulation and energy expenditure decrease (Kamegai *et al.*, 2001; Naka-zato *et al.*, 2001; Shintani *et al.*, 2001; Tschop *et al.*, 2000; Wren *et al.*, 2001), gastric secretion stimula-tion (Asakawa *et al.*, 2001; Fukumoto *et al.*, 2008; Masuda *et al.*, 2000), gastric emptying acceleration (Dass *et al.*, 2003; Depoortere *et al.*, 2008; Fujino *et al.*, 2003, Peeters, 2006), glucose homeostasis modulation (Broglio *et al.*, 2005; Delhanty & van der Lely, 2011; Gauna *et al.*, 2005; Murata *et al.*, 2002). Ghrelin can also modulate cardiovascular functions (Isgaard & Johansson, 2005; Soeki *et al.*, 2008), inflammation (Chang *et al.*, 2003; Chen *et al.*, 2008; Dembinski *et al.*, 2003; Dixit *et al.*, 2004; Dixit *et al.*, 2009; Li *et al.*, 2004; Nagaya *et al.*, 2001; Sehirli *et al.*, 2008; Xia *et al.*, 2004), reproductive function (Garcia *et al.*, 2007), bone formation (Fukushima *et al.*, 2005) and cell proliferation in various cell types (De Vriese *et al.*, 2005; De Vriese & Delporte, 2007b; Korbonits *et al.*, 2004). Figure 1 summa-rizes the different physiological actions of ghrelin. Figure 2 illustrates the mechanism by which ghrelin induces appetite and food intake.

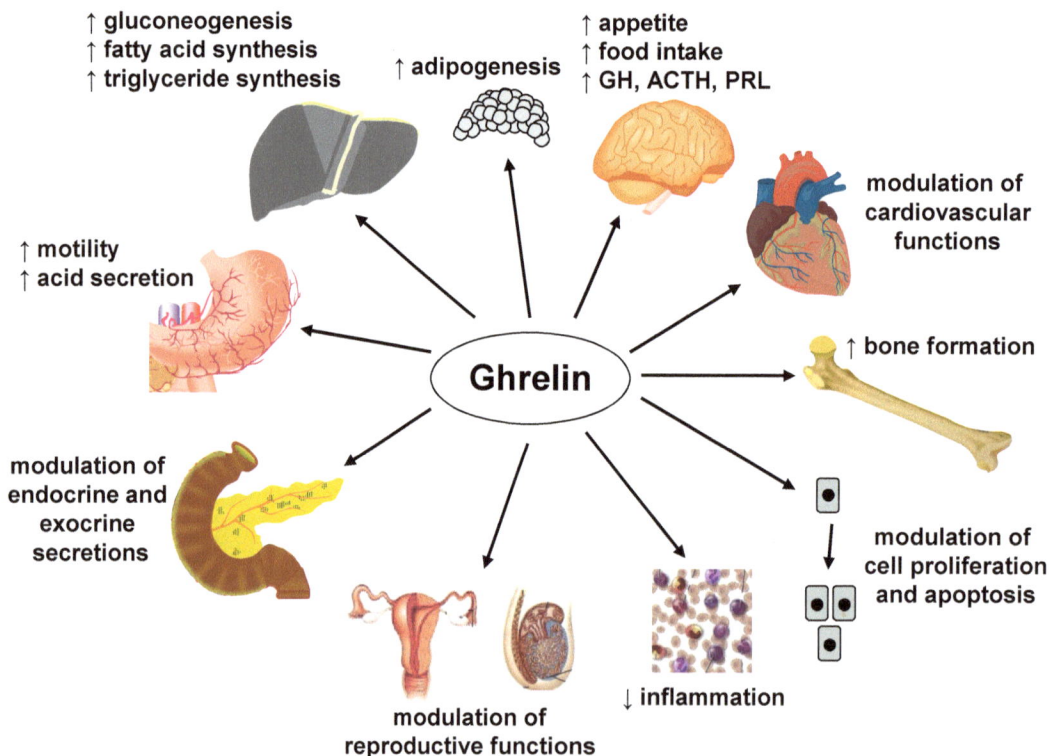

Figure 1: The major pleiotropic biological actions of ghrelin. GH: growth hormone; ACTH: adre-nocorticotrophic hormone; PRL: prolactin.

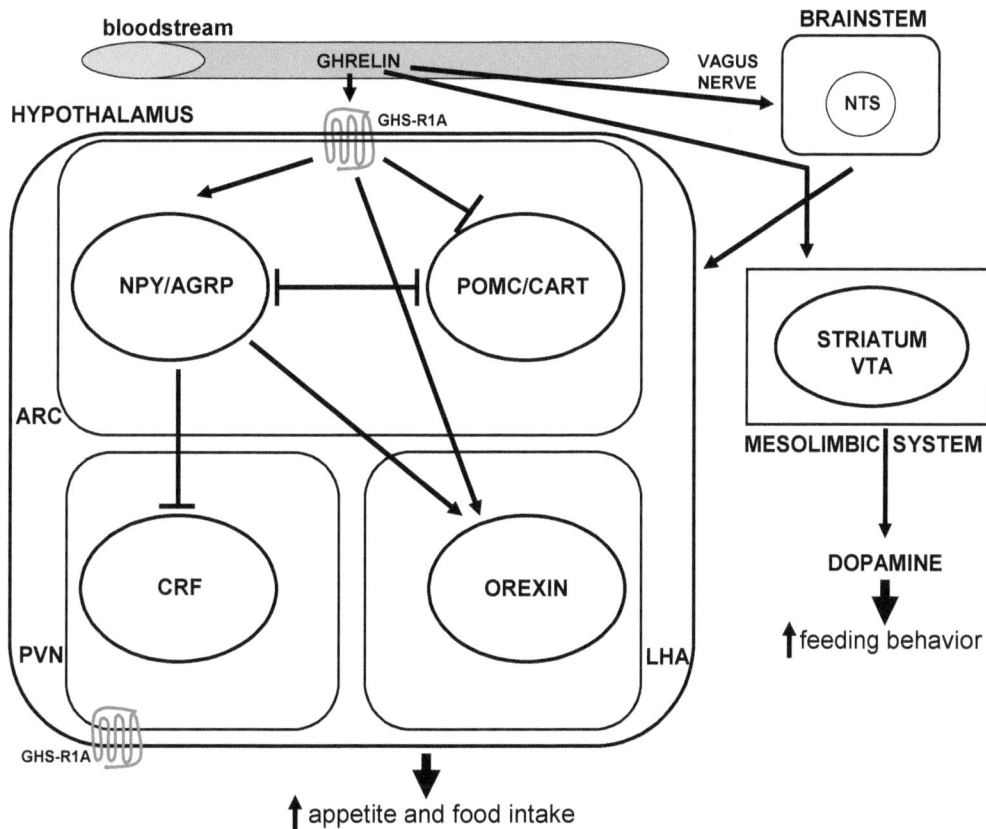

Figure 2: Central nervous system mechanisms involved in the appetite-inducing effect of ghrelin. AGRP: agouti related-protein; ARC: arcuate nucleus; CRF: corticotrophin-releasing factor; LHA: lateral hypothalamic area; NPY: neuropeptides Y; NTS: nucleus of the solitary tract; POMC: propiomelanocortin; PVN: paraventricular nucleus; VTA: ventral tegmental area. Arrows indicate stimulation, while lignes with bars indicate inhibition.

1.6   Ghrelin, Ghrelin Receptor and GOAT Polymorphisms

Ghrelin and GHSR genes both map to chromosome 3p26 locus, a region that has been shown to be linked to obesity (Kissebah *et al.*, 2000; Yeh *et al.*, 2005). Polymorphisms of ghrelin and GHSR genes have been found in both coding and non-coding regions.

The association between preproghrelin, GHSR or GOAT genes polymorphism and several pathological conditions has been extensively investigated and recently reviewed in depth elsewhere (Gueorguiev & Korbonitis, 2013; Liu *et al.*, 2011; Ukkola, 2011; Yi *et al.*, 2011). This chapter will then only focus on main general findings in this complex area of research.

1.6.1   Eating Disorders

The potential link between ghrelin and GHSR genes polymorphism and obesity has been investigated in numerous studies (Bing *et al.*, 2005; Dardennes *et al.*, 2007; Gueorguiev *et al.*, 2009; Gjesing *et al.*, 2010; Hinney *et al.*, 2002; Korbonits *et al.*, 2002; Larsen *et al.*, 2005; Liu *et al.*, 2011; Martin *et al.*, 2008;

Miraglia del Giudice *et al.*, 2004; Ukkola *et al.*, 2001; Seim *et al.*, 2011; Vivenza *et al.*, 2004; Wang *et al.*, 2004).

Preproghrelin Leu72Met polymorphism in exon 2 was associated with the early onset of obesity and higher body mass index (BMI) (Miraglia del Giudice *et al.*, 2004; Kornbonits *et al.*, 2002; Miraglia del Giudice *et al*, 2004; Ukkola *et al.*, 2001; Ukkola *et al.*, 2002). However, other studies showed that the prevalence of 72Met allele was similar in children and adults control and obese cohorts (Miraglia del Giudice *et al.*, 2004; Hinney *et al.*, 2002; Jo *et al.*, 2005; Ukkola *et al.*, 2001). A single nucleotide polymorphism (SNP) 3056T>C in intron 2, correlated to higher BMI and fat mass, might play a role in eating disorders (Ando *et al.*, 2007). However, another study showed no association between 3056T>C SNP and several obesity parameters (Takezawa *et al.*, 2009). Several other studies revealed the existence of other preproghrelin SNP that could be linked to obesity (De Vriese *et al.*, 2009; Liu *et al.*, 2011; Ukkola, 2011).

Several GHSR SNPs have been identified (De Vriese *et al.*, 2009; Liu *et al.*, 2011; Ukkola, 2011). However, studies evaluating the link between GHSR SNPs and obesity have led to contradictory data (Baessler *et al.*, 2005; Gjesing *et al.*, 2010; Gueorguiev *et al.*, 2009; Wang *et al.*, 2004). Newer approaches addressing the possibility of using GHSR SNPs as markers to predict therapy, for example in dietary and exercise regimens aiming for weight reduction (Mager *et al.*, 2008), could be very useful in the context of targeted molecular therapy.

Genetic factors could explain more than 50% of the variance observed in eating behaviour in normal subjects and subjects with eating disorders. Contradictory data exist concerning the association of several ghrelin SNP (such as Leu72Met, Arg51Gln and Gln90Leu) with bulimia nervosa and anorexia nervosa (Ando *et al.*, 2007; Cellini *et al.*, 2006; Kindler *et al.*, 2011; Monteleone *et al.*, 2006; Monteleone *et al.*, 2007). Only one study has investigated the association between GHSR polymorphism and eating disorders (bulimia nervosa and anorexia nervosa) and suggested no association between the 171T>C SNP and eating disorders (Miyasaka *et al.*, 2006). Also, a single study has reported that GOAT polymorphism (genotype G/G at SNP rs10096097) could be associated with anorexia nervosa (Muller *et al.*, 2010).

1.6.2   Type 2 Diabetes

With the discovery of ghrelin and GHSR-1a expression in pancreas, it has been suggested that ghrelin and GHSR gene SNP could be linked to glucose metabolism (Gnanapavan *et al.*, 2002). Relationships between ghrelin and both insulin and glucose metabolism are complex and have been previously reviewed in depth (Chanclon *et al.*, 2012; Dezaki and Yada, 2012; Sangiao-Alvarellos and Cordido, 2010; Verhulst and Depoortere, 2012). Studies have evaluated the association between ghrelin or GHSR SNPs and type 2 diabetes by association with either glucose and insulin levels following fasting or oral glucose tolerance test, or with type 2 diabetes prevalence. In this context, studies led to contradictory data concerning the possible association between ghrelin or GHSR SNPs and type 2 diabetes (Berthold *et al.*, 2009; Liao *et al.*, 2013; Liu *et al.*, 2011).

1.6.3   Cardiovascular Diseases

While Arg51Gln ghrelin SNP was shown to be associated with hypertension (Poykko *et al.*, 2003), discrepant data exist concerning the association of Leu72Met ghrelin SNP with hypertension (Bing *et al.*, 2005; Ukkola *et al.*, 2002) or with coronary artery disease (Tang *et al*, 2008; Zhang *et al.*, 2011). Haplotype analysis revealed that the presence of certain alleles (such as -501A>C) could influence hypertensive risk in the absence or presence Leu72Met (Berthold *et al.*, 2012; Ukkola *et al.*, 2012). Variants of GHSR have also been shown to be linked or not linked to left ventricular hypertrophy, and myocardial infarction

(Baessler *et al.*, 2006; Baessler *et al.*, 2007). A study of the ghrelin expression level and variant -501A>C SNP with cardiac hypertrophy (Ukkola *et al.*, 2012), suggested an association with left ventricular mass index, independent of blood pressure, in a cohort of 1037 middle-aged subjects.

If further studies support associations of ghrelin or ghrelin receptor variants with susceptibility to develop various cardiovascular ailments, this may provide a diagnostic tool for prophylactic medicine and even therapeutic strategies targeting ghrelin expression and/or effect.

1.6.4   Cancer

Ghrelin and GHSR variants association with susceptibility to various cancers, tumour development and progression, has explored as well.

Ghrelin and GHS-R are expressed in various tumours such as adrenal, breast, endometrial, gastrointestinal, liver, lung, ovarian, pancreatic, parathyroid, pituitary, prostate, renal, salivary gland, testicular and thyroid tumours, astrocytoma and leukaemia (Chopin *et al.*, 2012; De Vriese *et al.*, 2005; De Vriese *et al.*, 2007b; Gueorguiev and Korbonits, 2013; Majchrzak *et al.*, 2012). Depending on the tumour type ghrelin has been shown to promote or inhibit cell proliferation, promote angiogenesis and tumour invasion, inhibit apoptosis, and exhibit immunomodulatory and anti-inflammatory effects (Chopin *et al.*, 2012; Majchrzak *et al.*, 2012).

No association has been found between the most common variants, e.g. Leu72Met and Arg51Gln preproghrelin SNPs, and polycystic ovary syndrome (Wang *et al.*, 2009). The T allele of preproghrelin rs27647 SNP appears to confer a protective borderline effect to colorectal risk (Campa *et al.*, 2010).

A recent study (Motawi *et al*, 2013), in hepatitis C Egyptian patients, suggested an association of A allele at position 346 of ghrelin and susceptibility to HCC in the hepatitis C patients. The role of ghrelin in cancer cachexia has been discussed above (see 2.3.1). Epigenetic changes, a hallmark in cancer, in GHS-R gene promoter region, have been identified in breast cancer and can discriminate between invasive ductal carcinoma and normal breast tissue (Botla *et al.*, 2012; Ordway *et al.*, 2007). Hypermethylation of the GHS-R gene promoter region leads to decreased GHS-R1A expression in breast cancer (Botla *et al.*, 2012; Ordway *et al.*, 2007), as well as several rodent tumour cell lines from hypothalamus, pituitary, heart and liver (Inoue *et al.*, 2011). Epigenetic changes in GHS-R promoter region could therefore play a role in the sensitivity of cells to ghrelin, and significantly impact various disease phenotypes. Further studies are yet required to test this hypothesis; indeed leverage on epigenetic gene modifications is an increasing area of investigation as a potential therapeutic approach.

1.6.5   Conclusions

Ghrelin and GHSR genes SNP and gene variants may be involved in modifying susceptibility to environmental pressures of weight gain or loss in humans and various pathologies, that may be considered related, such as type 2 diabetes, eating disorders, cardiovascular diseases and cancer. However, the current status of the increasing divergent data obtained by genetic association studies are likely to be due to differences in allele frequencies between populations, study designs, cohort sizes and methodologies. Therefore, future studies are warranted to properly examine the association of preproghrelin or GHRS gene SNP and variants, with pathological conditions, aiming at designing studies of appropriate statistical power.

Nevertheless, the now obvious multifactor aspects of metabolism and pathogenesis will require integrating ghrelin in a network of signalling, whereby the final response results from the integration of the various signals in response to the environmental and metabolic cues. This integration of network signals therefore may explain, on the one hand, why leverage on one signal only yields subtle effects; and on the other hand, why leverage of a given signal on various "signal network patterns" may result in different, even opposing, observed effects. Therefore, the understanding of ghrelin's (and its receptors) effects must eventually be set within a proper "systems biology frame", i.e. crosstalk between ghrelin and its partners taken concomitantly into account.

2   Clinical Applications of Ghrelin

2.1   GH-Deficiency Disorders

Ghrelin possesses a strong and dose-dependent growth hormone (GH) releasing effect, both in vivo and in vitro, in humans and animals by acting on the GHS-R1a receptor present on pituitary somatotropic cells (Date *et al.*, 2000a; Hataya *et al.*, 2001; Malagon *et al.*, 2003; Takaya *et al.*, 2000). Des-acyl ghrelin is unable to stimulate GH secretion under physiological conditions, as it cannot bind to GHS-R. However, over-expression of des-acyl ghrelin in transgenic animals results in a small phenotype, maybe by modulation the GH-insulin growth factor 1 axis (Ariyasu *et al.*, 2005). Ghrelin induces GH secretion from somatotropic cells by activating the cGMP signal transduction pathway but also the nitric oxide synthase pathway (Rodriguez-Pacheco *et al.*, 2008). Combined administration of ghrelin and GH-releasing hormone (GHRH) displays synergistic effects, rather than additive effects, on GH release. Ghrelin action on GH release seems to be mediated by the hypothalamus as patients presenting organic lesions in the hypothalamus region are not able to release GH in response to ghrelin (Popovic *et al.*, 2003). Ghrelin can be used as a provocative test for the diagnosis of GH deficiency in lean and overweight adults, but not in obese patients as obesity strongly reduces GH response to ghrelin (Gasco *et al.*, 2012). In a mouse model of ghrelinoma, adult mice have elevated ghrelin and IGF-1 levels but normal GH levels. However, GH levels were higher after GHRH injection, suggesting that chronic elevation of ghrelin activates GH-IGF-I axis (Iwakura *et al.*, 2009).

GHS-R mutations that segregate with short stature have been reported (Pantel *et al.*, 2006). As ghrelin is decreased after dexamethasone administration in children with idiopathic short stature (ISS), the existence of a feedback link among ghrelin, glucocorticoids and the GH/IGF-I axis has been suggested (Radetti *et al.*, 2008). Ghrelin secretion is elevated in children with lower IGF-I/IGFBP-3 ratio, suggesting that lower bioactivity of IGF-I is a stimulating factor for ghrelin synthesis (Stawerska *et al.* 2012a) However, in ISS patients, short stature does not appear to be frequently caused by abnormalities in ghrelin signaling (Iniguez *et al.*, 2011; Hess *et al.*, 2012). In children with growth hormone deficiency and neurosecretory dysfunction, ghrelin concentration is higher than in healthy controls and in children with ISS (Stawerska *et al.*, 2012b). The GH-releasing effect of ghrelin increases at puberty and decreases with age, but is independent of gender (Broglio *et al.*, 2003; Ghigo *et al.*, 2005). As aging is associated with progressive decrease in GH secretion, the effects of ghrelin should be studied in elderly patients. Administration of a GHS-R agonist, MK-0677, in elderly patients with hip fracture have not shown a significant increase in strength or function when compared to the placebo group, however a trend was observed (Bach *et al.*, 2004). In elderly subjects, ghrelin levels are positively correlated with serum IGF-1 levels, suggesting that the negative feedback mechanism does not function properly (Akamizu *et al.*, 2006). Although GHS-R1a expression remains stable during aging (Sun *et al.*, 2007) impairment of the ghrelin system could partially explain the age-related decrease of GH secretion.

2.2   Eating Disorders

2.2.1   Obesity

Obesity is an increasing global health problem that significantly increases the risk of comorbidities including cardiovascular, respiratory, neurological, gastrointestinal, endocrine and musculoskeletal diseases (Kushner and Roth, 2003). Obese patients, both children and adults, were found to have lower plasma ghrelin levels than in non-obese control subjects (Tschop *et al.*, 2001; Soriano-Guillen *et al.*, 2004). Ghrelin levels fluctuate in a compensatory manner to body weight variations, suggesting that the decreased levels of ghrelin could represent an adaptation to reduce the hunger stimulus (Soriano-Guillen *et al.*, 2004). Ghrelin levels decrease with weight gain resulting from overfeeding (Williams *et al.*, 2006), pregnancy (Palik *et al.*, 2007), olanzapine treatment (Hosojima *et al.*, 2006), or high fat diet (Robertson *et al.*, 2004; Otukonyong *et al.*, 2005). Conversely, ghrelin levels increase with weight loss resulting from food restriction (Purnell *et al.*, 2007), long-term chronic exercise but not acute exercise (Kraemer & Castracane, 2007). Votruba *et al.* confirmed that fasting ghrelin concentration is negatively correlated with body mass index but suggested that morning ghrelin concentrations are not affected by short-term overfeeding (Votruba *et al.*, 2009). Wadden *et al.* investigated the response of acylated ghrelin after 7 days of overfeeding. Surprisingly, fasting ghrelin concentration was significantly increased in response to the positive energy challenge and independent of obesity status (Wadden *et al.*, 2012). This increase may counteract the rising insulin resistance. However, acylated ghrelin was negatively correlated with BMI in normal weight and overweight subjects (Wadden *et al.*, 2012). Besides, Rodriguez *et al.* reported that circulating concentrations of acylated ghrelin were increased, whereas desacyl ghrelin levels were decreased in obesity and obesity-associated type-2 diabetes (Rodriguez *et al.*, 2009). A meta-analysis of clinical studies evaluating ghrelin levels in obesity concluded that total and active ghrelin in normal weight groups were significantly higher than the obese groups (Zhang *et al.*, 2011). Overnutrition during early life induces an increase in body weight of young mice that persisted until adulthood and decreases acylated ghrelin circulating levels (Soares *et al.*, 2012). In addition, GHSR-1a signaling pathway was upregulated in white adipose tissue of these obese young mice, leading to positive modulation of content and phosphorylation of protein involved in cell energy storage and use (Soares *et al.*, 2012). Moreover, subjects homozygous for the obesity-associated gene have dysregulated circulating ghrelin levels of acylated ghrelin and attenuated posprandial appetite reduction (Karra *et al.*, 2013). Finally, it has been suggested that the postprandial rise in insulin secretion or the secretion of glucagon-like peptide 1 (GLP-1) and gastric inhibitory peptide (GIP) may mediate the postprandial decrease of ghrelin (Mohlig *et al.*, 2002; Perez-Tilve *et al.*, 2007). Hagemann *et al.* showed that GLP-1 at supraphysiological levels reduces the rise in ghrelin levels in the late postprandial period and suggested that this might contribute to its anorexic effects (Hagemann *et al.*, 2007). Considering the multiple factors that may affect ghrelin responsiveness, further larger studies are required to clarify its role in human obesity.

Prader-Willi syndrome (PWS) is a genetic neurodevelopmental disorder characterized by mental retardation and hyperphagia leading to severe obesity. Ghrelin has been implicated as a potential cause of the insatiable appetite and the obesity of these patients. In PWS patients, plasma ghrelin levels are higher than in healthy subjects and do not decrease after a meal, which is consistent with increased hunger (Cummings *et al.*, 2002a; DelParigi *et al.*, 2002; Purtell *et al.*, 2011). Other studies showed that ghrelin levels decreased postprandially in adult patients with PWS, but to a lesser extent than in obese and lean subjects (Gimenez-Palop *et al.*, 2007; Paik *et al.*, 2007). This reduced postprandial ghrelin suppression may be explained by a low postprandial release of PYY, an anorexigenic peptide that decreases postprandial ghrelin levels (Gimenez-Palop *et al.*, 2007). Interestingly, PWS children having not yet developed hyperphagia or excessive obesity (5 years of age and younger) have normal ghrelin levels (Erdie-Lalena *et al.*, 2006; Haqq *et al.*, 2008; Goldstone *et al.*, 2012). Ghrelin levels could increase with the onset of hyperphagia (Erdie-Lalena *et al.*, 2006; Haqq *et al.*, 2008). However, Fiegerlova *et al.*, showed that plasma ghrelin levels in children with PWS were elevated at all age levels, including the first years of life, thus preceding the development of obesity (Feigerlova *et al.*, 2008).

Gastric bypass surgery is an effective treatment for morbid obesity. However, the influence of this type of surgery on ghrelin levels needs to be clarified. Some studies found a decrease (Chan *et al.*, 2006; Cummings *et al.*, 2002b; Fruhbeck *et al.*, 2004; Korner *et al.*, 2006; Chronaiou *et al.*, 2012), no change (Couce *et al.*, 2006; Mancini *et al.*, 2006; Stenstrom *et al.*, 2006) or an increase of ghrelin secretion (Haider *et al.*, 2007; Mingrone *et al.*, 2006; Stratis *et al.*, 2006; Barazzoni *et al.*, 2013, Cigdem Arica *et al.*, 2013). These different outcomes may depend on the different surgical techniques used across centers, but also on how, where and when the postoperative samples were taken. Ghrelin levels are affected more by lowered caloric intake and the resulting weight loss, rather than gastric bypass surgery. Fasting ghrelin displays an inversely significant correlation with body mass index in both stable body weight conditions and after gastric bypass (Ybarra *et al.*, 2009). However, as ghrelin's signals for feeding is conveyed mostly by the vagal afferent system, vagal nerve transection during gastric bypass could explain the controversial outcomes (Date *et al.*, 2012). Preservation of the celiac branch of the vagus nerve during laparoscopy-assisted distal gastrectomy leads to significantly lower postprandial plasma ghrelin levels compared to a group in which the celiac branch of the vagus nerve was not preserved (Takigushi *et al.*, 2013). Samat et al. suggest that postprandial ghrelin suppression is associated with weight loss and enhanced insulin sensitivity following gastric bypass surgery in obese adults with type 2 diabetes (Samat *et al.*, 2013).

2.2.2   Anorexia Nervosa

Anorexia nervosa is characterized by very low body weight and an aversion to body weight increase, and is associated with gastrointestinal, metabolic and psychological complications. No effective pharmacological treatments are currently available for this disorder. Gut-brain peptides involved in hunger regulation have been though to be involved in the pathogenesis of this disorder (Inui, 2001). In particular, the possible role of ghrelin in this disorder has been investigated.

High total plasma ghrelin levels have been found in patients with anorexia nervosa, which is consistent with a state of chronic negative energy balance and could be a result of an adaptation to prolonged lack of nutrient intake (Otto *et al.* 2001; Janas-Kozik *et al.*, 2007; Germain *et al.*, 2009; Ogiso *et al.*, 2011). A meta-analysis concluded that persons with anorexia nervosa had higher baseline concentrations of ghrelin, but that ghrelin release after a meal is not different (Prince *et al.*, 2009). Only a few studies have separately measured both acyl ghrelin and des-acyl ghrelin levels and mostly showed that the ratio of des-acyl ghrelin to acyl ghrelin tend to be higher in patients with anorexia nervosa than in control subjects (Hotta *et al.*, 2004; Nakahara *et al.*, 2008; Koyama *et al.*, 2010; Ogiso *et al.*, 2011). Ghrelin administration to patients with anorexia nervosa led to contradictory data in terms of hunger scores, appetite, body weight and/or energy expenditure (Hotta *et al.*, 2009; Miljic *et al.*, 2006). Patients with anorexia nervosa had a blunted anabolic response after ghrelin administration as compared to healthy controls (Broglio *et al.*, 2004; Miljic *et al.*, 2006). This could be explained by impaired GH/IGF-1 axis observed in anorectic patients, leading to GH resistance (Ohlsson *et al.*, 1998).

Increased GOAT mRNA levels in response to long-term chronic malnutrition (Gonzalez *et al.*, 2008) could represent the underlying mechanism responsible for increased acylated ghrelin levels in anorexia nervosa (Soriano-Guillen *et al.*, 2004). Moreover, a single nucleotide polymorphism of GOAT might be associated with anorexia nervosa (Müller *et al.*, 2011). Personalized medicine targeting GOAT could therefore represent a novel therapeutic approach for the treatment of anorexia nervosa.

Suppression of the central ghrelin signaling system via GHS-R1a could reduce hyperactive behavior in patients suffering from anorexia nervosa, suggesting that the ghrelin receptor could provide a therapeutically relevant target for treatment of anorexia nervosa as well (Verhagen *et al.*, 2011).

2.3 Muscle Waisting Conditions

2.3.1 Cachexia

Cachexia is characterized by weight loss, muscle atrophy, fatigue and loss of appetite. Cachexia appears in about half of all cancer patients, and in chronic diseases, and is associated with increased morbidity and mortality. Cytokines, involved in the aetiology of cancer cachexia, elicit effects mimicking leptin signalling and suppressing orexigenic ghrelin and neuropeptide Y signalling. Treatment of cachexia is a multifactorial approach. Ghrelin is known to stimulate GH secretion and appetite, but also to exert anti-inflammatory actions as well, and may represent a therapeutic strategy for the treatment of certain types of cachexia (Nagaya *et al.*, 2005; Garcia *et al.*, 2007). Intravenous administration of ghrelin increases appetite and stimulates food intake (Wren *et al.*, 2001). Ghrelin increases food intake by activating hypothalamic NPY/AGRP neurons, stimulating the production of NPY and AGRP (Coiro *et al.*, 2006; Kohno *et al.*, 2007; Kohno *et al.*, 2008). Ghrelin also inhibits POMC neurons, preventing the release of the anorexigenic peptide α-MSH (Riediger *et al.*, 2003). Plasma ghrelin levels are elevated in patients suffering from cachexia associated with chronic heart failure, lung cancer, chronic liver disease and prostate cancer (Nagaya *et al.*, 2001; Shimizu *et al.*, 2003; Tacke *et al.*, 2003; Malendowicz *et al.*, 2009). Although cachexia involves elevated levels of ghrelin, the beneficial effects of ghrelin on appetite in cachexia have been evaluated in several clinical trials. In rodent models of cancer-cachexia, ghrelin administration significantly increases weight and food intake and partially reverses cachexia associated with the cancer (Hanada *et al.*, 2003; Wang *et al.*, 2006; DeBoer *et al.*, 2007). A randomized, placebo-controlled trial in cancer patients with impaired appetite has shown that ghrelin could increase energy intake (Neary *et al.*, 2004). One concern regarding the use of ghrelin in cancer patients is that ghrelin may stimulate tumor growth by increasing growth factors such as GH and IGF-1. Short and long term clinical trials have shown that ghrelin was well tolerated and safe in patients with advanced cancer (Strasser *et al.*, 2008; Lundholm *et al.*, 2010). However, large scale clinical trials are needed to confirm the safety of ghrelin treatment. In cachexia associated with chronic heart failure, ghrelin administration resulted in an increase in food intake and body weight, with improvement in the exercise capacity and left ventricular function (Nagaya *et al.*, 2004). In patients with chronic obstructive pulmonary disease (COPD), repeated administration of ghrelin increased food intake, body weight, lean body mass, and peripheral and respiratory muscle strength (Nagaya *et al.*, 2005; Miki *et al.*, 2012). In peritoneal dialysis patients with end stage renal disease, a chronic condition frequently associated with nutritional dysfunction, ghrelin treatment increases food intake (Wynne *et al.*, 2005; Ashby *et al.*, 2009). Using a nephrectomised rat model of renal cachexia, Deboer et al. demonstrated that ghrelin treatment improved lean body mass accrual and decreased circulating inflammatory cytokines (Deboer *et al.*, 2008).

2.3.2 Sarcopenia

Ghrelin seems to be an important modulator of physiological functions associated with aging. Endogenous ghrelin signalling seems to become less efficient during aging (Baranowska *et al.*, 2006). Chronic restoration of the GH/IGF-1 axis with the ghrelin mimetic MK-0677 increased lean mass in elderly patients, suggesting that MK-0677 compensates for a deficit in endogenous ghrelin signalling (Smith *et al.* 2005). Sarcopenia is characterized by an age-related decline in muscle mass and strength. The loss of muscle mass is typically offset by increases in fat mass. The pathogenesis of sarcopenia is a multifactorial process including physical activity, nutritional intake, oxidative stress, and hormonal changes (Sakuma & Yamaguchi, 2012). IGF-1 seems to be the most important mediator of muscle growth and repair and it is proven that age-associated decline in GH levels in combination with lower IGF-1 levels contributes to the development of sarcopenia (Ferrucci *et al.*, 2002; Philippou *et al.*, 2007). Treatment with ghrelin may reduce the muscle atrophy related to age-dependent decrease in GH (Nass *et al.*, 2008). In healthy adults, plasma ghrelin concentrations are inversely related to body mass index, but also to skeletal muscle mass (Tai *et al.*, 2009). In a model of chronic kidney disease, ghrelin treatment resulted in improved lean body mass build up that was related in part to a decrease in muscle protein degradation (Deboer *et al.*, 2008). Ghrelin inhibited skeletal muscle protein breakdown in rats with thermal injury (Balasubramaniam *et al.*, 2009). Ghrelin administration improved body weight gain and skeletal muscle catabolism associated with angiotensin II-induced cachexia in mice, by improving the nutritional status and IGF-1 signalling in the skeletal muscle. Early restoration of IGF-1 mRNA in the skeletal muscle by ghrelin might lead to improvements of muscle catabolism at later periods (Sugiyama *et al.*, 2012). Des-acyl ghrelin seems also to reduce muscle cachexia produced by injury and proinflammatory cytokines (Sheriff *et al.*, 2012). Both ghrelin and des-acyl ghrelin inhibit dexamethasone-induced skeletal muscle atrophy by acting on a yet unidentified receptor in a GH-independent manner (Porporato *et al*, 2013).

2.4   Gastrointestinal Hypomotility Disorders

Gastric acid secretion is stimulated by intravenous injection of ghrelin (Asakawa *et al.*, 2001; Masuda *et al.*, 2000), acting most likely via the vagus nerve (Masuda *et al.*, 2000). Contradictory data exist concerning the effect of intracerebroventricular administration of ghrelin (Date *et al.*, 2001; Levin *et al.*, 2005; Sibilia *et al.*, 2002). Furthermore, simultaneous administration of ghrelin and gastrin induce a synergic effect on gastric acid secretion (Fukumoto *et al.*, 2008).

Gastric motility is stimulated by ghrelin inducing the migrating motor complex and accelerating gastric emptying (Dass *et al.*, 2003; Depoortere *et al*, 2005; Fujino *et al.*, 2003; Peeters, 2005; Peeters, 2013). Due to its prokinetic effect, ghrelin can reverse gastric postoperative ileus (Trudel *et al.*, 2002) and improve diabetic gastroparesis (Murray *et al.*, 2005; Qiu *et al.*, 2008). GHS-R agonists have been shown to increase gastrointestinal motility in rodents (Shimizu *et al.*, 2006; Fraser *et al.*, 2008). Stimulation of the GHS-R increases upper gastrointestinal motility in both a basal state and in a model of opiate-induced bowel dysfunction. Ghrelin and ghrelin agonists may provide an integrated approach for the treatment of multiple gastrointestinal hypomotility-related disorders (Charoenthongtrakul *et al.*, 2009).

The gastroprotective effects of ghrelin against experimental-induced ulcers involve a cross talk between nitric oxide and prostaglandins (Konturek *et al.*, 2004; Peeters, 2005; Sibilia *et al.*, 2003; Sibilia *et al.*, 2008).

2.5   Diabetes

Glucose metabolism is regulated by ghrelin (Verhulst and Depoortere, 2012). Despite controversial data, most data suggest that ghrelin decreases insulin secretion by altering insulin sensitivity, leading to increased circulating glucose levels (Broglio *et al.*, 2001; Verhulst and Depoortere, 2012). The pathways involved in the inhibitory effect of ghrelin on insulin secretion include enhanced insulinoma-associated protein 2ß (Doi *et al.*, 2006) and activation of AMPK-uncoupling protein (UCP2) (Andrews *et al.*, 2008; Zhang *et al.*, 2001). Ghrelin activates glycogenolysis and increases hepatic triglyceride content (Heijboer *et al.*, 2006). In a mouse model of ghrelinoma, insulin secretion by glucose tolerance tests was significantly attenuated whereas insulin sensitivity determined by insulin tolerance tests was preserved; indicating that chronic elevation of ghrelin suppresses insulin secretion and leads to glucose intolerance (Iwakura *et al.*, 2009). As ghrelin has diabetogenic effects, ghrelin antagonists may be suited for treatment of type-2 diabetes by increasing insulin secretion in pancreatic β-cells and by improving insulin sensitivity in peripheral tissues (Verhulst and Depoortere, 2012).

2.6   Inflammation

Ghrelin exerts anti-inflammatory effects by inhibiting the production of pro-inflammatory cytokines (Chang *et al.*, 2003; Dembinski *et al.*, 2003; Dixit *et al.*, 2004; Xia *et al.*, 2004). Ghrelin inhibits inflammation under different pathological conditions such as colonic inflammation pancreatitis, sepsis, arthritis, pain, diabetic nephropathy, inflammatory bowel disease (Warzecha *et al.*, 2010; Granado *et al.*, 2005; Chorny *et al.*, 2008; Deboer *et al.*, 2011; Cheyuo *et al.*, 2012; Baatar *et al.*, 2011; Das, 2011; Sibilia *et al.*, 2012; Tschuchimochi *et al.*, 2013; De Boer, 2011).

The protective effects of ghrelin on the development of experimental pancreatitis have limited clinical value as it requires ghrelin administration prior to pancreatic damage (Warzecha *et al.*, 2010). The beneficial effects consist of improved pancreatic blood flow, reduction of IL1ß, and stimulation of pancreatic cell proliferation (Warzecha *et al.*, 2010). In sepsis, increased norepinephrine release causes hepatocellular dysfunction and upregulation of proinflammatory cytokines, such as TNF. Ghrelin treatment in sepsis reduced norepinephrine and TNF levels by upregulation MAPK phosphatase 1 (Jacob *et al.*, 2010). Furthermore, ghrelin improves organ blood flow by inhibiting NF-kB (Wu *et al.*, 2007) and inhibits the production of HMGB1 by activated macrophages (Chorny *et al.*, 2008). In an animal model of arthritis, ghrelin reduced IL6 levels and the symptoms of arthritis (Granado *et al.*, 2005). Des-acyl ghrelin and GHS, but not ghrelin, are able to decrease IL6 and IL1ß levels induced by insoluble fibrillary ß-amyloid protein deposition in mouse microglia by a mechanism independent of the activation of GHS-R1a (Bulgarelli *et al.*, 2009). Both ghrelin and desacyl ghrelin exhibit anti-hyperalgesic and anti-inflammatory effects by acting on a ghrelin receptor distinct from the GHS-R1a (Sibilia *et al.*, 2012). Ghrelin has been shown to prevent the development of experimental diabetic nephropathy in mice via the activation of GHS-R1a (Tsuchimochi *et al.*, 2013). Inflammatory bowel disease, in particular Crohn's disease, could be improved by ghrelin administration (DeBoer, 2011). However, human clinical trials should be performed to assess the usefulness of ghrelin in this disease. Furthermore, the A-501C single nucleotide polymorphism of the ghrelin gene was found to be associated with early onset of rheumatoid arthritis (Ozgen *et al.*, 2011). It remains controversial whether the A-501C single nucleotide polymorphism of the ghrelin gene alters ghrelin levels as it causes decreased ghrelin mRNA expression in PBMCs, but no modification of plasma ghrelin concentration (Mager *et al.*, 2008). Ghrelin might therefore act by an autocrine pathway within the immune microenvironment. Additional *in vivo* studies, including human clinical trials, are necessary to ascertain the therapeutic potential of ghrelin, GHS, and/or des-acyl ghrelin in inflammatory-related diseases.

2.7 Gastrectomy and Esophagectomy

Patients who have undergone total gastrectomy and esophagectomy experience body weight loss. Plasma ghrelin levels are decreased after such surgical procedures and are correlated with body weight loss (Ariyasu *et al.*, 2001; Takachi *et al.*, 2006; Doki *et al.*, 2006). Furthermore, reduced plasma ghrelin levels following esophagectomy is a new predictor of prolonged systemic inflammatory response syndrome (Yamamoto *et al.*, 2013). Ghrelin treatment of patients undergoing gastrectomy or esophagectomy induced higher food intake and appetite, as compared to patients treated with placebo (Adachi *et al.*, 2010; Yamamoto *et al.*, 2010). Ghrelin administration may therefore be useful to minimize the side effects of such surgical procedure. However, further studies are required to evaluate the beneficial effects of ghrelin treatment on the systemic inflammatory response syndrome as well.

2.8 Epilepsy

In epilepsy, contradictory data suggest that ghrelin could or could not prevent induced seizures (Portelli *et al.*, 2012; Biagini *et al.*, 2011; Casillas-Espinosa *et al.*, 2012). In mice, GHS-R deletion, inverse agonists, or desensitization leads to the attenuation of limbic seizures and epileptiform activity, suggesting that both agonists and inverse agonists are capable of exerting anticonvulsant effects (Portelli *et al.*, 2012). Besides, des-acyl ghrelin and a synthetic analogue of ghrelin were found to prevent progression to *status epilepticus*, suggesting that the desoctanoylated form of ghrelin possesses anticonvulsive properties (Biagini *et al.*, 2011). Ghrelin also protects neurons from apoptosis in induced epilepsy (Zhang *et al.*, 2013). Further studies are needed to clarify the role of ghrelin in this pathology.

2.9 Bone

Ghrelin induces bone formation by stimulating osteoblastic cell proliferation and differentiation, inhibiting cell apoptosis, and increasing bone mineral density (Delhanty *et al.*, 2013; Liang *et al.*, 2013; Fukushima *et al.*, 2005; Maccarinelli *et al.*, 2005). In rats, chronic central administration of ghrelin increases bone mass, through a mechanism independent of appetite regulation (Choi *et al.*, 2013). Per os ghrelin administration is capable of increasing new bone formation and stimulate intramembranous bone repair of calvarial bone defects in rats (Deng *et al.*, 2008). In human, mean plasma level of ghrelin was positively correlated with bone mineral density in perimenopausal, postmenopausal and premenopoausal subjects, while it was significantly decreased in perimenopausal and postmenopausal subjects as compared to premenopausal subjects (Nouh *et al.*, 2012). Ghrelin levels were associated with trabecular bone mass density, but not with total or cortical bone mass density in elderly wowen, while they were not associated with those parameters in men (Napoli *et al.*, 2011). In obese adolescent girls, Campos *et al.* showed that ghrelin is a negative predictor for bone mineral density and content (Campos *et al.*, 2013). In a randomised, double-blind, placebo-controlled study, ghrelin infusion had no acute effect on markers of bone turnover in healthy controls and post-gastrectomy subjects, but was inversely correlated with bone resorption (Huda *et al.*, 2007). Further studies are required to better understand the role of ghrelin in bone formation and investigate its potential use to treat elderly patients suffering from osteoporosis or at risk.

2.10   Cancer

Ghrelin and GHS-R are expressed in various tumors such as adrenal, breast, endometrial, gastrointestinal, liver, lung, ovarian, pancreatic, parathoid, pituitary, prostate, renal, salivary gland, testicular and thyroid tumors, astrocytoma and leukemia (Chopin *et al.*, 2012; De Vriese *et al.*, 2005; De Vriese *et al.*, 2007b; Gueorguiev and Korbonits, 2013; Majchrzak *et al.*, 2012). Depending on the tumor type ghrelin has been shown to promote or inhibit cell proliferation, promote angiogenesis and tumor invasion, inhibit apoptosis, and exhibit immunomodulatory and anti-inflammatory effects (Chopin *et al.*, 2012; Majchrzak *et al.*,

2012). The role of ghrelin in cancer cachexia has been discussed above (see 2.3.1). Hiura *et al.* showed that cisplatin-based chemotherapy significantly reduced plasma ghrelin levels and feeding activity (Hiura *et al.*, 2012). Short-term administration of exogenous ghrelin at the start of cisplatin-based chemotherapy with esophageal cancer patients stimulated food intake and minimized adverse effects (Hiura *et al.*, 2012). Epigenetic changes, typical features in cancer, in GHS-R gene promoter region have been identified in breast cancer and can discriminate between invasive ductal carcinoma and normal breast tissue (Botla *et al.*, 2012; Ordway *et al.*, 2007). Hypermethylation of the GHS-R gene promoter region leads to decreased GHS-R1A in breast cancer (Botla *et al.*, 2012; Ordway *et al.*, 2007), as well as several rodent tumor cell lines from hypothalamus, pituitary, heart and liver (Inoue *et al.*, 2011). Epigenetic changes in GHS-R promoter region could therefore play a role in the sensitivity of cells to ghrelin, and significantly impact various disease phenotypes. Further studies are still yet required to test this hypothesis more extensively.

3   Pharmacological Tools Modulating Ghrelin Action

Figure 3 illustrates the pharmacological tools modulating ghrelin action and their respective pharmacological targets. Figure 4 summarizes the major clinical applications of the pharmacological tools modulating ghrelin action.

3.1   Ghrelin Vaccine and Spiegelmers

Ghrelin neutralization may be useful to treat diseases associated with high ghrelin levels such as Prader Willi Syndrome characterized by severe obesity.

Vaccination against ghrelin aims at blocking the effects of ghrelin. In rats, injection of ghrelin hapten immunoconjugates led to the production of antibodies directed against the acylated form of ghrelin, reduced body weight with a preferential reduction of fat mass resulting from altered feeding efficiency (Zorrilla *et al.*, 2006). In pigs, ghrelin vaccine reduced food intake and body weight (Vizcarra *et al.*, 2007). Vaccination of normal weight and diet-induced obese mice induced high antibody response, decreased acute food intake, increased energy expenditure, but no change in body weight (Andrade *et al.*, 2013). In humans, clinical phase I/II trial using CYT 009-Ghr Qb vaccine (Cytos Biotechnology AG) lack to demonstrate any weight loss effect despite antibody response. Specific monoclonal antibodies directed against acyl ghrelin neutralize the peptide, inhibiting *in vivo* GHS-R1a activation, and blocking ghrelin-induced food intake in mice (Lu *et al.*, 2009).

Ghrelin neutralization was also obtained using spiegelmers, antisense polyethylene glycol-modified L-oligonucleotides, specifically binding ghrelin. In diet-induced obese mice, spiegelmer NOX-B11-2 decreased food intake and body weight (Asakawa *et al.*, 2003; Shearman *et al.*, 2006). Spiegelmer NOX-B11-3 inhibited ghrelin-induced GH release in rats (Helmling *et al.*, 2004), but had no effect on the fasting-induced neuronal activation in the hypothalamic arcuate nucleus (Becskei *et al.*, 2008).

To date, the clinical usefulness of ghrelin vaccine and ghrelin spiegelmers for the treatment of obesity remains to be proven (Monteiro, 2011).

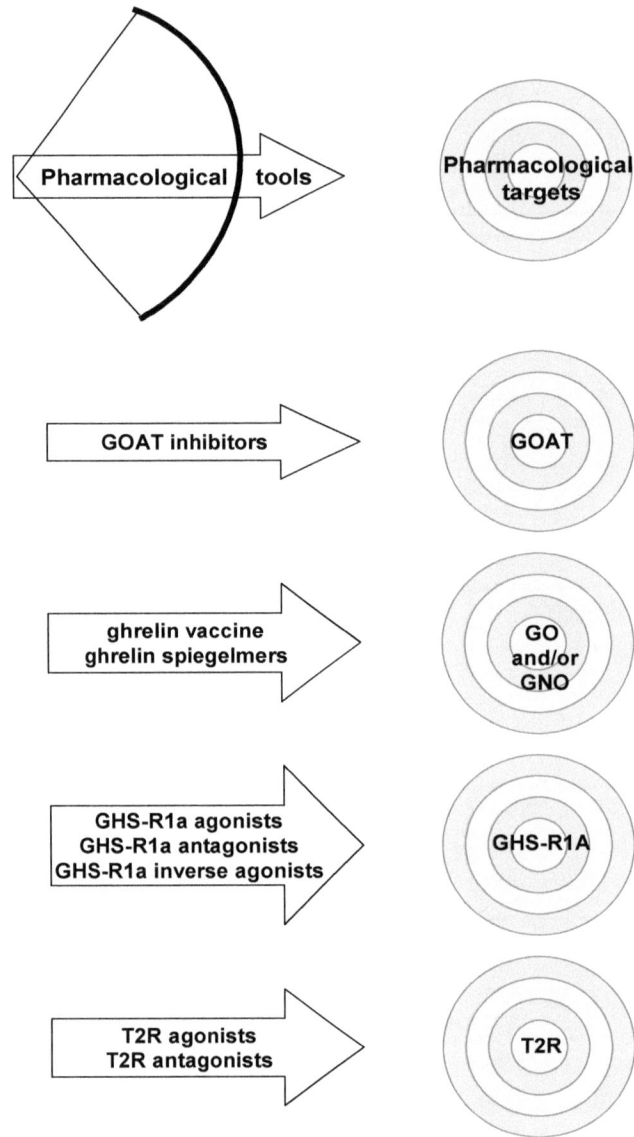

Figure 3: Pharmacological tools modulating ghrelin and their pharmacological targets. GHS-R1a: ghrelin receptor type 1A; GNO: non-octanoylated ghrelin; GO: octanoylated ghrelin; GOAT: ghrelin *O*-acyl transferase; T2R: bitter taste receptor.

3.2   Pharmacological Tools Targeting GHS-R1A

3.2.1   GHS-R1A Agonists

Hexapeptide KwFwLL-NH(2) with d-tryptophane at position 4 with 1-naphthyl-d-alanine (d-1-Nal) and 2-naphthyl-d-alanine (d-2-Nal) is a high potent agonist (Els *et al.*, 2012). The peptide [K[16](NODAGA)]ghrelin(1–28) behaved as a GHS-R1a agonist (Chopra, 2012; NODAGA: 1,4,7-triazacyclononane,1-glutaric acid-4,7-acetic acid).

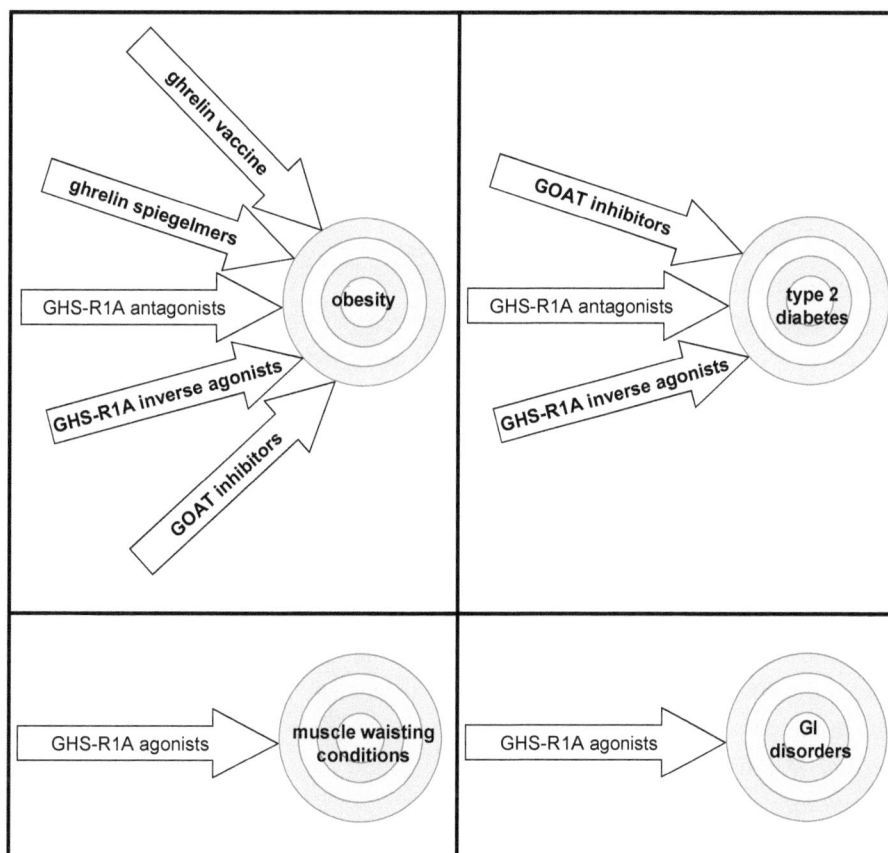

Figure 4: Major clinical applications of the pharmacological tools modulating ghrelin action. GHS-R1a: ghrelin receptor type 1A; GI: gastrointestinal; GOAT: ghrelin *O*-acyl transferase.

Series of novel GHS-R1a agonists were generated based on the conformationally constrained D-Trp-Phe-D-Trp (wFw) core of the prototype inverse agonist [D-Arg(1),D-Phe(5),D-Trp(7,9),Leu(11)]substance P (Siversten *et al.*, 2011). Semagacestat, a γ-secretase inhibitor belonging to a class of drugs being developed as therapeutic agents for Alzheimer's disease, and its precursor were identified as GHS-R1a agonists (Schellenkens *et al.*, 2013). A phase IIa study using TZP-102, a GHS-R1a agonist, relieved gastroparesis symptoms without modification in gastric emptying (Ejskjaer *et al.*, 2013). TZP-101 (ulimorelin) is a potent GHS-R1a agonist *in vitro*, in gastric emptying studies *in vivo*, and in gastrointestinal motily but is unexpectedly unable to induce GH release in rats in vivo (Bochicchio *et al.*, 2011; Hoveyda *et al.*, 2011; Wo *et al.*, 2011). This compound has progressed to phase III human clinical trial for the treatment of postoperative ileus.

3.2.2   GHS-R1A Antagonists

GHS-R1A antagonists have been developed for the treatment of type 2 diabetes, obesity (in particular Prader Willi Syndrome) and metabolic syndrome. [D-Lys-^{3}]GHRP-6, a peptide GHS-R1a antagonist, decreased food intake in lean and obese mice, and reduced weight gain (Shearman *et al.*, 2006; Beck *et al.*, 2004). Piperidine-substituted quinazolinone derivatives represent a class of small GHS-R1a antagonist molecules (Rudolph *et al.*, 2007). Phenyl or phenoxy groups are optimal substituents at position 6 of the quinazolinone core, and the replacement of phenyl groups in position 2 by small alkyl substituents are beneficial (Rudolph *et al.*, 2007). YIL-781, a piperidine-substituted quinazolinone derivative, is a potent GHS-R1a antagonist improving glucose-stimulated insulin secretion, reducing food intake and weight loss in diet-induced obese mice (Esler *et al.*, 2007).

GHS analogs carrying a trisubstituted 1,2,4-triazole structure - such as JMV2866, JMV2844 and JMV2959 - act as GHS-R1a antagonists (Demange *et al.*, 2007; Moulin *et al.*, 2008; Moulin *et al.*, 2013). Additional GHS-R1a antagonists of global similar structure were identified using homogenous time-resolved fluorescence-based assay screening (Leyris *et al.*, 2011). Piperazine-bisamide analogs represent potent GHS-R1a antagonists. One of these analogs featured high potency and inhibited GH release *ex vivo* (Yu *et al.*, 2010). Some carbohydrazide derivatives are potent and selective GHS-R1a antagonists (Sabbatini *et al.*, 2010). Among these compounds, GSK1614343 was shown to be a potent competitive antagonist of rat GHS-R1a, but unexpectedly produced an increase in food intake and body weight in both rats and dogs (Perdona *et al.*, 2011; Costantini *et al.*, 2011).

BIM-28163 was identified as a ghrelin antagonist blocking ghrelin-induced GH secretion, but un-expectedly induced body weight gain (Halem *et al.*, 2004; Hassouna *et al.*, 2013). Other GHS-R1a ana-logs developed to treat weight disorders, including obesity, are still considered as preclinical compounds (TZP-301, from Tranzyme Pharma, and EX-1350, from Elixir Pharmaceuticals) (Depoortere *et al.*, 2009). Some benzodiazepine antagonists of the GHS-R1a blocked the intracellular calcium signaling induced by ghrelin (Mihalic *et al.*, 2012), but their effects remain to be evaluated *in vivo*.

New indolinone derivatives of ghrelin were identified as new chiral class of ghrelin antagonists (Puleo *et al.*, 2012). One of these new derivatives, compound 14f, inhibited gastric emptying and food intake, and improved glucose tolerance (Puleo *et al.*, 2012). *In vitro* cDNA display was used to screen a peptide library for successful GHS-R1A antagonist identification. Such approaches led to the identifica-tion of a new short L-amino acid peptide G5-1 that antagonizes GHS-R1A (Ueno *et al.*, 2012).

In conclusions, several classes of GHS-R1a antagonists have been identified and could represent interesting pharmacological leads for the treatment of obesity as well as type 2 diabetes and metabolic syndrome. However, long-term animal and human studies still remain necessary to appropriately evaluate the beneficial properties of ghrelin antagonists in the context of obesity.

3.2.3   GHS-R1A Inverse Agonists

GHS-R1A inverse agonists have also been developed for the treatment of type 2 diabetes, obesity (in par-ticular Prader Willi Syndrome) and metabolic syndrome.

As GHS-R1a possesses high constitutive activity, it was suggested that inverse GHS-R1a agonists, decreasing its constitutive activity, may be useful for the treatment of obesity (Holst *et al.*, 2003; Holliday *et al.*, 2007; Damian *et al.*, 2012). In the hypothalamus, long term fasting increased GHS-R1a expression and concomitant signaling causing increased appetite and decreased energy expenditure. Therefore, re-duction of the GHS-R1a constitutive activity by an inverse agonist could increase the sensitivity to ano-rexigenic hormones like leptin or PYY, and prevent food intake between meals (Holst and Schwartz, 2004).

[D-Arg[1], D-Phe[5], D-Trp7,9, Leu11]substance P was identified as an inverse agonist on GHS-R1a (Holst *et al.*, 2006). Hexapeptides KwFwLL-NH(2) with β-(3-benzothienyl)-d-alanine (d-Bth), 3,3-diphenyl-d-alanine (d-Dip) and 1-naphthyl-d-alanine (d-1-Nal) at position 2 resulted in highly potent and efficient inverse agonists (Els *et al.*, 2012). The peptide N^{α}-NODAGA-KwFwLL-CONH$_2$ behaved as a GHS-R1A inverse agonist (Chopra, 2012; NODAGA: 1,4,7-triazacyclononane,1-glutaric acid-4,7-acetic acid). Spirocyclic piperidine-azetidine compounds were identified as GHS-R1a inverse agonists (Kung *et al.*, 2012).

In conclusion, GHR-R1a inverse agonists represent interesting pharmacological tools to inhibit GHS-R1a basal activity. However, further studies are necessary to evaluate the long-term use of these compounds in animal models, and finally their usefulness in the treatment of obesity and related diseases in humans.

3.3   Inhibitors of Ghrelin *O*-acyltransferase

Ghrelin O-acyltransferase (GOAT) represents an interesting pharmacological target to modulate acyl ghrelin levels (Guallillo *et al.*, 2008).

Inhibitors of GOAT have been developed. A pentapeptide, corresponding to the first five N-terminal amino acids of ghrelin with its C-terminal end amidated, competitively inhibited GOAT activity through an end-product inhibition mechanism. The inhibition of GOAT is better achieved when pentapeptides contain an octanoyl group linked to serine-3 by an amide linkage (Yang *et al.*, 2008). GOAT was also inhibited by peptide-based bisubstrate analog, GO-CoA-Tat, in cultured cells and in mice (Barnett *et al.*, 2010). Intraperitoneal administration of GO-CoA-Tat improved glucose tolerance and reduced body weight gain in mice (Barnett *et al.*, 2010). GO-CoA-Tat also decreased circulating octanoyl ghrelin levels and body weight gain in mice fed with high fat diet (Teubner *et al.*, 2013).

In conclusion, GOAT inhibitors represent extremely promising drugs for the treatment of obesity, diabetes and metabolic syndrome. However, attention must be paid to increasing des-acylated ghrelin, as this could lead to side effects linked to the yet uncharted, but increasing recognized roles of the un-acylated form of ghrelin.

3.4   New Pharmacological Tools

Gavage of bitter taste receptor (T2R) agonists was shown to increase plasma acyl ghrelin in mice through the stimulation of α-gustducin, the α-subunit of a trimeric G-protein complex involved in taste signal transduction (Janssen *et al.*, 2011). Immunofluorescence studies revealed that the stomach endocrine cells expressing ghrelin displayed up to 90-95% colocalization with α-gustducin. Furthermore, gavage of T2R-agonists increased food intake in wild-type mice but not in α-gustducin or GHS-R1a knock out mice (Janssen *et al.*, 2011). It is presently unclear if the transduction pathways induced following T2R activation could affect ghrelin acylation by GOAT and/or ghrelin release.

T2R could therefore represent yet another new interesting pharmacological target to modulate ghrelin secretion. Indeed, the potential use of T2R antagonists for the treatment of obesity remains to be evaluated.

Acknowledgements

This work was supported by grant 3.4502.09 from the Fund for Medical Scientific Research (FRSM, Belgium).

References

Adachi, S., Takiguchi, S., Okada, K., Yamamoto, K., Yamasaki, M., Miyata, H., Nakajima, K., Fujiwara, Y., Hosoda, H., Kangawa, K., Mori, M., & Doki, Y. (2010). Effects of ghrelin administration after total gastrectomy: a prospective, randomized, placebo-controlled phase II study. Gastroenterology, 138, 1312-1320.

Ando, T., Ichimaru, Y., Konjiki, F., Shoji, M., & Komaki, G. (2007). Variations in the preproghrelin gene correlate with higher body mass index, fat mass, and body dissatisfaction in young Japanese women. Am J Clin Nutr, 86, 25-32.

Andrade, S., Pinho, F., Ribeiro, A.M., Carreira, M., Casanueva, F.F., Roy, P., & Monteiro, M.P. (2013).Immunization against active ghrelin using virus-like particles for obesity treatment. Curr Pharm Des, ahead of print.

Andrews, Z. B., Liu, Z. W., Walllingford, N., Erion, D. M., Borok, E., Friedman, J. M., Tschop, M. H., Shanabrough, M., Cline, G., Shulman, G.I., Coppola, A., Gao, X.B., Horvath, T.L., & Diano, S. (2008). UCP2 mediates ghrelin's action on NPY/AgRP neurons by lowering free radicals. Nature, 454, 846-851.

Akamizu, T., Shinomiya, T., Irako, T., Fukunaga, M., Nakai, Y., Nakai, Y., & Kangawa, K. (2005). Separate Measurement of Plasma Levels of Acylated and Desacyl Ghrelin in Healthy Subjects Using a New Direct ELISA Assay. J Clin Endocrinol Metab, 90, 6-9.

Akamizu, T., Murayama, T., Teramukai, S., Miura, K., Bando, I., Irako, T., Iwakura, H., Ariyasu, H., Hosoda, H., Tada, H., Matsuyama, A., Kojima, S., Wada, T., Wakatsuki, Y., Matsubayashi, K., Kawakita, T., Shimizu, A., Fukushima, M., Yokode, M., & Kangawa, K. (2006). Plasma ghrelin levels in healthy elderly volunteers: the levels of acylated ghrelin in elderly females correlate positively with serum IGF-I levels and bowel movement frequency and negatively with systolic blood pressure. J Endocrinol, 182, 333-344.

Ariyasu, H., Takaya, K., Tagami, T., Ogawa, Y., Hosoda, K., Akamizu, T., Suda, M., Koh, T., Natsui, K., Toyooka, S., Shirakami, G., Usui, T., Shimatsu, A., Doi, K., Hosoda, H., Kojima, M., Kangawa, K., & Nakao, K. (2001). Stomach Is a Major Source of Circulating Ghrelin, and Feeding State Determines Plasma Ghrelin-Like Immunoreactivity Levels in Humans. J Clin Endocrinol Metab, 86, 4753-4758.

Ariyasu, H., Takaya, K., Iwakura, H., Hosoda, H., Akamizu, T., Arai, Y. Kangawa, K., & Nakao K. (2005). Transgenic mice overexpressing des-acyl ghrelin show small phenotype. Endocrinology, 146, 355-64.

Asakawa, A., Inui, A., Kaga, T., Yuzuriha, H., Nagata, T., Ueno, N., Makino, S., Fujimiya, M., Niijima, A., Fujino, M. A., & Kasuga, M. (2001). Ghrelin is an appetite-stimulatory signal from stomach with structural resemblance to motilin. Gastroenterology, 120, 337-345.

Asakawa, A., Inui, A., Kaga, T., Katsuura, G., Fujimiya, M., Fujino, M. A., & Kasuga, M. (2003). Antagonism of ghrelin receptor reduces food intake and body weight gain in mice. Gut, 52, 947-952.

Ashby, D.R., Ford, H.E., Wynne, K.J., Wren, A.M., Murphy, K.G., Busbridge, M., Brown, E.A., Taube, D.H., Ghatei, M.A., Tam, F.W., Bloom, S.R., & Choi, P. (2009). Sustained appetite improvement in malnourished dialysis patients by daily ghrelin treatment. Kidney Int, 76, 199-206.

Baatar, D., Patel, K., & Taub, D.D. (2011). The effects of ghrelin on inflammation and the immune system. Mol Cell Endocrinol, 20, 340, 44-58.

Bach, M.A., Rockwood, K., Zetterberg, C., Thamsborg, G., Hébert, R., Devogelaer, J.P., Christiansen, J.S., Rizzoli, R., Ochsner, J.L., Beisaw, N. Gluck, O., Yu, L., Schwab, T., Farrington, J., Taylor, A.M., Ng, J., & Fuh, V. MK 0677 Hip Fracture Study Group. (2004). The effects of MK-0677, an oral growth hormone secretagogue, in patients with hip fracture. J Am Geriatr Soc, 52, 516-523.

Baessler, A., Hasinoff, M.J., Fischer, M., Reinhard, W., Sonnenberg, G.E., Olivier, M., Erdmann, J., Schunkertt, H., Doering, A., Jacob, H.J., Commuzzie, A.G., Kissebah, A.H. & Kwitek, A.E. (2005). Genetic linkage and association of the growth hormone secretagogue receptor (ghrelin receptor) gene in human obesity. Diabetes, 54, 259-267.

Baessler, A., Kwitek, A.E., Fischer, M., Koehler, M., Reinhard, W., Erdmann, J., Riegger, G., Doering, A., Schunkert, H., & Hengstenberg, C. (2006). Association of the ghrelin receptor gene region with left ventricular hypertrophy in the general population: results of the MONICA/KORA Augsburg echocardiographic substudy. Hypertension, 47, 920-927.

Baessler, A., Fischer, M., Mayer, B., Koehler, M., Wiedmann, S., Stark, K., Doering, A., Erdmann, J., Riegger, G., Schunkert, H., Kwitek, A.E. & Hengstenberg, C. (2007). Epistatic interaction between haplotypes of the ghrelin ligand and receptor genes influence susceptibility to myocardial infaraction and coronary artery disease. Hum Mol Genet, 16, 887-899.

Balasubramaniam, A., Joshi, R., Su, C., Friend, L.A., Sheriff, S., Kagan, R.J. & James, J.H. (2009). Ghrelin inhibits skeletal muscle protein breakdown in rats with thermal injury through normalizing elevated expression of E3 ubiquitin ligases MuRF1and MAFbx. Am J Physiol Regul Integr Comp Physiol, 296, R893-R901.

Baragli, A., Ghè, C., Arnolett.i, E., Granata, R., Ghigo, E., & Muccioli, G. (2011). Acylated and unacylated ghrelin attenuate isoproterenol-induced lipolysis in isolated rat visceral adipocytes through activation of phosphoinositide 3-kinase γ and phosphodiesterase 3B. Biochim Biophys Acta, 1811, 386-396.

Baranowska, B., Bik, W., Baranowka-Bik, A., Wolinska-Witort, E., Szybinska, A., Martynska, L., & Cmielowska. (2006). Neuroendocrine control of metabolic homeostasis in Polish centenarians. J Physiol Pharmacol, 57 suppl 6, 55-61.

Barnett, B.P., Hwang, Y., Taylor, M.S., Kirchner, H., Pfluger, P.T., Bernard, V., Lin, Y.Y., Bowers, E.M., Mukherjee, C., Song, W.J., Longo, P.A., Leahy, D.J., Hussain, M.A., Tschöp, M.H., Boeke, J.D., & Cole, P.A. (2010). Glucose and weight control in mice with a designed ghrelin O-acyltransferase inhibitor. Science, 330, 1689-1692.

Beaumont, N. J., Skinner, V. O., Tan, T. M., Ramesh, B. S., Byrne, D. J., MacColl, G. S., Keen, J. N., Bouloux, P. M., Mikhailidis, D. P., Bruckdorfer, K. R., Vanderpump, M. P., & Srai, K. S. (2003). Ghrelin can bind to a species of high density lipoprotein associated with paraoxonase. J Biol Chem, 278, 8877-8880.

Beck, B., Max, J. P., Fernette, B., & Richy, S. (2004). Adaptation of ghrelin levels to limit body weight gain in the obese Zucker rat. Biochem Biophys Res Commun, 318, 846-851.

Becskei, C., Bilik, K.U., Klussmann, S., Jarosch, F., Lutz, T.A., & Riediger, T. (2008). The anti-ghrelin Spiegelmer NOX-B11-3 blocks ghrelin- but not fasting-induced neuronal activation in the hypothalamic arcuate nucleus. J Neuroendocrinol, 20, 85-92.

Berthold, H.K., Gianakidou, E., Krone, W., Mantzoros, C.S., & Gouni-Berthold, I. (2009). The Leu72Met polymorphism of the ghrelin gene is associated with a decreased risk for type 2 diabetes. Clin Chim Acta, 399,112-116.

Berthold, H.K., Gianakidou, E., Krone, W., Trégouët, D.A., & Gouni-Berthold, I. (2012). Influence of ghrelin gene polymorphisms on hypertension and atherosclerotic disease. Hypertens Res, 33, 155-160.

Biagini, G., Torsello, A., Marinelli, C., Gualtieri, F., Vezzali, R., Coco, S., Bresciani, E., & Locatelli, V. (2011). Beneficial effects of desacyl-ghrelin, hexarelin and EP-80317 in models of status epilepticus. Eur J Pharmacol, 670, 130-136.

Bing, C., Ambye, L., Fenger, M., Jorgensen, T., Borch-Johnsen, K., Madsbad, S., & Urhammer, S. A. (2005). Large-scale studies of the Leu72Met polymorphism of the ghrelin gene in relation to the metabolic syndrome and associated quantitative traits. Diabet Med, 22, 1157-1160.

Bochicchio, G., Charlton, P., Pezzullo, J.C., Kosutic, G., & Senagore, A. (2012). Ghrelin agonist TZP-101/ulimorelin accelerates gastrointestinal recovery independently of opioid use and surgery type: covariate analysis of phase 2 data. World J Surg, 36, 39-45.

Botla, S.K., Gholami, A.M., Malekpour, M., Moskalev, E.A., Fallah, M., Jandaghi, P., Aghajani, A., Bondar I.S., Omranipour, R., Malekpour, F., Mohajeri, A., Babadi, A.J., Sahin, O., Bubnov, V.V., Najmabadi, H., Hoheisel, J.D., & Riazalhosseini, Y. (2012). Diagnostic value of GHSR DNA methylation pattern in breast cancer. Breast Cancer Res Treat, 135, 705-713.

Broglio, F., Arvat, E., Benso, A., Gottero, C., Muccioli, G., Papotti, M., van der Lely, A. J., Deghenghi, R., & Ghigo, E. (2001). Ghrelin, a natural GH secretagogue produced by the stomach, induces hyperglycemia and reduces insulin secretion in humans. J Clin Endocrinol Metab, 86, 5083-5086.

Broglio, F., Benso, A., Castiglioni, C., Gottero, C., Prodam, F., Destefanis, S. Gauna, C., van der Lely, A.J., Deghenghi, R., Bo, M., Arvat, E., & Ghigo, E. (2003). The endocrine response to ghrelin as a function of gender in humans in young and elderly subjects. J Clin Endocrinol Metab. 88, 1537-1542.

Broglio, F., Gianotti, L., Destefanis, S., Fassino, S., Abbate Daga, G., Mondelli, V., Lanfranco, F., Gottero, C., Gauna, C., Hofland, L., Van der Lely, A.J., & Ghigo, E. (2004). The endocrine response to acute ghrelin administration is blunted in patients with anorexia nervosa, a ghrelin hypersecretory state. Clin Endocrinol, 60, 592-599.

Broglio, F., Prodam, F., Me, E., Riganti, F., Lucatello, B., Granata, R., Benso, A., Muccioli, G., & Ghigo, E. (2005). Ghrelin: endocrine, metabolic and cardiovascular actions. J Endocrinol Invest, 28, 23-25.

Bulgarelli, I., Tamiazzo, L., Bresciani, E., Rapetti, D., Caporali, S., Lattuada, D., Locatelli, V., & Torsello, A. (2009). Desacyl-ghrelin and synthetic GH-secretagogues modulate the production of inflammatory cytokins in mouse microglia cellls stimulated by β-amyloid fibrils. J Neurosci Res, 87, 27187-2727.

Campa, D., Pardini, B., Naccarati, A., Vodickova, L., Novotny, J., Steinke, V., Rahner, N., Holinsky-Feder, E., Morak, M., Schackert, H.K., Görgens, H., Kötting, Betz, B., Kloor, M., Engel, C., Büttner, R., Propping, P., Försti, A., Hemminki, K., Barale, R., Vodicka, P., & Canzian, F. (2010). Polymorphims of genes coding for ghrelin and its receptor in relation to colorectal cancer risk: a two-step gene-wide case-control study. BMC Gastroenterol, 10, 112.

Casillas-Espinosa, P.M., Powell, K.L., & O'Brien, T.J. (2012). Regulators of synaptic transmission: roles in the pathogenesis and treatment of epilepsy. Epilepsia, 53 Suppl 9, 41-58.

Cellini, E., Nacmias, B., Brecelj-Anderluh, M., Badia-Casanovas, A., Bellodi, L., Boni, C., Di Bella, D., Estivill, X., Fernandez-Aranda, F., Foulon, C., Friedel, S., Gabrovsek, M., Gorwood, P., Gratacos, M., Guelfi, J., Hebebrand, J., Hinney, A., Holliday, J., Hu, X., Karwautz, A., Kipman, A., Komel, R., Rotella, C. M., Ribases, M., Ricca, V., Romo, L., Tomori, M., Treasure, J., Wagner, G., Collier, D. A., & Sorbi, S. (2006). Case-control and combined family trios analysis of three polymorphisms in the ghrelin gene in European patients with anorexia and bulimia nervosa. Psychiatr Genet, 16, 51-52.

Cheyuo, C., Jacob, A., & Wang, P.. (2012). Ghrelin-mediated sympathoinhibition and suppression of inflammation in sepsis. Am J Physiol, 302, E265-E272.

Chan, C.B. & Cheng, C.H.K. (2004). Identification and functional characterization of two alternatively spliced growth hormone secretagogue receptor transcripts from the pituitary of black seabream Acanthopagrus schlegeli. Mol Cell Endocrinol, 214, 81-95.

Chan, J.L., Mun, E.C., Stoyneva, V., Mantzoros, C.S., & Goldfine, A.B. (2006). Peptide YY levels are elevated after gastric bypass surgery. Obesity, 14, 194-198.

Chanclon, B., Martinez-Fuentes, A.J., & Gracia-Navarro, F. (2012). Role of SCT, CORT and ghrelin and its receptors at the endocrine pancreas. Front Endocrinol, 3, 114.

Chang, L., Zhao, J., Yang, J., Zhang, Z., Du, J., & Tang, C. (2003). Therapeutic effects of ghrelin on endotoxic shock in rats. Eur J Pharmacol, 473, 171-176.

Charoenthongtrakul, S., Giuliana, D., Longo, K.A., Govek, E.K., Nolan, A., Gagne, S., Morgan, K., Hixon, J., Flynn, N., Murphy, B.J., Hernández, A.S., Li, J., Tino, J.A., Gordon, D.A., DiStefano, P.S., & Geddes, B.J. (2009). Enhanced gastrointestinal motility with orally active ghrelin receptor agonists. J Pharmacol Exp Ther, 329, 1178-1786.

Chen, J., Liu, X., Shu, Q., Li, S., & Luo, F. (2008). Ghrelin attenuates lipopolysaccharide-induced acute lung injury through no pathway. Med Sci Monit, 14, BR141-BR146.

Choi, H.J., Ki, K.H., Jang, J.Y., Jang, B.Y., Song, J.A., Baek, W.Y., Kim, J.H., An, J.H., Kim, S.W., Kim, S.Y., Kim, J.E., & Shin, C.S. (2013). Chronic central administration of increases bone mass through a mechanism independent of appetite regulation. PLoS One, 8, e65505.

Chopin, L.K., Seim, I., Walpole, C.M. & Herington, A.C. (2012). The ghrelin axis-Does it have an appetite for cancer progression? Endocrine Rev, 33, 849-891.

Chopra A. (2012). ^{68}Ga-Labeled NODAGA-conjugated ghrelin receptor agonists and inverse agonists. Molecular Imaging and Contrast Agent Database (MICAD) [Internet]. Bethesda (MD): National Center for Biotechnology Information (US).

Chorny, A., Anderson, P., Gonzalez-Rey, E., & Delgado M. (2008). Ghrelin protects against experimental sepsis by inhibiting high-mobility group box 1 release and by killing bacteria. J Immunol, 180, 8369-8377.

Chow, K.B., Sun, J., Chu, K.M., Tai Cheung, W., Cheng, C.H., &Wise, H. (2012). The truncated ghrelin receptor polypeptide (GHS-R1b) is localized in the endoplasmic reticulum where it forms heterodimers with ghrelin receptors (GHS-R1a) to attenuate their cell surface expression. Mol Cell Endocrinol, 348, 247-254.

Chronaiou, A., Tsoli, M., Kehagias, I., Leotsinidis, M., Kalfarentzos, F., & Alexandrides, T.K. (2012). Lower ghrelin levels and exaggerated postprandial peptide-YY, glucagon-like peptide-1, and insulin responses, after gastric fundus resection, in patients undergoing Roux-en-Y gastric bypass: a randomized clinical trial. Obes Surg, 22, 1761-1770.

Coiro, V., Saccani-Jotti, G., Rubino, P., Manfredi, G., Melani, A., & Chiodera, P. (2006). Effects of ghrelin on circulating neuropeptide Y levels in humans. Neuro Endocrinol Lett, 27, 755-757.

Costantini, V.J., Vicentini, E., Sabbatini, F.M, Valerio, E., Lepore, S., Tessari, M., Sartori, M., Michielin, F., Melotto, S., Bifone, A., Pich, EM., & Corsi, M. (2011). GSK1614343, a novel ghrelin receptor antagonist, produces an unexpected increase of food intake and body weight in rodents and dogs. Neuroendocrinology, 94, 158-168.

Couce, M.E., Cottam, D., Esplen, J., Schauer, P., & Burguera, B. (2006). Is ghrelin the culprit for weight loss after gastric bypass surgery? A negative answer. Obes. Surg. 16, 870-878.

Cummings, D.E., Purnell, J.Q., Frayo, R.S., Schmidova, K., Wisse, B.E., & Weigle, D.S. (2001). A preprandial rise in plasma ghrelin levels suggests a role in meal initiation in humans. Diabetes, 50, 1714-1719.

Cummings, D.E., Clement, K., Purnell, J.Q., Vaisse, C., Foster, K.E., Frayo, R.S., Schwartz, M.W., Basdevant, A., & Weigle, D.S. (2002a). Elevated plasma ghrelin levels in Prader Willi syndrome. Nat. Med. 8, 643-644.

Cummings, D.E., Weigle, D.S., Frayo, R.S., Breen, P.A., Ma, M.K., Dellinger, E.P., & Purnell, J.Q. (2002b). Plasma ghrelin levels after diet-induced weight loss or gastric bypass surgery. N. Engl. J. Med. 346, 1623-1630.

Cummings, D.E. (2006). Ghrelin and the short- and long-term regulation of appetite and body weight. Physiol Behav, 89, 71-84.

Damian, M., Marie, J., Leyris, J.P., Fehrentz, J.A., Verdié, P., Martinez, J., Banères, J.L., & Mary, S. (2012). High constitutive activity is an intrinsic feature of ghrelin receptor protein: a study with a functional monomeric GHS-R1a receptor reconstituted in lipid discs. J Biol Chem, 287, 3630-3641.

Dardennes, R. M., Zizzari, P., Tolle, V., Foulon, C., Kipman, A., Romo, L., Iancu-Gontard, D., Boni, C., Sinet, P. M., Therese, B. M., Estour, B., Mouren, M. C., Guelfi, J. D., Rouillon, F., Gorwood, P., & Epelbaum, J. (2007). Family trios analysis of common polymorphisms in the obestatin/ghrelin, BDNF and AGRP genes in patients with Anorexia nervosa: association with subtype, body-mass index, severity and age of onset. Psychoneuroendocrinology, 32, 106-113.

Das, U.N. (2011). Relationship between gut and sepsis. World J Diabetes, 15, 1-7.

Dass, N.B., Munonyara, M., Bassil, A.K., Hervieu, G.J., Osbourne, S., Corcoran, S., Morgan, M., & Sanger, G.J. (2003). Growth hormone secretagogue receptors in rat and human gastrointestinal tract and the effects of ghrelin. Neuroscience, 120, 443-453.

Date, Y., Kojima, M., Hosoda, H., Sawaguchi, A., Mondal, M. S., Suganuma, T., Matsukura, S., Kangawa, K., & Nakazato, M. (2000a). Ghrelin, a Novel Growth Hormone-Releasing Acylated Peptide, Is Synthesized in a Distinct Endocrine Cell Type in the Gastrointestinal Tracts of Rats and Humans. Endocrinology, 141, 4255-4261.

Date, Y., Murakami, N., Kojima, M., Kuroiwa, T., Matsukura, S., Kangawa, K., & Nakazato, M. (2000b). Central effects of a novel acylated peptide, ghrelin, on growth hormone release in rats. Biochem Biophys Res Commun, 275, 477-480.

Date, Y., Nakazato, M., Murakami, N., Kojima, M., Kangawa, K., & Matsukura S. (2001). Ghrelin acts in the central nervous system to stimulate gastric acid secretion. Biochem Biophys Res Commun, 280, 904-907.

Date, Y., Nakazato, M., Hashiguchi, S., Dezaki, K., Mondal, M. S., Hosoda, H., Kojima, M., Kangawa, K., Arima, T., Matsuo, H., Yada, T., & Matsukura, S. (2002). Ghrelin is present in pancreatic alpha-cells of humans and rats and stimulates insulin secretion. Diabetes, 51, 124-129.

Davis, J.F., Perello, M., Choi, D.L., Magrisso, I.J., Kirchner, H., Pfluger, P.T., Tschoep, M., Zigman, J.M., & Benoit, S.C. (2012). GOAT induced ghrelin acylation regulates hedonic feeding. Horm Behav, 62, 598-604.

Deboer, M.D., Zhu, X.X., Levasseur, P., Meguid, M.M., Suzuki, S., Inui, A., Taylor, J.E., Halem, H.A., Dong, J.Z., Datta, R., Culler, M.D., & Marks, D.L. (2007). *Ghrelin treatment causes increased food intake and retention of lean body mass in a rat model of cancer cachexia. Endocrinology, 148, 3004-3012.*

Deboer, M.D., Zhu, X., Levasseur, P.R., Inui, A., Hu, Z. Han, G. Mitch, W.E., Taylor, J.E., Halem, H.A., Dong, J.Z., Datta, R., Culler, M.D., & Marks, D.L. (2008). *Ghrelin treatment of chronic kidney disease: improvements in lean body mass and cytokine profile. Endocrinology, 149, 827-835.*

Deboer, M.D. (2011). *Use of ghrelin as a treatment for inflammatory bowel disease: mechanistic considerations. Int J Pept, 2011, 189242.*

Delhanty, P.J. & van der Lely, A.J. (2011). *Ghrelin and glucose homeostasis. Peptides, 32, 2309-2318.*

Delhanty, P.J., van der Eerden, B.C., & van Leeuwen, J.P. (2013). *Biofactors, doi:10.1002/biof.1120.*

DelParigi, A., Tschop, M., Heiman, M. L., Salbe, A. D., Vozarova, B., Sell, S. M., Bunt, J. C., & Tataranni, P. A. (2002). *High circulating ghrelin: a potential cause for hyperphagia and obesity in prader-willi syndrome. J. Clin. Endocrinol. Metab. 87, 5461-5464.*

Demange, L., Boeglin, D. Moulin, A., Mousseaux, D., Ryan, J., Bergé, G., Gagne, D., Heitz, A., Perrissoud, D., Locatelli, V., Torsello, A., Galleyrand, J.C., Fehrentz, J.A., & Martinez, J. (2007). *Synthesis and pharmacological in vitro and in vivo evaluations of novel triazole derivatives as ligands of the ghrelin receptor. J Med Chem, 50, 1939-1957.*

Dembinski, A., Warzecha, Z., Ceranowicz, P., Tomaszewska, R., Stachura, J., Konturek, S.J., & Konturek, P.C. (2003). *Ghrelin attenuates the development of acute pancreatitis in rat. J Physiol Pharmacol, 54, 561-573.*

Deng, F., Ling, L., Ma, J., Liu, C., & Zhang, W. (2008). *Stimulation of intramembranous bone repair in rats by ghrelin. Exp Physiol, 93, 872-879.*

Depoortere, I., De Winter, B., Thijs, T., De Man, J., Pelckmans, P., & Peeters, T. (2005). *Comparison of the gastroprokinetic effects of ghrelin, GHRP-6 and motilin in rats in vivo and in vitro. Eur J Pharmacol, 515, 160-168.*

Depoortere, I., Thijs, T., Moechars, D., De, S. B., Ver, D. L., & Peeters, T. L. (2008). *Effect of peripheral obestatin on food intake and gastric emptying in ghrelin-knockout mice. Br J Pharmacol, 153, 1550-1557.*

Depoortere, I. (2009) *Targeting the ghrelin receptor to regulate food intake. Regul Pept, 156, 13-23.*

De Vriese, C., Gregoire, F., Lema-Kisoka, R., Waelbroeck, M., Robberecht, P., & Delporte, C. (2004). *Ghrelin degradation by serum and tissue homogenates: identification of the cleavage sites. Endocrinology, 145, 4997-5005.*

De Vriese, C., Gregoire, F., De Neef, P., Robberecht, P., & Delporte, C. (2005). *Ghrelin is produced by the human erythroleukemic HEL cell line and involved in an autocrine pathway leading to cell proliferation. Endocrinology, 146, 1514-1522.*

De Vriese, C., Hacquebard, M., Gregoire, F., Carpentier, Y., & Delporte, C. (2007a). *Ghrelin interacts with human plasma lipoproteins. Endocrinology, 148, 2355-2362.*

De Vriese, C. & Delporte, C. (2007b). *Autocrine proliferative effect of ghrelin on leukemic HL-60 and THP-1 cells. J Endocrinol, 192, 199-205.*

De Vriese, C., Perret, J., & Delporte, C. (2009). *Ghrelin: a peptide involved in the control of appetite. In Appetite and Nutritional Assesmet, Ed. S.J. Ellsworth & R.C. Schuster, Nova Science Publishers, 1-48.*

Dezaki, K., & Yada, T. (2012). *Islet β-cell ghrelin signaling for inhibition of insulin secretion. Methods Enzymol, 514, 317-331.*

Dixit, V.D., Schaffer, E.M., Pyle, R.S., Collins, G.D., Sakthivel, S. K., Palaniappan, R., Lillard, J.W., Jr., & Taub, D.D. (2004). *Ghrelin inhibits leptin- and activation-induced proinflammatory cytokine expression by human monocytes and T cells. J Clin Invest, 114, 57-66.*

Dixit, V.D., Yang, H., Cooper-Jenkins, A., Giri, B.B., Patel, K., & Taub, D.D. (2009). *Reduction of T cell-derived ghrelin enhances proinflammatory cytokine expression: implications for age-associated increases in inflammation. Blood, 113, 5202-5205.*

Doi, A., Shono, T., Nishi, M., Furuta, H., Sasaki, H., & Nanjo, K. (2006). A-2beta, but not IA-2, is induced by ghrelin and inhibits glucose-stimulated insulin secretion. Proc Natl Acad Sci USA, 103, 885-890.

Doki, Y., Takachi, K., Ishikawa, O., Miyashiro, I., Sasaki, Y., Ohigashi, H., Nakajima, H., Hosoda, H., Kangawa, K., Sasakuma, F., Motoori, M., & Imaoka, S. (2006). Ghrelin reduction after esophageal substitution and its correlation to postoperative body weight loss in esophageal cancer patients. Surgery, 139, 797-805.

Ejskjaer, N., Wo, J.M., Esfandyari, T., Mazen Jamal, M. Dimcevski, G., Tarnow, L., Malik, R.A., Hellström, P.M., Mondou, E., Quinn, J., Rousseau, F., & McCallum, R.W. (2013). A phase 2a, randomized, double-blind 28-day study of TZP-102 a ghrelin receptor agonist for diabetic gastroparesis. Neurogastroenterol Motil, 25, e140-e150.

Els, S., Schild, E., Petersen, P.S., Kilian, T.M., Mokrosinski, J., Frimurer, T.M., Chollet, C., Schwartz, T.W., Holst, B., & Beck-Sickinger, A.G. (2012). An aromatic region to induce a switch between agonism and inverse agonism at the ghrelin receptor. J Med Chem, 55, 7437-7449.

Erdie-Lalena, C.R., Holm, V.A., Kelly, P.C., Frayo, R.S., & Cummings, D.E. (2006). Ghrelin levels in young children with Prader-Willi syndrome. J. Pediatr. 149, 199-204.

Esler, W.P., Rudolph, J., Claus, T.H., Tang, W., Barucci, N., Brown, S.E., Bullock, W., Daly, M., Decarr, L., Li, Y., Milardo, L., Molstad, D., Zhu, J., Gardell, S.J., Livingston, J.N., & Sweet, L.J. (2007). Small-molecule ghrelin receptor antagonists improve glucose tolerance, suppress appetite, and promote weight loss. Endocrinology, 148, 5175-5185.

Feigerlova, E., Diene, G., Conte-Auriol, F., Molinas, C., Gennero, I., Salles, J.P., Arnaud, C., & Tauber, M. (2008). Hyperghrelinemia precedes obesity in Prader-Willi syndrome. J Clin Endocrinol Metab 93, 2800-2805.

Ferrucci, L., Russo, C.R., Lauretani, F., Bandinelli, S., & Guralnik, M. (2002). A role for sarcopenia in late-life osteoporosis. Ageing Clin Exp Res 14, 1-4.

Fraser, G.L., Hoveyda, H.R., & Tannenbaum, G.S. (2008). Pharmacological demarcation of the growth hormone, gut motility and feeding effects of ghrelin using a novel ghrelin receptor agonist. Endocrinology; 149, 6280-6288.

Fruhbeck, G., Diez, C.A., & Gil, M.J. (2004). Fundus functionality and ghrelin concentrations after bariatric surgery. N. Engl. J. Med. 350, 308-309.

Fujino, K., Inui, A., Asakawa, A., Kihara, N., Fujimura, M., & Fujimiya, M. (2003). Ghrelin induces fasted motor activity of the gastrointestinal tract in conscious fed rats. J Physiol, 550, 227-240.

Fukumoto, K., Nakahara, K., Katayama, T., Miyazato, M., Kangawa, K., & Murakami, N. (2008). Synergistic action of gastrin and ghrelin on gastric acid secretion in rats. Biochem Biophys Res Commun, 374, 60-63.

Fukushima, N., Hanada, R., Teranishi, H., Fukue, Y., Tachibana, T., Ishikawa, H., Takeda, S., Takeuchi, Y., Fukumoto, S., Kangawa, K., Nagata, K., & Kojima, M. (2005). Ghrelin directly regulates bone formation. J Bone Miner Res, 20, 790-798.

Garcia, M.C., Lopez, M., Alvarez, C.V., Casanueva, F., Tena-Sempere, M., & Dieguez, C. (2007). Role of ghrelin in reproduction. Reproduction, 133, 531-540.

Gasco, V., Beccuti, G., Baldini, C., Prencipe, N., Di Giacomo, S., Berton, A., Guaraldi, F., Tabaro, I., Maccario, M., Ghigo, E. & Grottoli, S. (2012). Acylated ghrelin as a provocative test for the diagnosis of GH deficiency in adults. Eur J Endocrinol, 168, 23-30.

Gauna, C., Delhanty, P.J., Hofland, L.J., Janssen, J.A., Broglio, F., Ross, R.J., Ghigo, E., & van der Lely, A.J. (2005). Ghrelin stimulates, whereas des-octanoyl ghrelin inhibits, glucose output by primary hepatocytes. J Clin Endocrinol Metab, 90, 1055-1060.

Germain, N., Galusca, B., Grouselle, D., Frere, D., Tolle, V., Zizzari, P., Lang, F., Epelbaum, J., & Estour, B. (2009). Ghrelin/obestatin ratio in two populations with low bodyweight: constitutional thinness and anorexia nervosa. Psychoneuroendocrinology, 34, 413-419.

Ghelardoni, S., Carnicelli, V., Frascarelli, S., Ronca-Testoni, S., & Zucchi, R. (2006). Ghrelin tissue distribution: comparison between gene and protein expression. J Endocrinol Invest, 29, 115-121.

Ghigo, E., Broglio, F., Arvat, E., Maccario, M., Papotti, M., & Muccioli, G (2005). *Ghrelin: more than a natural GH secretagogue and/or orexigenic factor. Clin Endocrinol, 62, 1-17.*

Gimenez-Palop, O., Gimenez-Perez, G., Mauricio, D., Gonzalez-Clemente, J. M., Potau, N., Berlanga, E., Trallero, R., Laferrere, B., & Caixas, A. (2007). *A lesser postprandial suppression of plasma ghrelin in Prader-Willi syndrome is associated with low fasting and a blunted postprandial PYY response. Clin Endocrinol, 66, 198-204.*

Gjesing, A.P., Larsen, L.H., Torekov, S.S., Hainerova, I.A., Kapur, R., Johansen, A., Albrechtsen, A., Boj? S., Holst, B., Harper, A., Urhammer, S.A., Borch-Johnsen, K., Pisinger, C., Echwald., S.M., Eiberg, H., Astrup, A., Lebl, J., Ferrer, J., Schwartz, T.W., Hansen, T., & Pedersen, O. (2010). *Family and population-based studies of variation within the ghrelin receptor locus in relation to measures of obesity. PLoS One,5, e10084.*

Gnanapavan, S., Kola, B., Bustin, S. A., Morris, D. G., McGee, P., Fairclough, P., Bhattacharya, S., Carpenter, R., Grossman, A. B., & Korbonits, M. (2002). *The Tissue Distribution of the mRNA of Ghrelin and Subtypes of Its Receptor, GHS-R, in Humans. J Clin Endocrinol Metab, 87, 2988.*

Goebel-Stengel, M., Hofmann, T., Elbelt, U., Teuffel, P., Ahnis, A., Kobelt, P., Lambrecht, N.W., Klapp, B.F., & Stengel, A. (2013). *The ghrelin activating enzyme ghrelin-O-acyltransferase (GOAT) is present in human plasma and expressed dependent on body mass index. Peptides, 43, 13-19.*

Goldstone, A.P., Holland, A.J., Butler, J.V., & Whittington, J.E. (2012). *Appetite hormones and the transition to hyperphagia in children with Prader-Willi syndrome. Int J Obes, 36, 1564-1570.*

Gonzalez, C., Vazquez, M., Lopez, M., & Dieguez, C. (2008). *Influence of chronic undernutrition and leptin on GOAT mRNA levels in rat stomach mucosa. J Mol Endocrinol, 41, 415-421.*

Granado, M., Priego, T., Martín, A.I., Villanúa, M.A., & López-Calderón, A. (2005). *Anti-inflammatory effect of the ghrelin agonist growth hormone-releasing peptide-2 (GHRP-2) in arthritic rats. Am J Physiol, 288, E486-E492.*

Gualillo, O., Lago, F., & Dieguez, C. (2008). *Introducing GOAT: a target for obesity and anti-diabetic drugs? Trends Pharmacol Sci, 29, 398-401.*

Gueorguiev, M. Lecoeur, C., Meyre, D., Benzinou, M., Mein, C.A, Hinney, A., Vatin, V., Weill, J., Heude, B., Hebebrand, J., Grossman, A.B., Kornonits, M., & Froguel., P. (2009). *Association studies on ghrelin and ghrelin receptor gene polymorphisms with obesity. Obesity, 17, 745-754.*

Gueorguiev, M. & Kornonits, M. (2013). *Genetics of ghrelin system. Endocr Rev, 25, 25-40.*

Gutierrez, J.A., Solenberg, P.J., Perkins, D. R., Willency, J.A., Knierman, M.D, Jin, Z., Witcher, D.R., Luo, S., Onyia, J. E., & Hale, J. E. (2008). *Ghrelin octanoylation mediated by an orphan lipid transferase. Proc Natl Acad Sci USA, 105, 6320-6325.*

Haider, D. G., Schindler, K., Prager, G., Bohdjalian, A., Luger, A., Wolzt, M., & Ludvik, B. (2007). *Serum retinol-binding protein 4 is reduced after weight loss in morbidly obese subjects. J Clin Endocrinol Metab 92, 1168-1171.*

Halem, H.A., Taylor, J.E., Dong, J.Z., Shen, Y., Datta, R., Abizaid, A., Diano, S., Horvath, T., Zizzari, P., Bluet-Pajot, M.T., Epelbaum, J., & Culler, M.D. (2004). *Novel analogs of ghrelin: physiological and clinical implications. Eur J Endocrinol, 151 Suppl 1, S71-S75.*

Hanada, T., Toshinai, K., Kajimura, N., Nara-Ashizawa, N., Tsukada, T., Hayashi, Y., Osuye, K., Kangawa, K., Matsukura, S., Nakazato, M. (2003). *Anti-cachectic effect of ghrelin in nude mice bearing human melanoma cells. Biochem Biophys Res Commun, 301, 275-279.*

Haqq, A.M., Grambow, S.C., Muehlbauer, M., Newgard, C.B., Svetkey, L.P., Carrel, A.L., Yanovski, J.A., Purnell, J.Q., & Freemark, M. (2008). *Ghrelin concentrations in Prader-Willi syndrome (PWS) infants and children: changes during development. Clin Endocrinol, 69, 911-920.*

Hassouna, R., Labarthe, A., Zizzari, P., Videau, C., Culler, M., Epelbaum, J., & Tolle, V. (2013). *Actions of Agonists and Antagonists of the ghrelin/GHS-R Pathway on GH Secretion, Appetite, and cFos Activity. Front Endocrinol, 4, 25.*

Hataya, Y., Akamizu, T., Takaya, K., Kanamoto, N., Ariyasu, H., Saijo, M., Moriyama, K., Shimatsu, A., Kojima, M., Kangawa, K., & Nakao, K. (2001). A low dose of ghrelin stimulates growth hormone (GH) release synergistically with GH-releasing hormone in humans. J Clin Endocrinol Metab, 86, 4552.

Heijboer, A.C., van den Hoek, A.M., Parlevliet, E.T., Havekes, L.M., Romijn, J.A., Pijl, H., & Corssmit, E.P. (2006). Ghrelin differentially affects hepatic and peripheral insulin sensitivity in mice. Diabetologia, 49, 732-738.

Helmling, S., Maasch, C., Eulberg, D., Buchner, K., Schroder, W., Lange, C., Vonhoff, S., Wlotzka, B., Tschop, M. H., Rosewicz, S., & Klussmann, S. (2004). Inhibition of ghrelin action in vitro and in vivo by an RNA-Spiegelmer. Proc Natl Acad Sci USA, 101, 13174-13179.

Hess, O., Admoni, O., Khayat, M. Elias, G., Almagor, T., Shalev, S.A., & Tenenbaum-Rakover, Y. (2012). Ghrelin and growth hormone secretagogue receptor (GHSR) genes are not commonly involved in growth or weight abnormalities in an Israeli pediatric population. J Pediatr Endocrinol Metab, 25, 537-540.

Hinney, A., Hoch, A., Geller, F., Schafer, H., Siegfried, W., Goldschmidt, H., Remschmidt, H., & Hebebrand, J. (2002). Ghrelin gene: identification of missense variants and a frameshift mutation in extremely obese children and adolescents and healthy normal weight students. J Clin Endocrinol Metab, 87, 2716-2719.

Holliday, N.D., Holst, B., Rodionova, E.A., Schwartz, T.W., & Cox, H.M. (2007). Importance of constitutive activity and arrestin-independent mechanisms for intracellular trafficking of the ghrelin receptor. Mol Endocrinol, 21, 3100-3112.

Holmes, E., Davies, I., Lowe, G., & Ranganath, L. R. (2009). Circulating ghrelin exists in both lipoprotein bound and free forms. Ann Clin Biochem, 46, 514-516.

Holst, B., Cygankiewicz, A., Jensen, T. H., Ankersen, M., & Schwartz, T. W. (2003) High Constitutive Signaling of the Ghrelin Receptor--Identification of a Potent Inverse Agonist. Mol Endocrinol, 17, 2201-2210.

Holst, B., & Schwartz, T. W. (2004). Constitutive ghrelin receptor activity as a signaling set-point in appetite regulation. Trends Pharmacol Sci, 25, 113-117.

Holst, B., Lang, M., Brandt, E., Bach, A., Howard, A., Frimurer, T. M., Beck-Sickinger, A., & Schwartz, T. W. (2006). Ghrelin Receptor Inverse Agonists: Identification of an Active Peptide Core and Its Interaction Epitopes on the Receptor. Mol Pharmacol, 70, 936-946.

Hosoda, H., Kojima, M., Matsuo, H., & Kangawa, K. (2000). Ghrelin and des-acyl ghrelin: two major forms of rat ghrelin peptide in gastrointestinal tissue. Biochem Biophys Res Commun, 279, 909-913.

Hosoda, H., Kojima, M., Mizushima, T., Shimizu, S., & Kangawa, K. (2003). Structural divergence of human ghrelin. Identification of multiple ghrelin-derived molecules produced by post-translational processing. J Biol Chem, 278, 64-70.

Hosoda, H., Doi, K., Nagaya, N., Okumura, H., Nakagawa, E., Enomoto, M., Ono, F., & Kangawa, K. (2004). Optimum collection and storage conditions for ghrelin measurements: octanoyl modification of ghrelin is rapidly hydrolyzed to desacyl ghrelin in blood samples. Clin Chem, 50, 1077-1080.

Hosojima, H., Togo, T., Odawara, T., Hasegawa, K., Miura, S., Kato, Y., Kanai, A., Kase, A., Uchikado, H., & Hirayasu, Y. (2006). Early effects of olanzapine on serum levels of ghrelin, adiponectin and leptin in patients with schizophrenia. J. Psychopharmacol. 20, 75-79.

Hotta, M., Ohwada, R., Katakami, H., Shibasaki, T., Hizuka, N., & Takano, K. (2004). Plasma levels of intact and degraded ghrelin and their responses to glucose infusion in anorexia nervosa. J Clin Endocrinol Metab, 89, 5707-5712.

Hotta, M., Ohwada, R., Akamizu, T., Shibasaki, T., Takano, K., Kangawa, K. (2009). Ghrelin increases hunger and food intake in patients with restricting-type anorexia nervosa: a pilot study. Endocr J, 56, 1119-1128.

Hoveyda, H.R., Marsault, E., Gagnon, R., Mathieu, A.P., Vézina, M., Landry, A., Wang, Z., Benakli, K., Beaubien, S., Saint-Louis, C., Brassard, M., Pinault, J.F., Ouellet, L., Bhat, S., Ramaseshan, M., Peng, X., Foucher, L., Beauchemin, S., Bhérer, P., Veber, D.F., Peterson, M.L., & Fraser, G.L. (2011). Optimization of the potency and pharmacokinetic properties of a macrocyclic ghrelin receptor agonist (Part I): Development of ulimorelin (TZP-101) from hit to clinic. J Med Chem, 54, 8305-8320.

Howard, A.D., Feighner, S.D., Cully, D.F., Arena, J.P., Liberator, P.A., Rosenblum, C.I., Hamelin, M., Hreniuk, D.L., Palyha, O.C., Anderson, J., Paress, P. S., Diaz, C., Chou, M., Liu, K.K., McKee, K.K., Pong, S.S., Chaung, L Y., El-brecht, A., Dashkevicz, M., Heavens, R., Rigby, M., Sirinathsinghji, D.J.S., Dean, D. ., Melillo, D. G., Patchett, A.A., Nargund, R., Griffin, P.R., DeMartino, J.A., Gupta, S.K., Schaeffer, J.M., Smith, R.G., & Van der Ploeg, L.H.T. (1996). A Receptor in Pituitary and Hypothalamus That Functions in Growth Hormone Release. Science, 273, 974-977.

Iñiguez, G., Román, R., Youlton, R., Cassorla, F., & Mericq, V. (2011). Ghrelin plasma levels in patients with idiopathic short stature. Horm Res Paediatr, 75, 94-100.

Inoue, H., Sakamoto, Y., Kangawa, N., Kimura, C., Ogata, T., Fujieda, K., Qian, Z.R., Sano, T., & Itakura, M. (2011). Analysis of expression and structure of the rat GH-secretagogue/ghrelin receptor 5ghsr) gene: roles of epigenetic modifications in transcriptional regulation. Mol Cell Endocrinol, 345, 1-15.

Inui, A. (2001). Ghrelin: an orexigenic and somatotrophic signal from the stomach. Nat Rev Neurosci, 2, 551-560.

Isgaard, J. & Johansson, I. (2005). Ghrelin and GHS on cardiovascular applications/functions. J Endocrinol Invest, 28, 838-842.

Iwakura, H., Ariyasu, H., Li, Y, Kanamoto, N., Bando, M., Yamada, G., Hosoda, H., Hosoda, K., Shimatsu, A., Nakao, K., Kangawa, K., & Akamizu, T., (2009). A mouse model of ghrelinoma exhibited activated growth hormone-insulin-like growth factor I axis and glucose intolerance. Am J Physiol Endocrinol Metab, 297, E802-E811.

Jacob, A., Rajan, D., Pathickal, B., Balouch, I., Hartman, A., Wu, R., Zhou, M., & Wang, P. (2010).The inhibitory effect of ghrelin on sepsis-induced inflammation is mediated by the MAPK phosphatase-1. Int J Mol Med, 25, 159-164.

Janas-Kozik, M., Krupka-Matuszczyk, I., Malinowska-Kolodziej, I., & Lewin-Kowalik, J. (2007). Total ghrelin plasma level in patients with the restrictive type of anorexia nervosa. Regul Pept, 140, 43-46.

Janssen, S., Laermans, J., Verhulst, P. J., Thijs, T., Tack, J., & Depoortere, I. (2011). Bitter taste receptors and alpha-gustducin regulate the secretion of ghrelin with functional effects on food intake and gastric emptying. Proc Natl Acad Sci USA, 108, 2094-2099.

Jo, D. S., Kim, S. L., Kim, S. Y., Hwang, P. H., Lee, K. H., & Lee, D. Y. (2005). Preproghrelin Leu72Met polymorphism in obese Korean children. J Pediatr Endocrinol Metab, 18, 1083-1086.

Kageyama, H., Funahashi, H., Hirayama, M., Takenoya, F., Kita, T., Kato, S., Sakurai, J., Lee, E. Y., Inoue, S., Date, Y., Nakazato, M., Kangawa, K., & Shioda, S. (2005). Morphological analysis of ghrelin and its receptor distribution in the rat pancreas. Regul Pept, 126, 67-71.

Kamegai, J., Tamura, H., Shimizu, T., Ishii, S., Sugihara, H., & Wakabayashi, I. (2001). Chronic central infusion of ghrelin increases hypothalamic neuropeptide Y and Agouti-related protein mRNA levels and body weight in rats. Diabetes, 50, 2438-2443.

Kindler, J., Bailer, U., de Zwaan, M., Fuchs, K;, Leisch, F., Grün, B., Strnad, A., Stojanovic, M., Windisch, J., Lennkh-Wolfsberg, C., El-Giamal., N., Sieghart, W., Kasper, S., & Aschauer, H. (2011). No association of the neuropeptide Y (Leu7Pro) and ghrelin gene (Arg51Gln, Leu72Met, Gln90Leu) single nucleotide polymorphisms with eating disorders. Nord J Psychiatry, 65, 203-207

Kirchner, H., Gutierrez, J. A., Solenberg, P. J., Pfluger, P. T., Czyzyk, T. A., Willency, J. A., Schurmann, A., Joost, H. G., Jandacek, R. J., Hale, J. E., Heiman, M. L., & Tschop, M. H. (2009). GOAT links dietary lipids with the endocrine control of energy balance. Nature Medicine, 15, 741-745.

Kissebah, A. H., Sonnenberg, G. E., Myklebust, J., Goldstein, M., Broman, K., James, R. G., Marks, J. A., Krakower, G. R., Jacob, H. J., Weber, J., Martin, L., Blangero, J., & Comuzzie, A. G. (2000). Quantitative trait loci on chromosomes 3 and 17 influence phenotypes of the metabolic syndrome. Proc Natl Acad Sci U S A, 97, 14478-14483.

Kojima, M., Hosoda, H., Date, Y., Nakazato, M., Matsuo, H., & Kangawa, K. (1999). Ghrelin is a growth-hormone-releasing acylated peptide from stomach. Nature, 402, 656-660.

Kojima, M., Hosoda, H., Matsuo, H., & Kangawa, K. (2001). Ghrelin: discovery of the natural endogenous ligand for the growth hormone secretagogue receptor. Trends Endocrinol Metab, 12, 118-122.

Kohno, D., Nakata, M., Maekawa, F., Fujiwara, K., Maejima, Y., Kuramochi, M., Shimazaki, T., Okano, H., Onaka, T., & Yada, T. (2007). Leptin suppresses ghrelin-induced activation of neuropeptide Y neurons in the arcuate nucleus via phosphatidylinositol 3-kinase- and phosphodiesterase 3-mediated pathway. Endocrinology, 148, 2251-2263.

Kohno, D., Sone, H., Minokoshi, Y., & Yada, T. (2008). Ghrelin raises [Ca2+]i via AMPK in hypothalamic arcuate nucleus NPY neurons. Biochem Biophys Res Commun, 366, 388-392.

Konturek, P.C., Brzozowski, T., Pajdo, R., Nikiforuk, A., Kwiecien, S., Harsch, I., Drozdowicz, D., Hahn, E.G., & Konturek, S.J. (2004) Ghrelin-a new gastroprotective factor in gastric mucosa. J Physiol Pharmacol, 55, 325-336.

Korbonits, M., Bustin, S. A., Kojima, M., Jordan, S., Adams, E. F., Lowe, D. G., Kangawa, K., & Grossman, A. B. (2001). The expression of the growth hormone secretagogue receptor ligand ghrelin in normal and abnormal human pituitary and other neuroendocrine tumors. J Clin Endocrinol Metab, 86, 881-887.

Korbonits, M., Gueorguiev, M., O'Grady, E., Lecoeur, C., Swan, D. C., Mein, C. A., Weill, J., Grossman, A. B., & Froguel, P. (2002). A variation in the ghrelin gene increases weight and decreases insulin secretion in tall, obese children. J Clin Endocrinol Metab, 87, 4005-4008.

Korbonits, M., Goldstone, A. P., Gueorguiev, M., & Grossman, A. B. (2004). Ghrelin--a hormone with multiple functions. Front Neuroendocrinol, 25, 27-68.

Korner, J., Inabnet, W., Conwell, I. M., Taveras, C., Daud, A., Olivero-Rivera, L., Restuccia, N. L., & Bessler, M. (2006). Differential effects of gastric bypass and banding on circulating gut hormone and leptin levels. Obesity, 14, 1553-1561.

Koyama, K.I., Yasuhara, D., Nakahara, T., Harada, T., Uehara, M., Ushikai, A., Asakawa, A., & Inui, A. (2010). Changes in acyl ghrelin, des-acyl ghrelin, and ratio of acyl ghrelin to total ghrelin with short-term refeeding in female inpatients with restricting-type anorexia nervosa. Horm Metab Res, 42, 595-598.

Kraemer, R.R. & Castracane, V.D. (2007). Exercise and humoral mediators of peripheral energy balance: ghrelin and adiponectin. Exp. Biol. Med. (Maywood), 232, 184-194.

Kung, D.W., Coffey, S.B., Jones, R.M., Cabral, S., Jiao, W., Fichtner, M., Carpino, P.A., Rose, C.R., Hank, R.F., Lopaze, M.G., Swartz, R., Chen, H.T., Hendsch, Z., Posner, B., Wielis, C.F., Manning, B., Dubins J., Stock, I.A., Varma, S., Campbell, M., DeBartola, D., Kosa-Maines, R., Steyn, S.J., McClure, K.F. (2012). Identification of spirocyclic piperidine-azetidine inverse agonists of the ghrelin receptor. Bioorg Med Chem Lett, 22, 4281-4287.

Kushner, R.F., & Roth, J.L. (2003). Assessment of the obese patient. Endocrinol Metab Clin North Am, 32, 915-933.

Lai, K.C., Cheng, C.H., & Leung, P.S. (2007). The ghrelin system in acinar cells: localization, expression, and regulation in the exocrine pancreas. Pancreas, 35, e1-e8.

Larsen, L. H., Gjesing, A. P., Sorensen, T. I., Hamid, Y. H., Echwald, S. M., Toubro, S., Black, E., Astrup, A., Hansen, T., & Pedersen, O. (2005). Mutation analysis of the preproghrelin gene: no association with obesity and type 2 diabetes. Clin Biochem, 38, 420-424.

Leyris, J.P., Roux, T., Trinquet, E., Verdié, P., Fehrentz, J.A., Oueslati, N., Douzon, S., Bourrier, E., Lamarque, L., Gagne, D., Galleyrand, J.C., M'kadmi, C., Martinez, J., Mary, S., Banères, J.L., & Marie, J. (2011). Homogeneous time-resolved fluorescence-based assay to screen for ligands targeting the growth hormone secretagogue receptor type 1a. Anal Biochem, 408, 253-262.

Levin, F., Edholm, T., Ehrström, M., Wallin, B., Schmidt, P.T., Kirchgessner, A.M., Hilsted, L.M., Hellström, P.M., & Näslund, E. (2005). Effect of peripherally administered ghrelin on gastric emptying and acid secretion in the rat. Regul Pept, 131, 59-65.

Li, B., Duysen, E. G., & Lockridge, O. (2008). The butyrylcholinesterase knockout mouse is obese on a high-fat diet. Chem Biol Interact, 175, 88-91.

Li, W.G., Gavrila, D., Liu, X., Wang, L., Gunnlaugsson, S., Stoll, L.L., McCormick, M.L., Sigmund, C.D., Tang, C., & Weintraub, N.L. (2004). Ghrelin inhibits proinflammatory responses and nuclear factor-kappaB activation in human endothelial cells. Circulation, 109, 2221-2226.

Liao, N., Xie, Z.K., Huang, J., & Xe, Z.F. (2013). Association between the ghrelin Leu72Met polymorphism and type 2 diabetes risk: a meta-analysis. Gene, 517, 179-183.

Liu, J., Prudom, C.E., Nass, R., Pezzoli, S.S., Oliveri, M.C., Johnson, M.L., Veldhuis, P., Gordon, D.A., Howard, A.D., Witcher, D.R., Geysen, H.M., Gaylinn, B.D., & Thorner, M.O. (2008). Novel ghrelin assays provide evidence for independent regulation of ghrelin acylation and secretion in healthy young men. J Clin Endocrinol Metab, 93, 1980-1987.

Liu, B., Garcia, E.A., & Korbonits, M. (2011) Genetic studies on the ghrelin, growth hormone secretagogue receptor (GHSR) and ghrelin O-acyl transferase (GOAT) genes. Peptides, 32, 1219l-2207.

Lu, S., Guan, J. L., Wang, Q. P., Uehara, K., Yamada, S., Goto, N., Date, Y., Nakazato, M., Kojima, M., Kangawa, K., & Shioda, S. (2002). Immunocytochemical observation of ghrelin-containing neurons in the rat arcuate nucleus. Neurosci Lett, 321, 157-160.

Lu, S.C., Xu, J., Chinookoswong, N., Liu, S., Steavenson, S., Gegg, C., Brankow, D., Lindberg, R., Veniant, M., & Gu, W. (2009). An acyl-ghrelin-specific neutralizing antibody inhibits the acute ghrelin-mediated orexigenic effects in mice. Mol Pharmacol, 75, 901-907.

Lundholm, K., Gunnebo, L., Körner, U., Iresjö, B.M., Engström, C., Hyltander, A., Smedh, U., & Bosaeus, I. (2010). Effects by daily long term provision of ghrelin to unselected weight-losing cancer patients: a randomized double-blind study. Cancer, 116, 2044-2052.

Maccarinelli, G., Sibilia, V., Torsello, A., Raimondo, F., Pitto, M., Gisutina, A., Netti, C. & Cocchi, D. (2005). Ghrelin regulates proliferation and differentiation of osteoblastic cells. J Endocrinol,184, 249-256.

Mager, U., Kolehmainen, M., de Mello, V. D., Schwab, U., Laaksonen, D. E., Rauramaa, R., Gylling, H., Atalay, M., Pulkkinen, L., & Uusitupa, M. (2008). Expression of ghrelin gene in peripheral blood mononuclear cells and plasma ghrelin concentrations in patients with metabolic syndrome. Eur J Endocrinol, 158, 499-510.

Majchrzak, K., Szyszko, K., Pawlowski, K.M., Motyl, T. & Krol., M. (2012). A role of ghrelin in cancerogenesis. Pol J Met Sci,, 15, 189-197.

Malagon, M.M., Luque, R.M., Ruiz-Guerrero, E., Rodriguez-Pacheco, F., Garcia-Navarro, S., Casanueva, F.F., Gracia-Navarro, F., & Castano, J.P. (2003). Intracellular signaling mechanisms mediating ghrelin-stimulated growth hormone release in somatotropes. Endocrinology, 144, 5372-5380.

Malendowicz, W., Ziolkowska, A., Szyszka, M., & Kwias, Z. (2009). Elevated blood active ghrelin and unaltered total ghrelin and obestatin concentrations in prostate carcinoma. Urol Int, 83, 471-475.

Mancini, M.C., Costa, A.P., de Melo, M. E., Cercato, C., Giannella-Neto, D., Garrido, A.B., Jr., Rosberg, S., Albertsson-Wikland, K., Villares, S.M., & Halpern, A. (2006). Effect of gastric bypass on spontaneous growth hormone and ghrelin release profiles. Obesity. (Silver Spring), 14, 383-387.

Martin, G. R., Loredo, J. C., & Sun, G. (2008). Lack of Association of Ghrelin Precursor Gene Variants and Percentage Body Fat or Serum Lipid Profiles. Obesity, 16, 908-912.

Masuda, Y., Tanaka, T., Inomata, N., Ohnuma, N., Tanaka, S., Itoh, Z., Hosoda, H., Kojima, M., & Kangawa, K. (2000). Ghrelin Stimulates Gastric Acid Secretion and Motility in Rats. Biochem Biophys Res Commun, 276, 905-908.

McKee, K.K., Palyha, O.C., Feighner, S.D., Hreniuk, D.L., Tan, C.P., Phillips, M.S., Smith, R.G., Van der Ploeg, L.H.T., & Howard, A.D. (1997). Molecular Analysis of Rat Pituitary and Hypothalamic Growth Hormone Secretagogue Receptors. Mol Endocrinol, 11, 415-423.

Mihalic, J.T., Kim, Y.J., Lizarzaburu, M., Chen, X., Deignan, J., Wanska, M.,Yu, M., Fu, J., Chen, X., Zhang, A., Connors, R., Liang, L., Lindstrom, M., Ma, J., Tang, L., Dai, K., & Li, L. (2012). Discovery of a new class of ghrelin receptor antagonists. Bioorg Med Chem Lett, 22, 2046-2051.

Miki, K., Maekura, R., Nagaya, N., Nakazato, M., Kimura, H., Murakami, S., Ohnishi, S., Hiraga, T., Miki, M., Kitada, S., Yoshimura, K., Tateishi, Y., Arimura, Y., Matsumoto, N., Yoshikawa, M., Yamahara, K., & Kangawa, K. (2012). Ghrelin treatment of cachectic patients with chronic obstructive pulmonary disease: a multicenter, randomized, double-blind, placebo-controlled trial. PLoS One, 7, e35708.

Miljic, D., Pekic, S., Djurovic, M., Doknic, M., Milic, N., Casanueva, F.F., Ghatei, M., & Popovic, V. (2006). Ghrelin has partial or no effect on appetite, growth hormone, prolactin, and cortisol release in patients with anorexia nervosa. J Clin Endocrinol Metab, 91, 1491-1495.

Mingrone, G., Granato, L., Valera-Mora, E., Iaconelli, A., Calvani, M. F., Bracaglia, R., Manco, M., Nanni, G., & Castagneto, M. (2006). Ultradian ghrelin pulsatility is disrupted in morbidly obese subjects after weight loss induced by malabsorptive bariatric surgery. Am. J. Clin. Nutr. 83, 1017-1024.

Miraglia del Giudice, E., Santoro, N., Cirillo, G., Raimondo, P., Grandone, A., D'Aniello, A., Di Nardo, M., & Perrone, L. (2004). Molecular screening of the ghrelin gene in Italian obese children: the Leu72Met variant is associated with an earlier onset of obesity. Int J Obes Relat Metab Disord, 28, 447-450.

Miyasaka, K., Hosoya, H., Sekime, A., Ohta, M., Amono, H., Matsushita, S., Suzuki, K., Higuchi, S., & Funakoshi, A. (2006). Association of ghrelin receptor gene polymorphism with bulimia nervosa in a Japanese population. J Neural Transm, 113, 1279-1285.

Monteiro, M.P. (2011). Anti-ghrelin vaccine for obesity: a feasible alternative to dieting? Expert Rev Vaccines, 10, 1363-1365.

Monteleone, P., Tortorella, A., Castaldo, E., Di Filippo, C., & Maj, M. (2007). The Leu72Met polymorphism of the ghrelin gene is significantly associated with binge eating disorder. Psychiatr Genet, 17, 13-16.

Moulin, A., Demange, L., Ryan, J., M'Kadmi, C., Galleyrand, J.C., Martinez, J., & Fehrentz, J.A. (2008). Trisubstituted 1,2,4-triazoles as ligands for the ghrelin receptor: on the significance of the orientation and substitution at position 3. Bioorg Med Chem Lett, 18, 164-168.

Moulin, A., Brunel, L., Boeglin., D., Demange, L., Ryan, J., M'Kadmi, C., Denoyelle, S., Martinez, J., & Fehrentz, J.A. (2013). The 1,2,4-triazole as a scaffold for the design of ghrelin receptor ligands: development of JMV 2959, a potent antagonist. Amino Acids, 44, 301-314.

Motawi, T.K., Shaker, O.G., Ismail, M.F., & Sayed, N.H. (2013). Genetic variants associated with the progression of hepatocellular carcinoma in hepatitis C Egyptian patients. Gene, 527, 516-520.

Muller, T.D., Perez-Tilve, D, Tong, J., Pfluger, P.T., & Tschöp. (2010). Ghrelin and its potential in the tretament of eating/wasting disorders and cachexia. J Cachexia Sarcopenia Muscle, 1, 159-167.

Muller, T.D., Tschop, M.H., Jarick, I., Ehrlich, S., Scherag, S., Herpertz-Dahlmann, B., Zipfel, S., Herzog, W., de Zwaan, M., Burghardt, R., Fleischhaker, C., Klampfl, K., Wewetzer, C., Herpertz, S., Zeeck, A., Tagay, S., Burgmer, M., Pfluger, P. T., Scherag, A., Hebebrand, J., & Hinney, A. (2011). Genetic variation of the ghrelin activator gene ghrelin O-acyltransferase (GOAT) is associated with anorexia nervosa. J Psychiatr Res, 45, 706-711.

Murata, M., Okimura, Y., Iida, K., Matsumoto, M., Sowa, H., Kaji, H., Kojima, M., Kangawa, K., & Chihara, K. (2002). Ghrelin modulates the downstream molecules of insulin signaling in hepatoma cells. J Biol Chem, 277, 5667-5674.

Murray, C.D., Martin, N.M., Patterson, M., Taylor, S.A., Ghatei, M.A., Kamm, M.A., Johnston, C., Bloom, S.R., & Emmanuel, A.V. (2005). Ghrelin enhances gastric emptying in diabetic gastroparesis: a double blind, placebo controlled, crossover study. Gut, 54, 1693-1698.

Nagaya, N., Uematsu, M., Kojima, M., Date, Y., Nakazato, M., Okumura, H., Hosoda, H., Shimizu, W., Yamagishi, M., Oya, H., Koh, H., Yutani, C., & Kangawa, K. (2001). Elevated circulating level of ghrelin in cachexia associated with chronic heart failure: relationships between ghrelin and anabolic/catabolic factors. Circulation, 104, 2034-2038.

Nagaya, N., Moriya, J., Yasumura, Y., Uematsu, M., Ono, F., Shimizu, W., Ueno, K., Kitakaze, M., Miyatake K., & Kangawa K. (2004). Effects of ghrelin administration on left ventricular function, exercise capacity, and muscle wasting in patients with chronic heart failure. Circulation, 110, 3674-3679.

Nagaya, N., Itoh, T., Murakami, S., Oya, H., Uematsu, M., Miyatake, K. & Kangawa, K. (2005). Treatment of cachexia with ghrelin in patients with COPD. Chest, 128, 1187-1193.

Nakahara, T., Harada, T., Yasuhara, D., Shimada, N., Amitani, H., Sakoguchi, T., Kamiji, M.M., Asakawa, A., & Inui, A. (2008). Plasma obestatin concentrations are negatively correlated with body mass index, insulin resistance index, and plasma leptin concentrations in obesity and anorexia nervosa. Biol Psychiatry, 64, 252-255.

Nakazato, M., Murakami, N., Date, Y., Kojima, M., Matsuo, H., Kangawa, K., & Matsukura, S. (2001). A role for ghrelin in the central regulation of feeding. Nature, 409, 194-198.

Napoli, N., Pedone, C., Pozzilli, P., Lauretani, F., Bandinelli, S., Ferrucci, L., & Incalzi, R.F. (2011). Effect of ghrelin on bone mass density: the InChianti study. Bone, 49, 257-267.

Nass, R., Pezzoli, S.S., Oliveri, M.C., Patrie, J.T., Harrell, F.E. Jr., Clasey, J.L., Heymsfield, S.B., Bach, M.A., Vance, M.L., & Thorner, M.O. (2008). Effects of an oral ghrelin mimetic on body composition and clinical outcomes in healthy older adults: a randomized trial. Ann Intern Med, 149, 601-611.

Neary, N.M., Small, C.J., Wren, A.M., Lee, J.L., Druce, M.R., Palmieri, C., Frost, G.S., Ghatei, M.A., Coombes, R.C., & Bloom, S.R. (2004). Ghrelin increases energy intake in cancer patients with impaired appetite: acute, randomized, placebo-controlled trial. J Clin Endocrinol Metab, 89, 2832-2836.

Nishi, Y., Hiejima, H., Hosoda, H., Kaiya, H., Mori, K., Fukue, Y., Yanase, T., Nawata, H., Kangawa, K., & Kojima, M. (2005). Ingested Medium-Chain Fatty Acids Are Directly Utilized for the Acyl Modification of Ghrelin. Endocrinology, 146, 2255-2264.

Nouh, O., Abd Elfattah, M.M., & Hassouna, A.A. (2012). Association between ghrelin levels and BMD: a cross sectional trial. Gynecol Endocrinol, 28, 570-572.

Ogiso, K., Asakawa, A., Amitani, H., & Inui, A. (2011). Ghrelin and anorexia nervosa: a psychosomatic perspective. Nutrition, 27, 988-993.

Ohgusu, H., Shirouzu, K., Nakamura, Y., Nakashima, Y., Ida, T., Sato, T., & Kojima, M. (2009). Ghrelin O-acyltransferase (GOAT) has a preference for n-hexanoyl-CoA over n-octanoyl-CoA as an acyl donor. Biochem Biophys Res Commun, 386, 153-158.

Ohgusu, H., Takahashi, T., & Kojima M. (2012). Enzymatic characterization of GOAT, ghrelin O-acyltransferase. Methods Enzymol, 514, 147-163.

Ohlsson, C., Bengtsson, B.A., Isaksson, O.G., Andreassen, T.T., & Slootweg, M.C. (1998). Growth hormone and bone. Endocr Rev, 19, 55-79.

Ordway, J.M., Budiman, M.A., Korshunova, Y., Maloney, R.K., Bedell, J.A., Citek, R.W., Bacher, B., Peterson, S., Rohlfing, T., Leon, J., McPherson, J.D., & Jeddeloh, J.A. (2007). Identification of novel high-frequency DNA methylation changes in breast cancer. PLoS One,, 2, e1314.

Otto, B., Cuntz, U., Fruehauf, E., Wawarta, R. Folwaczny, C., Riepl, R.L., Heiman, M.L., Lehnert, P., Fichter, M., & Tschöp, M. (2001). Weight gain decreases elevated plasma ghrelin concentrations of patients with anorexia nervosa. Eur J Endocrinol, 145, 669-673.

Otukonyong, E. E., Dube, M. G., Torto, R., Kalra, P. S., & Kalra, S. P. (2005). High-fat diet-induced ultradian leptin and insulin hypersecretion are absent in obesity-resistant rats. Obes Res, 13, 991-999.

Ozgen, M., Kocca, S.S., Etem E.O., Yuce, H., Aydin, S., & Isik, A. (2011). Ghrelin gene polymorphims in rheumatoid arthritis. Joint Bone Spine, 78, 368-373.

Paik, K. H., Lee, M. K., Jin, D. K., Kang, H. W., Lee, K. H., Kim, A. H., Kim, C., Lee, J. E., Oh, Y. J., Kim, S., Han, S. J., Kwon, E. K., & Choe, Y. H. (2007). Marked suppression of ghrelin concentration by insulin in Prader-willi syndrome. J. Korean Med. Sci. 22, 177-182.

Palik, E., Baranyi, E., Melczer, Z., Audikovszky, M., Szöcs, A., Winkler, G., & Cseh, K. (2007). Elevated serum acylated (biologically active) ghrelin and resistin levels associate with pregnancy-induced weight gain and insulin resistance. Diabetes Res Clin Pract, 76, 351-357.

Pantel, J., Legendre, M., Cabrol, S., Hilal, L., Hajaji, Y., Morisset, S., Nivot, S., Vie-Luton, M.P., Grouselle, D. de Kerdanet, M., Kadiri, A., Epelbaum, J., Le Bouc, Y., & Amselem, S. (2006), Loss of constitutive activity of the growth hormone secretagogue receptor in familial short stature. J Clin Invest 116, 760-768.

Peeters, T.L. (2005). Ghrelin: a new player in the control of gastrointestinal functions. Gut, 54, 1638-1649.

Peeters, T. L. (2006). Potential of ghrelin as a therapeutic approach for gastrointestinal motility disorders. Curr Opin Pharmacol, 6, 553-558.

Peeters, T.L. (2013). Ghrelin and the gut. Endocr Dev, 25, 41-48.

Perdonà, E., Faggioni, F., Buson, A., Sabbatini, F.M. Corti, C., & Corsi, M. (2011). Pharmacological characterization of the ghrelin receptor antagonist, GSK1614343 in rat RC-4B/C cells natively expressing GHS type 1a receptors. Eur J Pharmacol, 650, 178-183.

Philippou, A., Halapas, A., Maridaki, M., & Koutsilieris, M. (2007). Type I insulin-like growth factor receptor signaling in skeletal muscle regeneration and hypertrophy. J Musculoskelet Neuronal Interact, 7, 208-218.

Poporato, P.E., Filigheddu, N., Reano, S., Ferrara, M., Angelino, E., Gnocchi, V.F., Prodam, F., Ronchi, G., Fagoonee, S., Fornaro, M., Chianale, F., Baldanzi, G., Surico, N., Sinigaglia, F., Perroteau, I., Smith, R.G., Sun, Y., Geuna, S., & Graziani, A. (2013). Acylated and unacylated ghrelin impair skeletal muscle atrophy in mice. J Clin Invest, 123, 611-622.

Popovic, V., Miljic, D., Micic, D., Damjanovic, S., Arvat, E., Ghigo, E., Dieguez, C., & Casanueva, F.F. (2003). Ghrelin main action on the regulation of growth hormone release is exerted at hypothalamic level. J Clin Endocrinol Metab 88, 3450-3453.

Portelli, J., Michotte, Y., & Smolders, I.. (2012). Ghrelin: an emerging new anticonvulsant neuropeptide. Epilepsia, 53, 585-595.

Pöykkö, S.M., Ukkola, O., Kauma, H., Savolainen, M.J., & Kesäniemi, Y.A. (2003). Ghrelin Arg51Gln mutation is a risk for type 2 diabetes and hypertension in a random sample of middle-aged subjects. Diabetologia, 46, 455-458.

Prado, C. L., Pugh-Bernard, A. E., Elghazi, L., Sosa-Pineda, B., & Sussel, L. (2004). Ghrelin cells replace insulin-producing beta cells in two mouse models of pancreas development. Proc Natl Acad Sci USA, 101, 2924-2929.

Prince, A.C., Brooks, S.J., Stahl, D., & Treasure, J. (2009). Systematic review and meta-analysis of the baseline concentrations and physiological responses of gut hormones to food in eating disorders. Am J Clin Nutr, 89, 755-765.

Puleo, L., Marini, P., Avallone, R., Zanchet, M., Bandiera, S., Baroni, M., & Croci, T. (2012). Synthesis and pharmacological evaluation of indolinone derivatives as novel ghrelin receptor antagonists. Bioorg Med Chem, 20, 5623-5636.

Purnell, J.Q., Cummings, D., & Weigle, D.S. (2007). Changes in 24-h area-under-the-curve ghrelin values following diet-induced weight loss are associated with loss of fat-free mass, but not with changes in fat mass, insulin levels or insulin sensitivity. Int. J. Obes. (Lond), 31, 385-389.

Purtell, L., Sze, L., Loughnan, G., Smith, E., Herzog, H., Sainsbury, A. Steinbeck, K., Campbell, L.V., & Viardot, A. (2011). In adults with Prader-Willi syndrome, elevated ghrelin levels are more consistent with hyperphagia than high PYY and GLP-1 levels. Neuropeptides 45, 301-307.

Qiu, W.C., Wang, Z.G., Wang, W.G., Yan, J., & Zheng, Q. (2008). Gastric motor effects of ghrelin and growth hormone releasing peptide 6 in diabetic mice with gastroparesis. World J Gastroenterol, 14, 1419-1424.

Radetti, G., Prodam, F., Lauriola, S., Di Dio, G., D'Addato, G., Corneli, G., Bellone, S., & Bona, G. (2008). Acute ghrelin response to intravenous dexamethasone administration in idiopathic short stature or isolated idiopathic growth hormone-deficient children. J Endocrinol Invest 31, 224-228.

Rediger, A., Piechowski, C.L., Yi, C.X., Tarnow, P., Strotmann, R., Grüters, A., Krude, H., Schöneberg, T., Tschöp, M.H., Kleinau, G., & Biebermann, H. (2011). Mutually opposite signal modulation by hypothalamic heterodimerization of ghrelin and melanocortin-3 receptors. J Biol Chem, 286, 39623-39631.

Riediger, T., Traebert, M., Schmid, H.A., Scheel, C., Lutz, T.A., & Scharrer, E. (2003). Site-specific effects of ghrelin on the neuronal activity in the hypothalamic arcuate nucleus. Neurosci Lett 341, 151-155.

Rindi, G., Necchi, V., Savio, A., Torsello, A., Zoli, M., Locatelli, V., Raimondo, F., Cocchi, D., & Solcia, E. (2002). Characterisation of gastric ghrelin cells in man and other mammals: studies in adult and fetal tissues. Histochem Cell Biol, 117, 511-519.

Rodríguez-Pacheco, F., Luque, R.M., Tena-Sempere, M., Malagón, M.M., & Castaño, J.P. (2008). Ghrelin induces growth hormone secretion via a nitric oxide/cGMP signalling pathway. J Neuroendocrinol 20, 406-412.

Rodríguez, A., Gómez-Ambrosi, J., Catalán, V., Gil, M.J., Becerril, S., Sáinz, N., Silva, C., Salvador, J., Colina, I., & Frühbeck, G. (2009). Acylated and desacyl ghrelin stimulate lipid accumulation in human visceral adipocytes. Int J Obes 33, 541-552.

Rudolph, J., Esler, W. P., O'connor, S., Coish, P. D., Wickens, P. L., Brands, M., Bierer, D. E., Bloomquist, B. T., Bondar, G., Chen, L., Chuang, C.Y., Claus, T.H., Fathi, Z., Fu, W., Khire, U.R., Kristie, J.A., Liu, X.G., Lowe, D.B., McClure, A.C., Michels, M., Ortiz, A.A., Ramsden, P.D., Schoenleber, R.W., Shelekhin, T.E., Vakalopoulos, A., Tang, W., Wang. L., Yi, L., Gardell, S.J., Livingston, J.N., Sweet, L.J., & Bullock, W.H. (2007). Quinazolinone derivatives as orally available ghrelin receptor antagonists for the treatment of diabetes and obesity. J Med Chem, 50, 5202-5216.

Sabbatini, F.M., Di Fabio, R., Corsi, M., Cavanni, P., Bromidge, S.M., St Denis, Y., D'Adamo, L., Contini, S., Rinaldi, M., Guery, S., Savoia, C., Mundi, C., Perini, B., Carpenter, A.J., Dal Forno, G., Faggioni, F., Tessari, M., Pavone, F., Di Francesco, C., Buson, A., Mattioli, M., Perdona, E., & Melotto, S. (2010). Discovery process and characterization of novel carbohydrazide derivatives as potent and selective GHSR1a antagonists. Chem Med Chem, 5, 1450-1455.

Sakata, I., Nakamura, K., Yamazaki, M., Matsubara, M., Hayashi, Y., Kangawa, K., & Sakai, T. (2002). Ghrelin-producing cells exist as two types of cells, closed- and opened-type cells, in the rat gastrointestinal tract. Peptides, 23, 531-536.

Sakata, I., Yang, J., Lee, C.E., Osborne-Lawrence, S., Rovinsky, S.A., Elmquist, J.K., & Zigman, J.M. (2009). Colocalization of ghrelin O-acyltransferase and ghrelin in gastric mucosal cells. AmJ Physiol, 297, E134-E141.

Sakuma, K., & Yamaguchi, A. (2012). Sarcopenia and age-related endocrine function. Int J Endocrinol, 2012, 127362.

Sangiao-Alvarellos, S., & Cordido, F. (2012). Effect of ghrelin on glucose-insulin homeostasis: therapeutic implications. Int J Pept, 2010, 2010 pii 234709.

Satou, M., Nishi, Y., Yoh, J., Hattori, Y., & Sugimoto, H. (2010). Identification and Characterization of Acyl-Protein Thioesterase 1/Lysophospholipase I As a Ghrelin Deacylation/Lysophospholipid Hydrolyzing Enzyme in Fetal Bovine Serum and Conditioned Medium. Endocrinology, 151, 4765-4775.

Satou, M., & Sugimoto, H. (2012). The study of ghrelin deacetylation enzymes. Methods Enzymol, 514, 165-179.

Schellekens, H., van Oeffelen, W.E., Dinan, T.G., & Cryan, J.F. (2013). Promiscuous dimerization of the growth hormone secretagogue receptor (GHS-R1a) attenuates ghrelin-mediated signaling. J Biol Chem, 288, 181-191.

Sehirli, O., Sener, E., Sener, G., Cetinel, S., Erzik, C., & Yegen, B. C. (2008). Ghrelin improves burn-induced multiple organ injury by depressing neutrophil infiltration and the release of pro-inflammatory cytokines. Peptides, 29, 1231-1240.

Seim, I., Josh, P., Cunningham, P., Herington, A., & Chopin, L. (2011). Ghrelin axis genes, peptides and receptors: recent findings and future challenges. Mol Cell Endocrinol, 340, 3-9.

Shanado, Y., Kometani, M., Uchiyama, H., Koizumi, S., & Teno, N. (2004). Lysophospholipase I identified as a ghrelin deacylation enzyme in rat stomach. Biochem Biophys Res Commun, 325, 1487-1494.

Shearman, L. P., Wang, S. P., Helmling, S., Stribling, D. S., Mazur, P., Ge, L., Wang, L., Klussmann, S., Macintyre, D. E., Howard A.D., & Starck, A.M. (2006). Ghrelin neutralization by a ribonucleic acid-SPM ameliorates obesity in diet-induced obese mice. Endocrinology, 147, 1517-1526.

Sheriff, S., Kadeer, N., Joshi,R., Friend, L.A., James, J.H., & Balasubramaniam, A. (2012). Des-acyl ghrelin exhibits pro-anabolic and anti-catabolic effects on C2C12 myotubes exposed to cytokines and reduces burn-induced muscle proteolysis in rats. Mol Cell Endocrinol,35, 286-295.

Shimizu, Y., Nagaya, N., Isobe, T., Imazu, M., Okumura, H., Hosoda, H., Kojima, M., Kangawa, K., & Kohno, N. (2003). Increased plasma ghrelin level in lung cancer cachexia. Clin Cancer Res 9, 774-778.

Shimizu, Y., Chang, E.C., Shafton, A.D., Ferens, D.M., Sanger, G.J., Witherington, J., & Furness, J.B. (2006). Evidence that stimulation of ghrelin receptors in the spinal cord initiates propulsive activity in the colon of the rat. J Physiol 576, 329-338.

Shintani, M., Ogawa, Y., Ebihara, K., izawa-Abe, M., Miyanaga, F., Takaya, K., Hayashi, T., Inoue, G., Hosoda, K., Kojima, M., Kangawa, K., & Nakao, K. (2001). Ghrelin, an endogenous growth hormone secretagogue, is a novel orexigenic peptide that antagonizes leptin action through the activation of hypothalamic neuropeptide Y/Y1 receptor pathway. Diabetes, 50, 227-232.

Sibilia, V., Pagani, F., Guidobono, F., Locatelli, V., Torsello, A., Deghenghi, R., & Netti, C. (2002). Evidence for a central inhibitory role of growth hormone secretagogues and ghrelin on gastric acid secretion in conscious rats. Neuroendocrinology, 75, 92-97.

Sibilia, V., Rindi, G., Pagani, F., Rapetti, D., Locatelli, V., Torsello, A., Campanini, N., Deghenghi, R., & Netti, C. (2003). Ghrelin protects against ethanol-induced gastric ulcers in rats: studies on the mechanisms of action. Endocrinology, 144, 353-359.

Sibilia, V., Pagani, F., Rindi, G., Lattuada, N., Rapetti, D., De Luca, V., Campanini, N., Bulgarelli, I., Locatelli, V., Guidobono, F., & Netti, C. (2008). Central ghrelin gastroprotection involves nitric oxide/prostaglandin cross-talk. Brit J Phramacol, 154, 688-697.

Sibilia, V., Pagani, F., Mrak, E., Dieci, E., Tulipano, G., & Ferrucci, F. (2012). Pharmacological characterization of the ghrelin receptor mediating its inhibitory action on inflammatory pain in rats Amino Acids 43, 1751-1759.

Sivertsen, B., Lang, M., Frimurer, T.M., Holliday, N.D., Bach, A., Els, S., Engelstoft, M.S., Petersen, P.S., Madsen, A.N., Schwartz, T.W., Beck-Sickinger, A.G., & Holst, B. (2011). Unique interaction pattern for a functionally biased ghrelin receptor agonist. J Biol Chem, 286, 20845-20860.

Smith, R.G., Pong, S. S., Hickey, G., Jacks, T., Cheng, K., Leonard, R., Cohen, C.J., Arena, J. P., Chang, C.H., Drisko, J., Wyvratt, M., Fisher, M., Nargund, R., & Patchett, A. (1996). Modulation of pulsatile GH release through a novel receptor in hypothalamus and pituitary gland. Recent Prog Horm Res, 51, 261-285.

Smith, R.G., Jiang, H., & Sun, Y. (2005). Developments in ghrelin biology and potential clinical relevance. Trends Endocrinol Metab, 16, 436-442.

Soeki, T., Kishimoto, I., Schwenke, D. O., Tokudome, T., Horio, T., Yoshida, M., Hosoda, H., & Kangawa, K. (2008). Ghrelin suppresses cardiac sympathetic activity and prevents early left ventricular remodeling in rats with myocardial infarction. Am J Physiol, 294, H426-H432.

Soriano-Guillen, L., Barrios, V., Campos-Barros, A., & Argente, J. (2004). Ghrelin levels in obesity and anorexia nervosa: effect of weight reduction or recuperation. J Pediatr, 144, 36-42.

Stawerska, R., Smyczynska, J., Czkwianianc, E., Pisarek, H., Hilczer, M., & Lewinski, A. (2012a). Ghrelin concentration is correlated with IGF-I/IGFBP-3 molar ratio but not with GH secretion in children with short stature. Neuro Endocrinol Lett, 33, 412-418.

Stawerska, R., Smyczyńska, J., Czkwianianc, E., Hilczer, M., & Lewiński, A. (2012b). High concentration of ghrelin in children with growth hormone deficiency and neurosecretory dysfunction. Neuro Endocrinol Lett, 33, 331-339.

Stengel, A., Goebel, M., Wang, L., & Tachq, Y. (2010). Ghrelin, des-acyl ghrelin and nesfatin-1 in gastric X/A-like cells: Role as regulators of food intake and body weight. Peptides, 31, 357-369.

Stenstrom, B., Zhao, C. M., Tommeras, K., Arum, C. J., & Chen, D. (2006). Is gastrin partially responsible for body weight reduction after gastric bypass? Eur. Surg. Res. 38, 94-101.

Strasser, F., Lutz, T.A., Maeder, M.T., Thuerlimann, B., Bueche, D., Tschöp, M., Kaufmann, K., Holst, B., Brändle, M., von Moos, R., Demmer, R., & Cerny, T. (2008). Safety, tolerability and pharmacokinetics of intravenous ghrelin for cancer-related anorexia/cachexia: a randomised, placebo-controlled, double-blind, double-crossover study. Br J Cancer, 98, 300-308.

Stratis, C., Alexandrides, T., Vagenas, K., & Kalfarentzos, F. (2006). Ghrelin and peptide YY levels after a variant of biliopancreatic diversion with Roux-en-Y gastric bypass versus after colectomy: a prospective comparative study. Obes Surg 16, 752-758.

Sugiyama, M., Yamaki, A., Furuya, M., Inomata, N., Minamitake, Y., Ohsuye, K., & Kangawa, K. (2012). Ghrelin improves body weight loss and skeletal muscle catabolism associated with angiotensin II-induced cachexia in mice. Regul Pept, 178, 21-28.

Sun, Y., Garcia, J.M., & Smith, R.G. (2007). Ghrelin and growth hormone secretagogue receptor expression in mice during aging. Endocrinology, 148, 1323-1329.

Tacke, F., Brabant, G., Kruck, E., Horn, R., Schöffski, P., Hecker, H., Manns, M.P., & Trautwein, C. (2003). Ghrelin in chronic liver disease. J Hepatol, 38, 447-454.

Tai, K., Visvanathan, R., Hammond, A.J., Wishart, J.M., Horowitz, M., & Chapman, I.M. (2009). Fasting ghrelin is related to skeletal muscle mass in healthy adults. Eur J Nutr, 48, 176-183.

Takachi, K., Doki, Y., Ishikawa, O., Miyashiro, I., Sasaki, Y., Ohigashi, H., Murata, K., Nakajima, H., Hosoda, H., Kangawa, K., Sasakuma, F., & Imaoka S. (2006). Postoperative ghrelin levels and delayed recovery from body weight loss after distal or total gastrectomy. J Surg Res, 130, 1-7.

Takaya, K., Ariyasu, H., Kanamoto, N., Iwakura, H., Yoshimoto, A., Harada, M., Mori, K., Komatsu, Y., Usui, T., Shimatsu, A., Ogawa, Y., Hosoda, K., Akamizu, T., Kojima, M., Kangawa, K., & Nakao, K. (2000). Ghrelin strongly stimulates growth hormone release in humans. J Clin Endocrinol Metab, 85, 4908-4911.

Takezawa, J., Yamada., K., Morita, A., Aiba, N., & Watanabe, S. (2009).Preproghrelin gene polymorphisms in obese Japanese: association with diabetes mellitus in men and with metabolic syndrome parameters in women. Obesity Res Clin Practice, 3, 179-191.

Tang, N.P., Wang, L.S., Yang, L., Gu, H.J., Zhu, H.J., Zhou, B., Sun, Q.M., Cong, R.H., & Wang, B. (2008). Preproghrelin Leu72Met polymorphism in Chinese subjects with coronary disease and controls. Clin Chim Acta, 387, 42-47.

Teubner, B.J., Garretson, J.T., Hwang, Y., Cole, P.A., & Bartness, T.J. (2013). Inhibition of ghrelin O-acyltransferase attenuates food deprivation-induced increases in ingestive behavior. Horm Behav, 63, 667-673.

Trudel, L., Tomasetto, C., Rio, M.C., Bouin, M., Plourde, V., Eberling, P., & Poitras, P. (2002). Ghrelin/motilin-related peptide is a potent prokinetic to reverse gastric postoperative ileus in rat. Am J Physiol, 282, G948-G952.

Tschöp, M., Smiley, D. L., & Heiman, M. L. (2000). Ghrelin induces adiposity in rodents. Nature, 407, 908-913.

Tschöp, M., Weyer, C., Tataranni, P.A., Devanarayan, V., Ravussin, E., & Heiman, M.L. (2001). Circulating ghrelin levels are decreased in human obesity. Diabetes 50, 707-709.

Tsuchimochi, W., Kyorakun I., Yamaguchi, H., Toshinai, K., Shiomi, K., Kangawa, K., & Nakazato, M. (2013). Ghrelin prevents the development of experimental diabetic neuropathy in rodents. Eur J Pharmacol,702, 187-193.

Ueno, S., Yoshida, S., Mondal, A., Nishina, K., Koyama, M., Sakata, I., Miura, K., Hayashi, Y., Nemoto, N., Nishigaki, K., & Sakai, T. (2012). In vitro selection of a peptide antagonist of growth hormone secretagogue receptor using cDNA display. Proc Natl Acad Sci USA, 109, 11121-11116.

Ukkola, O., Ravussin, E., Jacobson, P., Snyder, E. E., Chagnon, M., Sjostrom, L., & Bouchard, C. (2001). Mutations in the preproghrelin/ghrelin gene associated with obesity in humans. J Clin Endocrinol Metab, 86, 3996-3999.

Ukkola, O., Ravussin, E., Jacobson, P., Perusse, L., Rankinen, T., Tschop, M., Heiman, M. L., Leon, A. S., Rao, D. C., Skinner, J. S., Wilmore, J. H., Sjostrom, L., & Bouchard, C. (2002). Role of ghrelin polymorphisms in obesity based on three different studies. Obes Res, 10, 782-791.

Ukkola, O. (2011). Genetic variants of ghrelin in metabolic disorders. Peptides, 32, 2319-2322.

Ukkola, O., Pääkklö, T., & Kesäniemi, Y.A. (2012). Ghrelin and its promoter variant associated with cardiac hypertrophy. J Hum Hypertens, 26, 452-457.

Verhagen, L.A., Egecioglu, E., Luijendijk, M.C., Hillebrand, J.J., Adan, R.A., & Dickson, S.L. (2011). Acute and chronic suppression of the central ghrelin signaling system reveals a role in food anticipatory activity. Eur Neuropsychopharmacol, 21, 384-392.

Verhulst, P.J., & Depoortere, I. (2012) Ghrelin's second life: from appetite stimulator to glucose regulator. World J Gastroenterol, 18, 3183-3195.

Vivenza, D., Rapa, A., Castellino, N., Bellone, S., Petri, A., Vacca, G., Aimaretti, G., Broglio, F., & Bona, G. (2004). Ghrelin gene polymorphisms and ghrelin, insulin, IGF-I, leptin and anthropometric data in children and adolescents. Eur J Endocrinol, 151, 127-133.

Vizcarra, J.A., Kirby, J.D., Kim, S.K., & Galyean, M.L. (2007). Active immunization against ghrelin decreases weight gain and alters plasma concentrations of growth hormone in growing pigs. Domest Anim Endocrinol, 33,176-189.

Volante, M., Allia, E., Gugliotta, P., Funaro, A., Broglio, F., Deghenghi, R., Muccioli, G., Ghigo, E., & Papotti, M. (2002). Expression of ghrelin and of the GH secretagogue receptor by pancreatic islet cells and related endocrine tumors. J Clin Endocrinol Metab, 87, 1300-1308.

Wang, H. J., Geller, F., Dempfle, A., Schauble, N., Friedel, S., Lichtner, P., Fontenla-Horro, F., Wudy, S., Hagemann, S., Gortner, L., Huse, K., Remschmidt, H., Bettecken, T., Meitinger, T., Schafer, H., Hebebrand, J., & Hinney, A. (2004). Ghrelin receptor gene: identification of several sequence variants in extremely obese children and adolescents, healthy normal-weight and underweight students, and children with short normal stature. J Clin Endocrinol Metab, 89, 157-162.

Wang, W., Andersson, M., Iresjö, B.M., Lönnroth, C., & Lundholm, K. (2006). Effects of ghrelin on anorexia in tumor-bearing mice with eicosanoid-related cachexia. Int J Oncol, 28, 1393-1400.

Wang., K., Wang., L., Zhao, Y., Shi, Y., Wang., L., & Chen Z.J. (2009) No association of the Arg51Gln and Leu72Met polymorphisms of the ghrelin gene and polycystic ovary syndrome. Hum Reprod, 24, 485-490.

Warzecha, Z., Ceranowicz, P., Dembinski, A., Cieszkowski, J., Kusnierz-Cabala, B., Tomaszewska, R., Kuwahara, A., & Kato, I. (2010). Therapeutic effect of ghrelin in the course of cerulein-induced acute pancreatitis in rats. J Physiol Pharmacol, 61, 419-427.

Wierup, N. & Sundler, F. (2005). Ultrastructure of islet ghrelin cells in the human fetus. Cell Tissue Res, 319, 423-428.

Wierup, N., Svensson, H., Mulder, H., & Sundler, F. (2002). The ghrelin cell: a novel developmentally regulated islet cell in the human pancreas. Regul Pept, 107, 63-69.

Williams, D.L., Grill, H.J., Cummings, D.E., & Kaplan, J.M. (2006). Overfeeding-induced weight gain suppresses plasma ghrelin levels in rats. J Endocrinol Invest, 29, 863-868.

Wo, J.M., Ejskjaer, N., Hellström, P.M., Malik, R.A., Pezzullo, J.C., Shaughnessy, L., Charlton, P., Kosutic, G., & McCallum, R.W. (2011). Randomised clinical trial: ghrelin agonist TZP-101 relieves gastroparesis associated with severe nausea and vomiting--randomised clinical study subset data. Aliment Pharmacol Ther, 33, 679-688.

Wren, A.M., Seal, L.J., Cohen, M.A., Brynes, A.E., Frost, G.S., Murphy, K.G., Dhillo, W.S., Ghatei, M.A., & Bloom, S.R. (2001). Ghrelin Enhances Appetite and Increases Food Intake in Humans. J Clin Endocrinol Metab, 86, 5992.

Wu, R., Dong, W., Zhou, M., Zhang, F., Marini, C.P., Ravikumar, T.S., & Wang, P. (2007). Ghrelin attenuates sepsis-induced acute lung injury and mortality in rats. Am J Respir Crit Care Med, 176, 805-813.

Wynne, K., Giannitsopoulou, K., Small, C.J., Patterson, M., Frost, G., Ghatei, M.A., Brown, E.A., Bloom, S.R., & Choi, P. (2005). Subcutaneous ghrelin enhances acute food intake in malnourished patients who receive maintenance peritoneal dialysis: a randomized, placebo-controlled trial. J Am Soc Nephrol, 16, 2111-2118.

Xia, Q., Pang, W., Pan, H., Zheng, Y., Kang, J. S., & Zhu, S. G. (2004). Effects of ghrelin on the proliferation and secretion of splenic T lymphocytes in mice. Regul Pept, 122, 173-178.

Yamamoto, K., Takiguchi, S., Miyata, H.,Miyazaki, Y., Hiura, Y., Yamasaki, M., Nakajima, K., Fujiwara, Y., Mori, M., Kangawa, K., & Doki, Y. (2013). Reduce plasma ghrelin levels on day 1 after esophagectomy: a ew predictor of prolonged systemic inflammatory response syndrome. Surg Todayy, 43, 48-54.

Yang, J., Brown, M. S., Liang, G., Grishin, N. V., & Goldstein, J. L. (2008). Identification of the Acyltransferase that Octanoylates Ghrelin, an Appetite-Stimulating Peptide Hormone. Cell, 132, 387-396.

Ybarra, J., Bobbioni-Harsch, E., Chassot, G., Huber, O., Morel, P., Assimacopoulos-Jeannet, F., & Golay, A. (2009). Persistent correlation of ghrelin plasma levels with body mass index both in stable weight conditions and during gastric-bypass-induced weight loss. Obes Surg, 19, 327-31.

Yeh, A. H., Jeffery, P. L., Duncan, R. P., Herington, A. C., & Chopin, L. K. (2005). Ghrelin and a novel preproghrelin isoform are highly expressed in prostate cancer and ghrelin activates mitogen-activated protein kinase in prostate cancer. Clin Cancer Res, 11, 8295-8303.

Yi, C.X., Heppner, K., & Tschöp, M.H. (2011). Ghrelin in eating disorders. Mol Cell Endocrinol, 340, 29-34.

Yu, M., Lizarzaburu, M., Beckmann, H., Connors, R., Dai, K., Haller, K., Li, C., Liang, L., Lindstrom, M., Ma, J., Motani, A., Wanska, M., Zhang, A., Li, L., & Medina, J.C. (2010). Identification of piperazine-bisamide GHSR antagonists for the treatment of obesity. Bioorg Med Chem Lett, 20, 1758-1762.

Zhang, W., Chen, M., Chen, X., Segura, B.J., Mulholland, M.W.. (2001). Inhibition of pancreatic protein secretion by ghrelin in the rat. J Physiol, 537, 231-236.

Zhang, N., Yuan, C., Li, Z., Li, J., Li, X., Li,C., Li, R., & Wang S.R. (2011). Meta-analysis of the relationship between obestatin and ghrelin levels and the ghrelin/obestatin ratio with respect to obesity. Am J Med Sci 341, 48-55.

Zhang, Q., Huang, W.D., Lv, X.Y., & Yang, Y.M. (2011). The association of ghrelin polymorphisms with coronary artery disease and ischemic chronic heart failure in an elderly Chinese population. Clin Biochem, 44, 386-390.

Zhang, R., Yang, G., Wang, Q., Guo, F., & Wang, H. (2013). Acylated ghrelin protects hippocampal neurons in pilocarpine-induced seizures of immature rats by inhibiting cell apoptosis. Mol Biol Rep, 40, 51-58.

Zhao, T.J., Liang, G., Li, R.L., Xie, X., Sleeman, M.W., Murphy, A.J., Valenzuela, D.M., Yancopoulos, G.D., Goldstein, J.L., & Brown, M.S. (2010). Ghrelin O-acyltransferase (GOAT) is essential for growth hormone-mediated survival of calorie-restricted mice. Proc Natl Acad Sc USA, 107, 7467-7472.

Zorrilla, E.P., Iwasaki, S., Moss, J.A., Chang, J., Otsuji, J., Inoue, K., Meijler, M.M., & Janda, K.D. (2006). Vaccination against weight gain. Proc Natl Acad Sci USA, 103, 13226-13331.

The Human Testis-Specific *PDHA2* Gene: Functional Role, Regulatory Mechanisms and Potential Therapeutic Target

Isabel Rivera
Research Institute for Medicines and Pharmaceutical Sciences (iMed.UL)
and Department of Biochemistry and Human Biology
Faculty of Pharmacy, University of Lisbon, Portugal

Ana Pinheiro
Research Institute for Medicines and Pharmaceutical Sciences (iMed.UL)
Faculty of Pharmacy, University of Lisbon, Portugal

Maria João Silva
Research Institute for Medicines and Pharmaceutical Sciences (iMed.UL)
and Department of Biochemistry and Human Biology
Faculty of Pharmacy, University of Lisbon, Portugal

Isabel Tavares de Almeida
Research Institute for Medicines and Pharmaceutical Sciences (iMed.UL)
Faculty of Pharmacy, University of Lisbon, Portugal

1   Introduction

Pyruvate Dehydrogenase Complex (PDC) Deficiency (PDCD) is a severe inborn error of metabolism that causes cell energy impairment, and predominantly results from mutations in *PDHA1* gene that encodes the crucial α subunit of the pyruvate dehydrogenase (PDH, aka E1). Albeit, there is a second isoform encoded by *PDHA2*, a testis-specific gene, whose putative activation in somatic tissues has been considered as a potential therapy for PDCD.

1.1   Structure and Function of the Pyruvate Dehydrogenase Complex

Pyruvate dehydrogenase complex (PDC) is a multienzyme system located in the mitochondrial matrix that fulfills a major role in aerobic energy metabolism (Robinson, 2001). This system (Figure 1) represents the critical link between glycolysis and the tricarboxylic acid cycle by catalyzing the conversion of pyruvate, mainly derived from dietary glucose, to acetyl-CoA, which is then further oxidized for energy production or serves as substrate for biosynthetic processes (Patel & Harris, 1995).

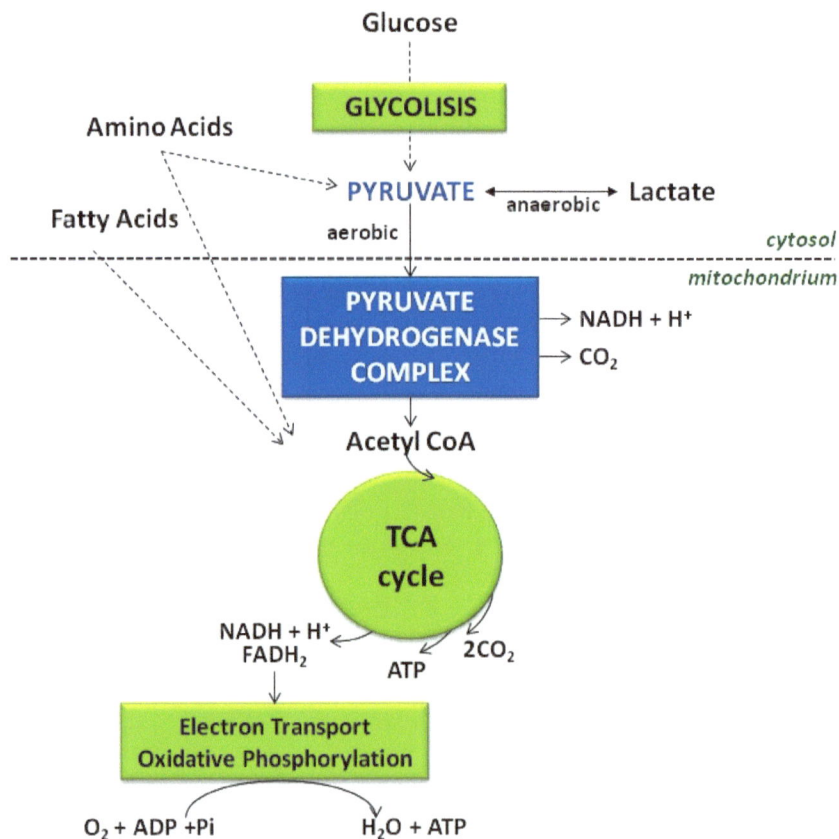

Figure 1: Cellular localization of pyruvate dehydrogenase complex (PDC) and its relationships with energy metabolism. PDC links glycolysis to tricarboxylic acid (TCA) cycle by converting pyruvate derived from carbohydrates (mainly glucose) into acetyl-CoA. Subsequently, acetyl-CoA is metabolized in the TCA cycle, which presents a central role in the chemical conversion of carbohydrates, fatty acids and amino acids into carbon dioxide, water and usable energy (ATP) by cooperation with the electron transport chain (adapted from Patel &Harris, 1995).

PDC is one of the largest and more intricate multienzyme structures ever known. The nuclear encoded mammalian complex, with a molecular mass of 9.5 million Da, is composed by multiple copies of three catalytic, one structural and two regulatory components: pyruvate dehydrogenase (E1), dihydrolipoyl acetyltransferase (E2), dihydrolipoyl dehydrogenase (E3); E3 binding protein (E3BP); pyruvate dehydrogenase kinase (PDK) and pyruvate dehydrogenase phosphatase (PDP).

Pyruvate dehydrogenase or E1 (EC 1.2.4.1) is the first component of PDC and performs the rate limiting reaction, the decarboxylation of pyruvate and the reductive acetylation of lipoyl moieties of E2 subunit. Mammalian E1 is a heterotetramer composed of two α and two β subunits (43 and 36 kDa, respectively) (Ciszak et al., 2001). This enzyme presents two catalytic sites, each requiring a thiamine pyrophosphate (TPP) molecule and a magnesium ion as cofactors. Each α subunit binds magnesium ion and pyrophosphate fragment, while each β subunit binds the pyrimidine fragment of TPP, thus originating one catalytic site at the interface of each α/β dimer (Ciszak et al., 2003). E1 subunit is also responsible for global PDC regulation, which relies on a mechanism of dephosphorylation (activation) / phosphorylation (inactivation) acting upon 3 specific serine residues in the E1α subunit (Korotchkina & Patel, 2001).

The E1α subunit exists as two isoforms encoded by two different genes, *PDHA1* and *PDHA2*, whose sequences display 87% identity and 93% homology. The *PDHA1* gene is located on Xp22.1, contains 11 exons, spans approximately 17 kb of genomic DNA and is selectively expressed in somatic tissues. Additionally, an autosomal *locus*, *PDHA2*, lies on chromosome 4 (4q22-23), completely lacks introns, spans 1.4 kb of genomic DNA and displays characteristics of a functional processed gene; it is expressed only in testis after the onset of spermatogenesis (Dahl et al., 1990). In marsupials, there is only one copy of the gene encoding the E1α subunit of PDC which, after the marsupials/eutherians divergence, was translocated to the little arm of chromosome X, thus corresponding to *PDHA1* gene. However, the X-inactivation during spermatogenesis originated the evolution, by retrotransposition to an autosome, of a second testis-specific gene, *PDHA2* (Fitzgerald et al., 1993; Fitzgerald et al., 1996).

Comparative analysis of PDHA1 and PDHA2 protein sequences revealed the presence of highly conserved sequences mainly in determinant regions, such as the thiamine pyrophosphate binding motif and the phosphorylation sites. The existence of 47 different amino acids, 26 of which correspond to non-homologous substitutions, could antecipate drastic differences between both isoform activities. Nevertheless, Korotchkina and coworkers (2006) proved that PDHA1 and PDHA2 proteins display similar kinetic properties and regulation mechanisms.

Besides serine phosphorylation/dephosphorylation, the main regulatory mechanism of PDC activity, at least PDHA2 protein is also subject to tyrosine phosphorylation, a post-translational modification that seems implicated in sperm capacitation (Kumar et al., 2006 and 2008).

PDC plays a crucial role in cell energy metabolism, particularly in those tissues that obtain almost all their energy from carbohydrates. This is the case of the brain, which is higly dependent on aerobic oxidation of glucose for energy production. Furthermore, also the spermatogenic cells are likely to be more dependent on PDC function.

1.2 Spermatogenesis, a Highly Energy Demanding Biological Process

Spermatogenesis is a complex biological process of cellular transformation that produces male haploid germ cells from diploid spermatogonial stem cells. This cell differentiation occurs within seminiferous tubule boundaries of the testis and involves different stages such as mitosis, meiosis and spermiogenesis. Briefly, spermatogenesis begins when primitive type A spermatogonia proliferate by mitosis into type A and type B cells. Type B cells then sequentially differentiate into primary spermatocytes, which after two stages of meiosis result in haploid round spermatids. Finally, round spermatids undergo marked morphological differentiation to become mature sperm.

During spermatogenesis, spermatogenic cells go through meiotic divisions and become haploid, so half the cells will not contain an X chromosome. In addition, the X chromosome is inactivated early in spermatogenesis, so even those cells containing an X chromosome appear not to express the X-linked genes. A significant number of testis-specific genes are autosomal intronless genes arising from retrotransposition of parental gene transcripts (Brosius, 1999), and a disproportionately large number of putative parental genes are found on the X chromosome (Emerson *et al.*, 2004). Though retrogenes generally give rise to pseudogenes, it has been suggested that the late stage of spermatogenesis must provide an appropriate environment facilitating retroposon transcription and gene expression from promoter-like sequences (Kato & Nozali, 2012).

The X chromosome location of the normally expressed E1α gene (*PDHA1*) could represent a serious setback for energy production in sperm. Nevertheless, this problem is by-passed by the existance of the autosomal retroprocessed *PDHA2* gene which thus allows the accomplishment of energy requirements in these cells. This complex process requires the coordinated expression of a number of testis-specific genes. The understanding of the regulatory mechanisms underlying these genes' expression is crucial and the testis-specific gene that codes for the E1α subunit was soon pointed out as a reliable model to elucidate gene regulation during spermatogenesis (Iannello *et al.*, 1995).

The first approach to understand E1α testis-specific gene was performed in mouse, rather than in human. The reason underlying this choice was not only due to the relatively easy access to mouse tissues, but also because germ cell differentiation in mouse development is synchronized as the mouse proceeds towards sexual maturity, which provides an excellent opportunity to examine the temporal expression of genes in mouse testis. As a consequence, the transcriptional and translational expression patterns of the testis-specific and somatic forms of E1α subunit genes have already been studied in detail in mouse testis (Takakubo & Dahl, 1992).

Briefly, *Pdha2* transcripts were found in all spermatocytes and spermatids stages with a particular increased level in pachytene spermatocytes. In contrast, the expression of *Pdha1* was only detected in those cells where *Pdha2* expression was not detected (spermatogonia, Leydig and Sertoli cells). Immunostaining with a specific anti-E1α antibody showed that the synthesis of E1α protein was dramatically increased in primary spermatocytes, reaching the highest abundance in pachytene spermatocytes. The amount of protein remained at high levels throughout spermiogenesis; however, it remarkably declined in epididymal spermatozoa. Also, spermatogonia, Leydig and Sertoli cells displayed low levels of E1α protein. These results suggest that the transcriptional switch from the somatic *Pdha1* to the testis-specific *Pdha2* gene occurs during the first meiotic prophase of spermatogenesis, and also that the E1α protein involved in the development of spermatogenic cells is coded for by the *Pdha2* gene (Takakubo & Dahl, 1992).

Moreover, two transcripts for *Pdha2* have been identified. In the early stages of *Pdha2* expression, a 2.0 kb mRNA is the only form evident; however, as spermatogenesis proceeds and the mouse enters sexual maturity, a second smaller transcript becomes apparent. This smaller 1.7 kb transcript is produced in haploid cells and results from the use of an alternative polyadenylation signal (Fitzgerald *et al.*, 1992; Iannello & Dahl, 1992). Although the functional implications of transcript shortening are not clearly understood, it was suggested it might facilitate long-term stability of the mRNA (Young *et al.*, 1998).

A recent study of *PDHA2* gene during human spermatogenesis (Pinheiro *et al.*, 2012a) showed that the switch from the X-linked (*PDHA1*) to the autosomic (*PDHA2*) gene expression occurs at the spermatocyte stage. The results clearly revealed that the protein is localized in the cytoplasm of almost all cell types, thus confirming previous reports. However, in secondary spermatocytes and round spermatids a nuclear localization is apparent. These data, allied to a study highlighting the crucial involvement of PDHA2 in the process of hamster sperm capacitation, reporting the simultaneous extramitochondrial localization and tyrosine phosphorylation of PDHA2 in human spermatozoa (Kumar *et al.*, 2006 and 2008), seem to suggest that PDHA2 might also have a potential role in human sperm capacitation. The activation of *PDHA2* gene expression is most probably a mechanism to ensure the continued expression of the protein, thus allowing germ cell viability and functionality.

1.3   Pyruvate Dehydrogenase Deficiency: Causes, Consequences and Treatment

Pyruvate Dehydrogenase Complex Deficiency (PDCD) is one of the most common genetic disorders associated with an abnormal mitochondrial metabolism. PDCD results from a reduction in the enzymatic activity of PDC and leads to energy deprivation, especially in the central nervous system (Blass *et al.*, 1970).

PDCD can be caused by mutations in any of the genes encoding the complex subunits. Though defects may occur in all of its proteins, the E1α subunit is predominantly the culprit. Concerning all PDCD reported mutations, around 70% are assigned to *PDHA1* gene (OMIM #312170), and more than a half are of missense type. As the majority of mutations occur in the X-linked *PDHA1* gene, an X-linked pattern of inheritance is observed, but the number of affected males and females is similar (Dahl *et al.*, 1992). PDCD is a rare disorder being most of mutations sporadic ones and the recurrence rate very low.

Nevertheless, the true occurrence of this disorder is unknown because mild mutations may be asymptomatic, especially in females. The variability of the phenotype in heterozygous females appears to be largely determined by differences in X-inactivation patterns (Brown *et al.*, 1994; Willemsen *et al.*, 2006). Moreover, it has been observed that male patients who survived the neonatal period and early infancy generally have a milder phenotype, which seems inconsistent with a general rule of most X-linked dominant diseases (i.e. hemizygous male patients usually have a more severe phenotype than heterozygous female patients). A possible explanation for this apparent discrepancy may be that males carrying a mutant *PDHA1* allele that leads to severe deficiency of the enzyme are selected antenatally and, consequently, only male patients who harbor a milder mutant *PDHA1* allele survive the neonatal period. In females, on the other hand, possession of a mutant allele leading to severe enzyme deficiency could still be consistent with a live birth, depending on the pattern of X-inactivation; such individuals would then present a more severe phenotype than male patients who have the mild phenotype (Wada *et al.*, 2004).

Not only PDCD results in severe energy impairment, but it is also one of the major causes of lactic acidosis in children. The clinical presentation is extremely heterogeneous, with a spectrum ranging from fatal lactic acidosis in the newborn period to a chronic neurodegenerative condition. The primary phenotypic manifestation is the impairment of neurological function and/or development, but a wide range of clinical characteristics may be observed: hypotonia, seizures, CNS degeneration and malformations, ataxia, respiratory alterations (apnea, hypoventilation), facial dysmorphic features (narrow head, frontal bossing, wide narrow bridge), peripheral and skeletal/cardiac neuropathy. Several authors classify the phenotype in three major categories, according to the observed severity: neonatal, infantile and benign (Brown *et al.*, 1994; Wexler *et al.*, 1997).

The current available therapy for PDCD relies on a palliative treatment aiming to stimulate PDC activity, to provide alternative fuels or to correct acidosis. However, it rarely influences the course of the disease and merely prevents the acute worsening of the syndrome. Ketogenic diets, that minimize carbohydrate and maximize fat daily intake, have been used to control lactic acidosis with minimal success. Although the ketogenic diet may reduce the blood levels of lactic acid and extend lifespan, CNS metabolic abnormalities persist, as evidenced by high lactic acid levels in the cerebrospinal fluid and progressive neurological degeneration. Moreover, due to the dependence of the brain on glucose as a fuel, this type of diet increases CNS vulnerability (Wexler *et al.*, 1997; Weber *et al.*, 2001).

In order to optimize PDC function, the standard care option is diet supplementation with cofactors, such as thiamine, carnitine, and lipoic acid. In selected PDCD cases, caused by the so-called thiamine-responsive mutations, high doses of thiamine are particularly effective and a more favorable outcome can be expected for these extremely rare patients (Robinson *et al.*, 1996). There is some evidence that dichloroacetate, which inhibits PDKs and thereby activates any residual functioning complex, will also reduce the metabolic disturbance in some patients but, again, this is rarely accompanied by any objective improvement in neurological performance (Berendzen *et al.*, 2006).

Despite these therapeutic approaches, all directed to correction of the phenotype, it is clear they are insufficient and that new avenues must be open, namely at the genotype level.

However, and specifically for most PDCD cases which are caused by mutations in the *PDHA1* gene, the potential therapy referred by several authors (Robinson *et al.*, 1996; Datta *et al.*, 1999) would be the somatic activation of the autosomic *PDHA2* gene that encodes the E1α subunit in spermatogenic cells. The activation of *PDHA2* gene in somatic cells would allow circumventing the absence or inactivation of the altered PDHA1 subunit.

1.4 DNA Methylation as a Pivotal Epigenetic Mechanism Regulating Tissue-Specific Gene Expression

DNA methylation is the most common eukaryotic DNA modification and probably the most extensively studied epigenetic mark. It plays important roles in embryonic development, transcription, chromatin structure, X chromosome inactivation, genomic imprinting, chromosome stability and in the silencing of retrotransposon, repetitive elements and tissue-specific genes (Lister *et al.*, 2009).

The patterns of DNA methylation are established and maintained by the interplay of different DNA methyltransferases (DNMTs) (Jurkowska *et al.*, 2011), which catalyze the transfer of the methyl group from S-adenosylmethionine to the cytosine in CpG dinucleotides, thus originating 5-methylcytosine (5mC) - the 5th base of the genome (Bestor, 2000). During early embryogenesis, *de novo* DNA methylation is mediated by DNMT3A and DNMT3B associated with DNMT3L (Okano *et al.*, 1999; Jia *et al.*, 2007). To maintain patterns of DNA methylation in daughter cells, the hemi-methylated DNA is methylated by DNMT1, which methylates the appropriate cytosine in newly synthesized DNA strands during successive replications (Goyal *et al.*, 2006). Other studies suggest that DNMT3A/B are also required for the maintenance of patterns of DNA methylation in somatic cells, particularly of repeat regions and imprinted genes (Jeong *et al.*, 2009).

After the studies of Datta and collaborators (1999) it emerged the idea that additional mechanisms, such as DNA methylation, could be underlying the human *PDHA2* transcriptional regulation, but yet no studies were further performed.

Nevertheless, the involvement of DNA methylation has already been proved to be operative in the mouse *Pdha2* gene. Actually, Iannello and co-workers, in 1997, showed a correlation between CpG hypomethylation within the core promoter and *Pdha2* transcription level. Although how CpG methylation inactivates the *Pdha2* promoter *in vivo* was still uncertain, one possibility was that it could alter the conformational arrangement of DNA by increasing its helical pitch, thereby affecting transcription factor binding to its cognate site (Iannello *et al.*, 1997).

A later study of this group proved that the methylation-dependent repression of the *Pdha2* core promoter is mediated regionally through the ATF/CREB consensus binding site (Iannello et al., 2000), a regulatory element that was never identified in the human *PDHA2* promoter. These authors found that targeting of the CpG dinucleotide within this *cis*-element significantly disrupted the ability of the basal promoter to activate gene expression *in vitro* and completely abolished promoter activity *in vivo*. Moreover, these CpG dinucleotides in the flanking region of the ATF/CREB binding site appeared to confer some conformational structure to the promoter, since mutations at these specific CpG dinucleotides resulted in elevated basal levels of transcription. This raised the possibility of a potential bifunctional role for CpG dinucleotides in either methylation-dependent or -independent processes (Iannello *et al.*, 2000).

Further studies during mouse spermatogenesis showed that the pattern of CpG methylation in the *Pdha2* promoter varied according to the spermatogenic cell type. And once more, evidence was shown that gene activation during spermatogenesis might involve both hypomethylation and the availability of specific transcription factors, being hypomethylation an essential step prior to the availability of transcription factors (Sp1, YY1, MEP-2 binding factor, and ATF/CREB factors) in order for *Pdha2* expression to occur (Iannello *et al.*, 1997).

In conclusion, methylation appears to be an important mechanism by which transcriptional repression of *Pdha2* in somatic mouse tissue is achieved. Activation of testis-specific genes, in particular those which are temporarily expressed during spermatogenesis, such as *Pdha2*, is likely to require various levels of regulation, such as DNA hypomethylation and conformational alterations, and accessibility or availability of specific transcription factors.

2   Structure, Function and Regulation of *PDHA2* Gene

2.1   Methylation Status of *PDHA2* Gene

In silico analysis of *PDHA2* gene sequence (GenBank accession no. M86808; for sequence numbering, nucleotide +1 was assigned to the adenosine of the initiation translation codon ATG), encompassing the beginning of 5'UTR (nt -643) until the end of 3'UTR (nt +1347), revealed the presence of 61 CpG sites whose distribution matches the criteria for the presence of two CpG islands. Island I spans 201 bp, beginning in the core promoter region and extending downstream into the open reading frame (nucleotides -128 to +73), contains nineteen CpG sites (9th to 27th), five of which inside the coding region. Island II spans 263 bp exclusively inside the coding region (nucleotides +197 to +460) and contains fourteen CpG sites (31st to 44th). Almost half the CpG sites are part of CpG islands, and the distribution of the remaining is the following one: eight are upstream island I, three are between the two islands and the other seventeen sites are located downstream island II (Figure 2) (Pinheiro *et al.*, 2010).

The methylation status of these two CpG islands shows several differences, either between islands or among tissues (Figure 3). Regarding CpG island I, all the nineteen sites are fully methylated, either in somatic tissues or in whole testis tissue. Additionally, a CpG site not included in CpG island I (7th site) and localized in the consensus binding sequence for the Sp1 transcription factor, also displays a

Figure 2: Schematic representation of the *PDHA2* gene showing the distribution of the 61 CpG sites and the localization of the 2 CpG islands.

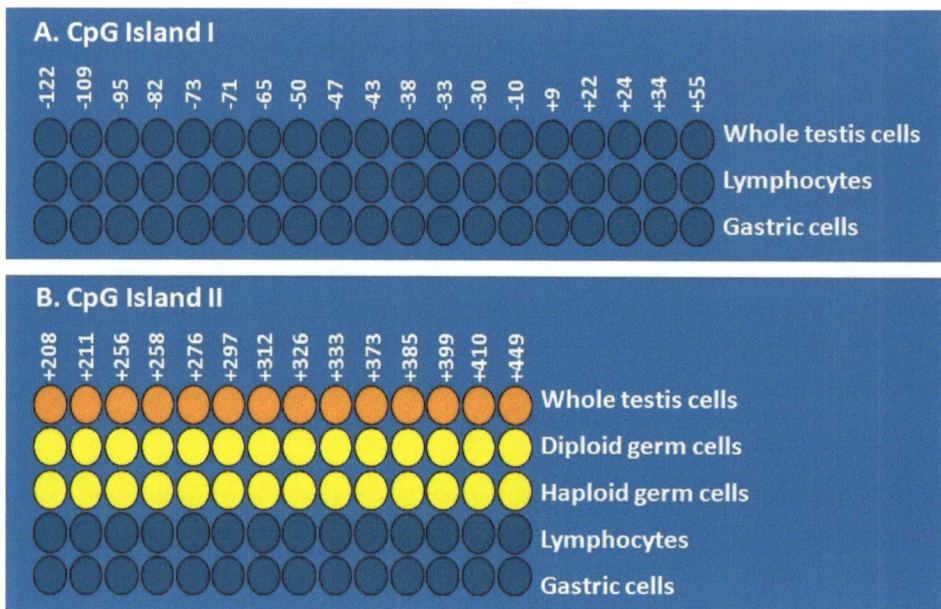

Figure 3: Methylation profiles of the 2 CpG islands present in the testis-specific *PDHA2* gene. A. CpG island I (19 sites); B. CpG island II (14 sites). Blue circles – full methylation; yellow circles – full demethylation; orange circles – half methylation.

completely methylated status in all types of tissues. The CpG island II presents, in somatic tissues, all the fourteen sites in a fully methylated status, while in whole testis tissue, a mixture of somatic and germ cells, methylated and unmethylated cytosines are present. Nevertheless, diploid and haploid germ cells display all the CpG sites fully demethylated (Pinheiro *et al.*, 2010).

2.2   *PDHA2* Gene Shows a Tissue-specific Expression

PDHA1 and *PDHA2* genes have distinct patterns of mRNA and protein expression, according to cell type. *PDHA1* gene is transcribed in all somatic tissues analysed til now, such as lymphocytes, fibroblasts, liver, whole testis, Sertoli cells and diploid and haploid germ cell fractions. Curiously, whole testis samples and both germ cell fractions reveal two additional smaller transcripts, while in pure somatic tissues only the wild-type messenger is visualized. *PDHA2* transcription is only detected in whole testis tissue and in diploid and haploid germ cell fractions (Pinheiro *et al.*, 2010).

During human spermatogenesis, *PDHA2* mRNA is first detected in spermatogonia and spermato-cytes (diploid germ cell fraction), its levels progressively increase in spermatids and testicular spermato-zoa (haploid germ cell fraction) reaching the highest levels in ejaculated spermatozoa. The X and Y chromosomes are subjected to meiotic sex chromosome inactivation (MSCI) at the pachytene level, and are later maintained in a repressive state during spermiogenesis. In this context and as expression of X-linked genes are still active in spermatogonia, a decline of *PDHA1* mRNA expression after the spermato-gonial stage is observed, being nearly undetectable in ejaculated sperm. Accordingly, a complementary expression pattern of the *PDHA2* gene in relation to *PDHA1* is observed as spermatogenesis progresses (Pinheiro *et al.*, 2012a).

Due to the high homology between PDHA1 and PDHA2 proteins, the detection of each PDHA iso-form by western blot analysis is hampered by the absence of specific antibodies. However, two-dimensional electrophoresis showed that somatic tissues only display the PDHA1 isoform, while the PDHA2 isoform is the only species observed in spermatozoa, but showing a shorter isoform with 32 kDa. Curiously, whole testis homogenate reveal the presence of both isoforms, the canonical PDHA1 with 43 kDa and the smaller PDHA2 with 32 kDa band, previously observed in germ cells (Pinheiro *et al.*, 2012a). Furthermore, immunohistochemistry in human testis sections reveals that PDHA proteins are localized in the cytoplasm, with the exception of secondary spermatocytes and round spermatids where a nuclear lo-calization is apparent. Spermatogonia display low levels of labeling, a strong staining is observed in pri-mary spermatocytes, secondary spermatocytes and round spermatids, and a low level of labeling is found in elongated spermatids. The supporting Sertoli cells display low levels of staining, whilst Leydig cells show mild levels and peritubular cells reveal an absence of staining (Pinheiro *et al.*, 2012a).

2.3   PDHA2 Gene Expression Correlates with Methylation Status

Comparing data originated from bisulfate sequencing with qRT-PCR and bidimensional electrophoresis analyses, reveals that *PDHA2* gene expression correlates with the methylation status of the coding region, being its full demethylation a pre-requisite to transcription initiation (Pinheiro *et al.*, 2010, 2012a and 2012b).

The methylation status of the CpG island I reveals similar results either for expressing testis tissue or for non-expressing somatic tissues, showing that all CpG sites are fully methylated, even those sites located in sequences thought to be important for regulation of *PDHA2* gene expression, namely the bind-ing sites for putative transcription factors (Datta *et al.*, 1999). The 7th CpG site, being part of the Sp1 binding sequence and located upstream of island I, revealed to be fully methylated in all types of tissues. The same result was observed for the 11th and 12th sites which closely flank the consensus binding se-quence for the MEP-2 transcription factor; previous studies by DNase footprinting analysis, using nuclear extracts of rat testis and liver, have shown that this region was protected in both situations (Datta *et al.*, 1999; Iannello *et al.*, 1993). Moreover, and most interestingly, it has been described a sequence that was protected only by rat testis extract (Datta *et al.*, 1999) and this sequence displays three CpG sites: sites 13th to 15th, all of them displaying full methylation, either in testis or in somatic samples that we have analyzed.

Therefore, the methylated status of the *PDHA2* core promoter region and the presence of the re-spective transcript in whole testis tissue and diploid and haploid germ cells suggest that the proteins re-sponsible for transcription initiation should not be sensitive to methylation of their binding sites, which has already been demonstrated for Sp1 transcription factors (Singal & Ginder, 1999). All these results underscore the notion that demethylation of the *PDHA2* core promoter region must not be a prerequisite for transcription initiation and, accordingly, must not be involved in the regulation of tissue-specific expression of *PDHA2* gene.

On the contrary, the exonic CpG island II displays distinct methylation status in somatic and testis cells, thus suggesting its importance for promoter activity. All the CpG sites are completely methylated in somatic tissues, which do not express the *PDHA2* transcript. The samples derived from whole testicular biopsy pieces show a mixture of methylated and unmethylated cytosines, which matches the fact that these samples contain not only germ cells but also somatic ones (Sertoli and Leydig cells). The samples prepared from a Sertoli cell only syndrome piece reveal the exclusively presence of methylated cytosines, thus correlating with the absence of *PDHA2* transcript.

The complete demethylation observed for all CpG sites in the exonic island II, either in diploid or haploid germ cells, showed a perfect correlation with this tissue-specific gene transcription and these results agree with previous observations by Dahl and collaborators of the *PDHA2* transcript being the predominant species in testis (Dahl *et al.*, 1990). Those authors suggested that not only those spermatocytes and spermatids with a Y chromosome, but also those with an X chromosome, express the testis-specific *PDHA2* gene. However, Pinheiro and collaborators (2010) could also detect residual levels of *PDHA1* transcript in these two cell types and this raises the question of its origin: only X chromosome containing cells or minimal transcriptional activity in all cells? The haploid germ cell samples used, being a mixture of X- and Y-chromosome cell types, preclude the complete elucidation of this point, though the results seem to point out the second hypothesis as the most likely (Pinheiro *et al.*, 2010).

2.4   *PDHA2* Gene Expression is Mainly Regulated by an Epigenetic Mechanism: Demethylation of its Coding Region

As previously seen, human *PDHA2* gene expression is restricted to post-meiotic germ cells suggesting the absence of positive modulating factors and/or the presence of repressors in somatic tissues. However, the lack of suitable human spermatogenic germ cell lines makes it difficult to easily elucidate the regulatory mechanisms involved upon *PDHA2* expression.

The first step towards understanding the regulation of a particular gene is the identification of regulatory elements and factors involved in basal expression. Functional analysis of the *PDHA2* gene promoter shows that *PDHA2* promoter-directed transcription of the luciferase reporter gene occurs in cultured somatic cells (HeLa, NT2 and SH-SY5Y), where *PDHA2* mRNA is undetectable. Deletion analysis further reveals that the region spanning from -122 to -6 is indispensable for basal expression of this TATA-less promoter. Moreover, and in each cell line, no significant differences are found among the reporter gene activities driven by all the other *PDHA2* deletion promoter constructs and, additionally, each construct displayed comparable reporter activities in the three different somatic cell lines (Pinheiro *et al.*, 2012b).

These observations suggest that the mechanisms involved in the repression of *PDHA2* expression in somatic cells are not operative when the core promoter or the 5' flanking region are transiently transfected into somatic cells. Moreover, these results corroborated the previous transactivation experiments described by Datta and colleagues (1999), who also observed *PDHA2* promoter-directed transcription in human hepatocellular carcinoma cells. Additionally, the same authors suggested the existence of a putative Sp responsive element that would be important for Sp1-dependent transcription initiation (Datta *et al.*, 1999). However, Pinheiro and collaborators using immunoprecipitation assays could not demonstrate any binding of Sp1 transcription factors to the proximal promoter of the *PDHA2* gene.

Additionally, and more importantly, the observation that *PDHA2* promoter reporter constructs presented high luciferase activity in all somatic cell lines, where the *PDHA2* mRNA cannot be detected, reinforces the idea that *PDHA2* tissue-specific expression may be under strict control of epigenetic mechanisms of regulation. Effectively, *in vitro* methylation of *PDHA2* promoter constructs with *Sss*I methylase results in a complete abrogation of luciferase activity (Pinheiro *et al.*, 2012b).

The involvement of epigenetics, namely DNA methylation and/or histone modifications, on the regulation of *PDHA2* gene expression was showed by treatment of eukaryotic cell lines with a potent inhibitor of the *de novo* methylation (5-Aza-2'-deoxycytidine or DAC) and with a pharmacological inhibitor of histone deacetylases (Trichostain A or TSA). Pinheiro and collaborators (2012b) showed that treatment of SH-SY5Y cell cultures with DAC induces *PDHA2* derepression with a concomitant accumulation of *PDHA2* transcript. On the other hand, inhibition of histone deacetylation does not elicit any induction of *PDHA2* expression, nor does it potentiate the DAC effect (Figure 4).

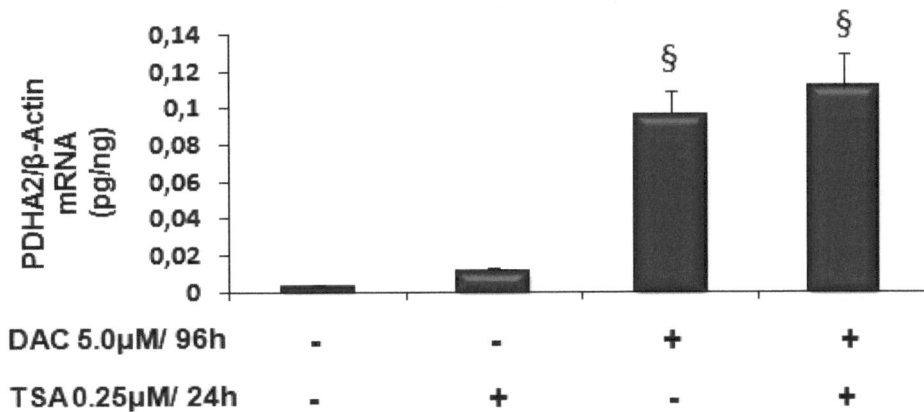

Figure 4: DAC increases *PDHA2* mRNA levels in SH-SY5Y cells. Real-time PCR analysis of *PDHA2* steady-state mRNA transcript levels in SH-SY5Y cells treated 5 μM DAC for 96 h and/or 0.25 μM TSA for 24 h. Values were normalized to the internal standard β-actin. Data represent means ± SEM of at least three independent experiments and was expressed as pg of *PDHA2* mRNA per ng of β-actin mRNA (§ $p < 0.01$).

Moreover, the accumulation of the *PDHA2* mRNA after DAC treatment correlates with an enrichment of RNA pol II at the *PDHA2* proximal promoter (+1 bp region), which likely triggers the observed increase in *PDHA2* mRNA levels. The fact that treatment with DAC alone elicits a significant effect upon *PDHA2* gene expression suggests that changes associated with methylation are sufficient to drive transcription initiation of this testis-specific gene in somatic cells (Pinheiro *et al.*, 2012b).

Once proved that DAC is able to induce *PDHA2* gene expression in cultured somatic cells, it was also shown that demethylation underlies *PDHA2* transcription. Effectively, DAC promotes a relevant demethylation of *PDHA2* coding region, which was fully methylated before treatment. However, the promoter CpG island I remains fully methylated, suggesting its insensibility to demethylation, at least by DAC treatment in the tested conditions (Pinheiro *et al.*, 2012b). These findings corroborate previous reported results, where was observed that *PDHA2* expressing tissues (i.e spermatogenic cells) present the coding region completely demethylated, while non-expressing tissues display it fully methylated

(Pinheiro *et al.*, 2010).

However, in 2011, Yamashita and colleagues identified multiple transcriptional start sites downstream of the canonical one (+248, +253 and +269), which are located precisely within the CpG island II region (nucleotides +197 to +460). Accordingly, this region could eventually harbor alternative promoter that would trigger the transcription of truncated *PDHA2* mRNAs. However, it was clearly shown that DAC induces transcription of full-length transcripts, data corroborated by the significant enrichment of RNA pol II at the proximal promoter (Pinheiro *et al.*, 2012b).

All these data confirm that methylation of the coding region is a key point in somatic cell silencing of *PDHA2* gene. Actually, DNA methylation appears to be particularly suitable for the regulation of germ line-specific genes, and this is probably related to the global demethylation process that occurs during the development of spermatogenic cells, which may provide the mechanism by which these germ line-specific genes are demethylated (Rocamora & Mezquita, 1989; del Mazo *et al.*, 1994). And, despite the fact that DNA methylation does not seem to be the primary control mechanism regulating the programmed expression of most tissue-specific genes resulting in tissue differentiation, there are several examples that indicate that DNA methylation can serve as the primary control mechanism for the expression of a number of germ line-specific genes (Choi & Chae, 1991; de Smet *et al.*, 1999; Kroft *et al.*, 2001).

Although the expression of previously referred genes proceeds *via* a promoter methylation-dependent mechanism, we also can find in the literature some references to human genes that are regulated by methylation of the coding region, namely monocarboxylate transporter MCT3 (Zhu *et al.*, 2005). Another particular interesting example is the mouse *Tact1/Actl7* gene (Hisano *et al.*, 2003), which is also intronless and testis-specific, like the *PDHA2* gene.

Indeed, it has already been described that methylation of the coding region, *per se*, can control gene expression by preventing promoter activity at the level of the chromatin structure. Indeed, CpG methylation induces a local repressive chromatin structure, mediated by the binding of methyl-CpG binding domain (MBD) proteins which recruit other proteins including sin3A and histone deacetylase; when a sufficient amount of CpGs is methylated, this repression is transmissible in *cis*, spreading for several hundred base pairs (Keshet *et al.*, 1985; Kass *et al.*, 1997; Bird & Wolfe, 1999). Accordingly, more or less distant methylated sequences, like the *PDHA2* coding region, can promote gene repression. Interestingly, and as stated by Nan and co-workers, this type of repression is greater if the promoter itself is methylated (Nan *et al.*, 1997), which is the case of *PDHA2* promoter.

Furthermore, it has also been postulated that methylation of the coding region can inhibit gene expression by interfering with the elongation step rather than with transcription initiation, by causing RNA pol II to pause or to prematurely terminate (Graessmann *et al.*, 1994; Choi *et al.*, 2009). Moreover, the inhibitory effect upon elongation is prominent when methylation occurs near the start codon (Hohn *et al.*, 1996). Pinheiro and collaborators (2012b) explored the elongation of *PDHA2* transcription by chromatin immunoprecipitation assays, but no significant particular differences were observed in the chromatin recovered before and after DAC treatment, namely when using the elongation marker H3K36me3. A recent report has shown a clear correlation between H3K36me3 marking and transcriptional activity in intron-containing genes; however, in intronless genes H3K36me3 is detected at much lower levels irrespective of expression levels (de Almeida *et al.*, 2011). Indeed, there are other examples showing that transcriptional elongation is differently controlled in intronless genes when compared to longer intron-containing genes (Medlin *et al.*, 2005). Accordingly, because *PDHA2* gene lacks introns, different approaches need to be designed.

3   Conclusion

PDHA2 gene activation in somatic tissues has been postulated as a conceptual therapy for PDC deficiencies caused by *PDHA1* gene mutations (Robinson *et al.*, 1996; Datta *et al.*, 1999). Accordingly, it is crucial to understand the mechanisms controlling human *PDHA2* tissue-specific expression, namely what factors are responsible for the silencing of this gene in somatic tissues, and its activation in spermatogenic ones (diploid and haploid germ cells). However, the lack of a suitable cell line to study the regulatory mechanisms underlying *PDHA2* gene expression has hampered this elucidation for a long time.

The opportunity to study its expression during human spermatogenesis, allowed us to suggest that the *PDHA2* gene most probably belongs, not only to a restricted group of germ line-specific genes that use DNA methylation as a primary silencing mechanism, but to a unique subset of those genes whose expression is regulated by the methylation status of the coding region. Unfortunately, literature is very scarce concerning the study of regulatory mechanisms underlying human testis-specific genes, thus hampering the identification of common regulatory strategies.

There are several proteins that present specific isoforms in male germ cells, such as phosphoglycerate kinase (PGK2) and lactate dehydrogenase (LDHC) among others, which curiously are mainly related to glycolysis and pyruvate metabolism (Eddy, 2002; Liu *et al.*, 2011). These testis-specific isoforms, besides compensating for other genes that may be inactivated in spermatogenesis, may also have additional structural or functional properties that serve unique roles in male germ cells. Then, the PDHA2 protein can have as well other properties beyond energy production, as in hamster sperm capacitation (Kumar *et al.*, 2008). Recently, Hereng and coworkers (2011) showed that, for fertilization, human spermatozoa rely substantially on ATP derived from glycolysis, and not from oxidative phosphorylation, thus reinforcing the previous hypothesis. These data open up new research lines to investigate PDHA2 protein function in sperm.

Furthermore, these new insights on the regulatory mechanism underlying *PDHA2* tissue-specific expression effectively open potential therapeutic avenues for PDC deficiency caused by *PDHA1* mutations. In 1996, Robinson and colleagues, following transfection studies with recombinant proteins, showed that PDHA2 is able to form functional heterotetramers with the E1β subunit. However, when both isoforms, PDHA1 and PDHA2, are produced in equal amounts, a reduction in PDC activity is observed, suggesting that the testis-specific protein is not fully compatible with the somatic isoform when the mixed tetramers were assembled. As previously referred, most disease-causing mutations in *PDHA1* gene are missense ones, originating absence or reduced protein levels. Consequently, the activation of *PDHA2* gene expression in somatic cells, originating a functional protein, could eventually contribute to correct or at least to ameliorate the PDCD phenotype.

Finally, a screening among our patients carrying mutations in *PDHA1* gene revealed the absence of *PDHA2* transcripts and hence protein in all blood samples, showing that the somatic activation of this testis-specific isoform is not a normal or natural compensatory mechanism. This observation is reinforced by a study on PGK deficiency due to PGK1 mutations which failed to show the somatic activation of its testis counterpart, PGK2 (Fermo *et al.*, 2012).

In summary, though some light has been shed upon regulation of *PDHA2* gene expression, a long way is still to be run concerning the elucidation of its real function(s) in spermatogenic cells, as well as the feasibility and effectiveness of its somatic activation as a new therapeutic approach in PDCD.

References

Berendzen, K., Theriaque, D.W., Shuster, J., Stacpoole, P.W. (2006). *Therapeutic potential of dichloroacetate for pyruvate dehydrogenase complex deficiency. Mitochondrion, 6(3), 126-135.*

Bestor, T.H. (2000). *The DNA methyltransferases of mammals. Human Molecular Genetics, 9(16), 2395-2402.*

Bird, A.P. & Wolffe, A.P. (1999) *Methylation-induced repression--belts, braces, and chromatin. Cell, 99, 451-454.*

Blass, J.P., Avigan, J., Uhlendorf, B.W. (1970). *A defect in pyruvate decarboxylase in a child with an intermittent movement disorder. Journal of Clinical Investigation, 49(3), 423-432.*

Brosius, J. (1999). *RNAs from all categories generate retrosequences that may be exapted as novel genes or regulatory elements. Gene, 238, 115-134.*

Brown, G.K., Otero, L.J., LeGris, M., Brown, R.M. (1994). *Pyruvate dehydrogenase deficiency. Journal of Medical Genetics, 31(11), 875-879.*

Choi, J.K., Bae, J.B., Lyu, J., Kim, T.Y., Kim, Y.J. (2009). *Nucleosome deposition and DNA methylation at coding region boundaries. Genome Biology, 10, R89.*

Choi, Y.C. & Chae, C.B. (1991). *DNA hypomethylation and germ cell-specific expression of testis-specific H2B histone gene. Journal of Biological Chemistry, 266, 20504-20511.*

Ciszak, E., Korotchkina, L.G., Hong, Y.S., Joachimiak, A., Patel, M.S. (2001). *Crystallization and initial X-ray diffraction analysis of human pyruvate dehydrogenase. Acta Crystallographica section D: Biological Crystallography, 57(Pt 3), 465-468.*

Dahl, H.H., Brown, G.K., Brown, R.M., Hansen, L.L., Kerr, D.S., Wexler, I.D., Patel, M.S., De Meirleir, L., Lissens, W., Chun, K., MacKay, N., Robinson, B.H. (1992). *Mutations and polymorphisms in the pyruvate dehydrogenase E1 alpha gene. Human Mutatation, 1(2), 97-102.*

Dahl, H.H., Brown, R.M., Hutchison, W.M., Maragos, C., Brown, G.K. (1990). *A testis-specific form of the human pyruvate dehydrogenase E1 alpha subunit is coded for by an intronless gene on chromosome 4. Genomics, 8(2), 225-232.*

Datta, U., Wexler, I.D., Kerr, D.S., Raz, I., Patel, M.S. (1999). *Characterization of the regulatory region of the human testis-specific form of the pyruvate dehydrogenase alpha-subunit (PDHA-2) gene. Biochimica & Biophysica Acta, 1447, 236-243.*

de Almeida, S.F., Grosso, A.R., Koch, F., Fenouil, R., Carvalho, S., Andrade, J., Levezinho, H., Gut, M., Eick, D., Gut, I., Andrau, J.C., Ferrier, P., Carmo-Fonseca, M. (2011). *Splicing enhances recruitment of methyltransferase HYPB/Setd2 and methylation of histone H3 Lys36. Nature Structure & Molecular Biology, 18, 977-983.*

de Smet, C., Lurquin, C., Lethe, B., Martelange, V., Boon, T. (1999). *DNA methylation is the primary silencing mechanism for a set of germ line- and tumor-specific genes with a CpG-rich promoter. Molecular and Cellular Biology, 19, 7327-7335.*

del Mazo, J., Prantera, G., Torres, M., Ferraro, M. (1994). *DNA methylation changes during mouse spermatogenesis. Chromosome Research, 2, 147-152.*

Eddy, E.M. (2002). *Male germ cell gene expression. Recent Progress in Hormone Research, 57, 103-128.*

Emerson, J.J., Kacsmann, H., Betran, E, Long, M. (2004). *Extensive gene traffic on the mammalian X chromosome. Science, 303, 537-540.*

Fermo, E., Bianchi, P., Chiarelli, L.R., Maggi, M., Mandarà, G.M., Vercelatti, C., Marcello, A.P., Barcellini, W., Cortelezzi, A., Valentini, G., Zanella, A. (2012). *A novel variant of phosphoglycerate kinase deficiency (p.I371K) with multiple tissue involvement: molecular and functional characterization. Molecular Genetics and Metabolism, 160(4), 455-461.*

Fitzgerald, J., Hutchison, W.M., Dahl, H.H. (1992). *Isolation and characterisation of the mouse pyruvate dehydrogenase E1 alpha genes. Biochimica & Biophysica Acta, 1131(1), 83-90.*

Fitzgerald, J., Wilcox, S.A., Graves, J.A., Dahl, H.H. (1993). A eutherian X-linked gene, PDHA1, is autosomal in marsupials: a model for the evolution of a second, testis-specific variant in eutherian mammals. Genomics, 18(3), 632-642.

Fitzgerald, J., Dahl, H.H., Jakobsen, I.B., Easteal, S. (1996). Evolution of mammalian X-linked and autosomal Pgk and Pdh E1 alpha subunit genes. Molecular Biology and Evolution, 13(7), 1023-1031.

Goyal, R., Reinhardt, R., Jeltsch, A. (2006). Accuracy of DNA methylation pattern preservation by the Dnmt1 methyltransferase. Nucleic Acids Research, 34(4), 1182-1188.

Graessmann, A., Sandberg, G., Guhl, E., Graessmann, M. (1994). Methylation of single sites within the herpes simplex virus tk coding region and the simian virus 40 T-antigen intron causes gene inactivation. Molecular and Cellular Biology, 14, 2004-2010.

Hereng, T.H., Elgstøen, K.B.P., Cederkvist, F.H., Eide, L., Jahnsen, T., Skålhegg, B.S., Rosendal, K.R. (2011). Exogenous pyruvate accelerates glycolysis and promotes capacitation in human spermatozoa. Human Reproduction, 26(12), 3249-3263.

Hisano, M., Ohta, H., Nishimune, Y., Nozaki, M. (2003). Methylation of CpG dinucleotides in the open reading frame of a testicular germ cell-specific intronless gene, Tact1/Actl7b, represses its expression in somatic cells. Nucleic Acids Research, 31, 4797-4804.

Hohn, T., Corsten, S., Rieke, S., Muller, M., Rothnie, H. (1996). Methylation of coding region alone inhibits gene expression in plant protoplasts. Proceedings of the National Academy of Sciences USA, 93, 8334-8339.

Iannello, R.C. & Dahl, H.H. (1992). Transcriptional expression of a testis-specific variant of the mouse pyruvate dehydrogenase E1 alpha subunit. Biology of Reproduction, 47(1), 48-58.

Iannello, R.C., Gould, J.A., Young, J.C., Giudice, A., Medcalf, R., Kola, I. (2000). Methylation-dependent silencing of the testis-specific Pdha-2 basal promoter occurs through selective targeting of an activating transcription factor/cAMP-responsive element-binding site. Journal of Biological Chemistry, 275(26), 19603-19608.

Iannello, R.C., Young, J., Sumarsono, S., Tymms, M., Kola, I. (1995). A model for understanding gene regulation during spermatogenesis: the mouse testis Pdha-2 promoter. Reproduction Fertility and Development, 7(4), 705-712.

Iannello, R.C., Young, J., Sumarsono, S., Tymms, M.J., Dahl, H.H., Gould, J., Hedger, M., Kola, I. (1997). Regulation of Pdha-2 expression is mediated by proximal promoter sequences and CpG methylation. Molecular and Cellular Biology, 17(2), 612-619.

Iannello, R.C., Kola, I., Dahl, H.-H.M. (1993). Temporal and tissue-specific interactions involving novel transcription factors and the proximal promoter of the mouse Pdha-2 gene. Journal of Biological Chemistry, 268 (1993) 22581-22590.

Jeong, S., Liang, G., Sharma, S., Lin, J.C., Choi, S.H., Han, H., Yoo, C.B., Egger, G., Yang, A.S., Jones, P.A. (2009). Selective anchoring of DNA methyltransferases 3A and 3B to nucleosomes containing methylated DNA. Molecular and Cellular Biology, 29(19), 5366-5376.

Jia, D., Jurkowska, R.Z., Zhang, X., Jeltsch, A., Cheng, X. (2007). Structure of Dnmt3a bound to Dnmt3L suggests a model for de novo DNA methylation. Nature, 449(7159), 248-251.

Jurkowski, T.P. & Jeltsch, A. (2011). Burning off DNA methylation: new evidence for oxygen-dependent DNA demethylation. Chembiochem, 12(17), 2543-2545.

Kass, S.U., Pruss, D., Wolffe, A.P. (1997). How does DNA methylation repress transcription?. Trends in Genetics, 13, 444-449.

Kato, Y. & Nozaki, M. (2012). Distinct DNA methylation dynamics of spermatogenic cell-specific intronless genes is associated with CpG content. PloSONE, 7(8), e43658.

Keshet, I., Yisraeli, J., Cedar, H. (1985). Effect of regional DNA methylation on gene expression. Proceedings of the National Academy of Sciences USA, 82, 2560-2564.

Korotchkina, L.G. & Patel, M.S. (2001). *Site specificity of four pyruvate dehydrogenase kinase isoenzymes toward the three phosphorylation sites of human pyruvate dehydrogenase. Journal of Biological Chemistry, 276(40), 37223-37229.*

Korotchkina, L.G., Sidhu, S., Patel, M.S. (2006). *Characterization of testis-specific isoenzyme of human pyruvate dehydrogenase. Journal of Biological Chemistry, 281(14), 9688-9696.*

Kroft, T.L., Jethanandani, P., McLean, D.J., Goldberg, E. (2001). *Methylation of CpG dinucleotides alters binding and silences testis-specific transcription directed by the mouse lactate dehydrogenase C promoter. Biology of Reproduction, 65, 1522-1527.*

Kumar, V., Rangaraj, N., Shivaji, S. (2006). *Activity of pyruvate dehydrogenase A (PDHA) in hamster spermatozoa correlates positively with hyperactivation and is associated with sperm capacitation. Biology of Reproduction, 75, 767–777.*

Kumar, V., Kota, V., Shivaji, S. (2008). *Hamster sperm capacitation: role of pyruvate dehydrogenase A and dihydrolipoamide dehydrogenase. Biology of Reproduction, 79; 190-199.*

Lister, R., Pelizzola, M., Dowen, R.H., Hawkins, R.D., Hon, G., Tonti-Filippini, J., Nery, J.R., Lee, L., Ye, Z., Ngo, Q.M., Edsall, L., Antosiewicz-Bourget, J., Stewart, R., Ruotti, V., Millar, A.H., Thomson, J.A., Ren, B., Ecker, J.R. (2009). *Human DNA methylomes at base resolution show widespread epigenomic differences. Nature, 462(7271), 315-322.*

Liu, F., Jin, S.H., Li, N., Liu, X., Wang, H.Y., Li, J.Y. (2011). *Comparative and functional analysis of testis-specific genes. Biological and Pharmaceutical Bulletin, 34(1), 28-35.*

Medlin, J., Scurry, A., Taylor, A., Zhang, F., Peterlin, B.M., Murphy, S. (2005). *P-TEFb is not an essential elongation factor for the intronless human U2 snRNA and histone H2b genes. EMBO Journal, 24, 4154-4165.*

Nan, X., Campoy, F.J., Bird, A. (1997). *MeCP2 is a transcriptional repressor with abundant binding sites in genomic chromatin. Cell, 88, 471-481.*

Okano, M., Bell, D.W., Haber, D.A., Li, E. (1999). *DNA methyltransferases Dnmt3a and Dnmt3b are essential for de novo methylation and mammalian development. Cell, 99(3), 247-257.*

Patel, M.S. & Harris R.A. (1995). *Mammalian alpha-keto acid dehydrogenase complexes: gene regulation and genetic defects. FASEB J, 9(12), 1164-1172.*

Patel, M.S. & Korochkina, L.G. (2003). *The Biochemistry of the Pyruvate Dehydrogenase Complex. Biochemistry and Molecular Biology Education, 31(1), 5-15.*

Pinheiro A., Faustino I., Silva M.J., Silva J., Sá R., Sousa M., Barros A., Tavares de Almeida I., Rivera I. (2010). *Human testis-specific PDHA2 gene: methylation status of a CpG island in the open reading frame correlates with transcriptional activity. Molecular Genetics and Metabolism, 99(4): 425-430.*

Pinheiro, A., Silva, M.J., Graça, I., Silva, J., Sá, R., Sousa, M., Barros, A., Tavares de Almeida, I., Rivera, I. (2012a). *Pyruvate dehydrogenase complex: mRNA and protein expression patterns of E1α subunit genes in human spermatogenesis. Gene, 506, 173-178.*

Pinheiro, A., Nunes, M.J., Milagre, I., Rodrigues, E., Silva, M.J., Tavares de Almeida, I., Rivera, I. (2012b). *Demethylation of the coding region triggers the activation of the human testis-specific PDHA2 gene in somatic tissues. PLoS ONE, 7(6), e38076.*

Robinson, B.H., MacKay, N., Chun, K., Ling, M. (1996). *Disorders of pyruvate carboxylase and the pyruvate dehydrogenase complex. Journal of Inherited Metabolic Disorders, 19, 452-462.*

Robinson, B.H. (2001). *Lactic Acidemia (Disorders of Pyruvate Carboxylase and Pyruvate Dehydrogenase). In The Metabolic and Molecular Bases of Inherited Disease. CR Scriver, AL Beaudet, WS Sly and D Valle. New York, McGraw-Hill Inc., 2275-2295.*

Rocamora, N. & Mezquita, C. (1989). *Chicken spermatogenesis is accompanied by a genomic-wide loss of DNA methylation. FEBS Letters, 247, 415-418.*

Singal, R. & Ginder, G.D. (1999). *DNA methylation. Blood, 93, 4059-4070.*

Takakubo, F. & Dahl, H.H. (1992). The expression pattern of the pyruvate dehydrogenase E1 alpha subunit genes during spermatogenesis in adult mouse. Experimental Cell Research, 199(1), 39-49.

Wada, N., Matsuishi, T., Nonaka, M., Naito, E., Yoshino, M. (2004). Pyruvate dehydrogenase E1alpha subunit deficiency in a female patient: evidence of antenatal origin of brain damage and possible etiology of infantile spasms. Brain and Development, 26(1), 57-60.

Weber, T.A., Antognetti, M.R., Stacpoole, P.W. (2001). Caveats when considering ketogenic diets for the treatment of pyruvate dehydrogenase complex deficiency. Journal of Pediatrics, 138(3), 390-395.

Wexler, I.D., Hemalatha, S.G., McConnell, J., Buist, N.R., Dahl, H.H., Berry, S.A., Cederbaum, S.D., Patel, M.S., Kerr, D.S. (1997). Outcome of pyruvate dehydrogenase deficiency treated with ketogenic diets. Studies in patients with identical mutations. Neurology, 49(6), 1655-1661.

Willemsen, M., Rodenburg, R.J., Teszas, A., van den Heuvel, L., Kosztolanyi, G., Morava, E. (2006). Females with PDHA1 gene mutations: a diagnostic challenge. Mitochondrion, 6(3), 155-159.

Yamashita, R., Sathira, N.P., Kanai, A., Tanimoto, K., Arauchi, T., Tanaka, Y., Hashimoto, S., Sugano, S., Nakai, K., Suzuki, Y. (2011). Genome-wide characterization of transcriptional start sites in humans by integrative transcriptome analysis. Genome Research, 21(5), 775-789.

Young, J.C., Gould, J.A., Kola, I., Iannello, R.C. (1998). Review: Pdha-2, past and present. Journal of Experimental Zoology, 282(1-2), 231-238.

Zhu, S., Goldschmidt-Clermont, P.J., Dong, C. (2005). Inactivation of monocarboxylate transporter MCT3 by DNA methylation in atherosclerosis. Circulation, 112, 1353-1361.

Prolactin Regulates Cyclin D1 Promoter Activity via Serine-threonine Kinase PAK1 and Adapter Protein Nck

Maria Diakonova, Peter Oladimeji, Leah Rider

Department of Biological Sciences
University of Toledo, USA

1   Introduction

1.1   Prolactin in Human Breast Cancer

Prolactin (PRL), a hormone of the growth hormone/cytokine family, exerts both endocrine and autocrine/paracrine effects and functions in both reproduction and as a cytokine (Bernichtein *et al.*, 2010; Ben-Jonathan *et al.*, 2008). Accumulating evidence from a variety of sources demonstrate a link between PRL and breast cancer (Tworoger and Hankinson, 2006; Clevenger, 2003). It has been shown that high circulating levels of PRL increase the risk of breast cancer in women (Tworoger and Hankinson, 2006; Hankinson *et al.*, 1999), PRL receptor (PRLR) is overexpressed in 95% of breast cancer cases and PRLR protein can be stabilized by oncogenic pathways (Swaminathan *et al.*, 2008; Meng *et al.*, 2004; Touraine *et al.*, 1998; Clevenger *et al.*, 1995; Ginsburg and Vonderhaar, 1995). The examination of transgenic mouse models provided experimental evidence that a sustained increase in the levels of circulating lactogenic hormones, in particular PRL, causes mammary cancer (Wennbo *et al.*, 1997; Tornell *et al.*, 1991). Moreover, human breast cancer cells are able to upregulate the local synthesis of PRL, suggesting that this hormone can act in an autocrine manner to promote the proliferation of neoplastic cells (Clevenger *et al.*, 1995; Ginsburg and Vonderhaar, 1995).

Initiation of PRL signaling involves PRL binding to PRLR and activation of the tyrosine kinase JAK2 which, in turn, phosphorylates the PRLR. Phosphorylated tyrosines (Tyr) within the receptor and JAK2 recruit an array of effector and/or signaling proteins. The best identified target of JAK2 is a family of transcription factors termed Signal Transducers and Activators of Transcription (STATs). STATs exist within the cytoplasm in a latent or inactive state; they are recruited by cytokine receptor complexes through an interaction involving a phosphotyrosine (on the cytokine receptor and/or the associated JAK) and the SH2 domain of the STAT protein (Reich, 2007; Schindler *et al.*, 2007; Lim and Cao, 2006). Three members of the STAT family participate in PRL signaling: STAT1, STAT3 and STAT5 (both A and B isoforms) (Schaber *et al.*, 1998; DaSilva *et al.*, 1996; Ball *et al.*, 1988). Additionally, phosphorylation of STAT6 during pregnancy has also been recently demonstrated (Khaled *et al.*, 2007). STAT5 was originally identified as mammary gland factor (Wakao *et al.*, 1994) and is the major STAT activated by PRL. JAK2/STAT5 pathway mediates most PRL action in lobuloalveolar development and lactation. However, the role of this pathway in the development and progression of breast cancer is more complex. Current data support the concept of dual roles of STAT5 as promoter of mammary tumorigenesis, and as suppressors of the progression of established breast cancer (Tan and Nevalainen, 2008; Wagner and Rui, 2008). JAK2 phopshorylation of STATs leads to their dimerization and translocation into the nucleus where they bind to specific response elements (GAS sequence) in the promoter of target genes, including promoter for cyclin D1 gene. The human cyclin D1 promoter contains two consensus GAS sites at -457 and -224. PRL induces STAT5 binding to the more distal GAS site (GAS1) to enhance cyclin D1 promoter activity (Brockman *et al.*, 2002). PRL also induces cyclin D1 promoter activity by removing a ubiquitous transcriptional factor Oct-1 from the GAS2 site in the cyclin D1 promoter (Brockman and Schuler, 2005). In addition, using mammary cells from JAK2 knockout mice, JAK2 has been shown to control expression of the cyclin D1 mRNA and regulate the accumulation of cyclin D1 protein in the nucleus by inhibiting signal transducers that mediate the phosphorylation and nuclear export of cyclin D1 (Sakamoto *et al.*, 2007).

1.2 Cyclin D1 As a Breast Cancer Oncogene

Cyclins regulate progression through the cell cycle and dysregulated expression of cyclins and/or cyclin-dependent kinases can lead to aberrant cellular growth, proliferation and tumorigenesis. D-type cyclins (i.e., cyclin D1, D2, and D3) are regulators of the cyclin-dependent kinases 4 and 6 (CDK4 and CDK6) and mediate the growth factor-induced progression through the G1 phase of the cell cycle (Sherr, 1995; Diehl, 2002). Activation of these kinases by D cyclins results in phosphorylation of retinoblastoma protein, leading to increased transcription of E2F-responsive genes, and subsequent mitosis. In addition, cyclin D1 regulates multiple other processes relevant to oncogenesis, including other actions in cell cycle progression, adhesion and migration, responses to DNA damage, protein synthesis, metabolism, and differentiation, in many cases, independently of CDK4/6 or its kinase activity (Arnold and Papanikolaou, 2005; Fu *et al.*, 2004; Coqueret, 2002) (Musgrove *et al.*, 2011). Cyclin D1 is the most extensively studied member of the D-type cyclins due to its suggested pivotal role as a protooncogene in a number of human malignancies including breast cancer ((Knudsen *et al.*, 2006; Lee and Sicinski, 2006; Sutherland and Musgrove, 2004; Suzuki *et al.*, 1999; Dickson *et al.*, 1995).

Among regulators of the cell cycle, cyclin D1 is a strong candidate target of PRL signaling since females deficient in cyclin D1 exhibit impaired mammary gland development similar to STAT5 knockout mice (Fantl *et al.*, 1995; Sicinski *et al.*, 1995). PRL is thought to influence cell proliferation and growth by altering the expression of cyclins D1 and B1 (Brockman and Schuler, 2005; Brockman *et al.*, 2002; Schroeder *et al.*, 2002). In addition to cyclins D1 and B1, a significant increase in cyclins A and E expression has been also detected in many breast cancers (Megha *et al.*, 1999; Keyomarsi and Pardee, 1993). The cyclin D1 gene is amplified or overexpressed in up to 50% of human breast cancers (Dickson *et al.*, 1995; McIntosh *et al.*, 1995), the overexpression of cyclin D1 in the mammary epithelium leads to the formation of tumors in transgenic mice after a latency of more than 1 year (Wang *et al.*, 1994), and interference of its nuclear export and proteolytic degradation has been shown to accelerate mammary carcinogenesis (Lin *et al.*, 2008). Moreover, the targeted ablation of cyclin D1 or the inhibition of its correct functional association with Cdk4/6 was suggested to completely prevent the onset of ErbB2-associated mammary cancer (Jeselsohn *et al.*, 2010; Landis *et al.*, 2006; Yu *et al.*, 2001). Interestingly, two independent mouse models have been recently established to demonstrate that lack of cycline D1 was associated with a compensatory upregulation of cyclin D3 indicating that cyclin D1 is an important but not essential mediator of PRL-induced mammary proliferation although is critical for differentiation and lactation (Asher *et al.*, 2012; Zhang *et al.*, 2011). How we mentioned earlier, not all actions of cyclin D–CDK4/CDK6 depend on substrate phosphorylation. Indeed, in addition to promotion of cell proliferation, cyclin D1 has been shown to regulate multiple other processes relevant to oncogenesis independently of CDK4/6 or its kinase activity (Musgrove *et al.*, 2011). One major non-catalytic function of the D-cyclins is transcriptional regulation. Cyclin D1 is tethered to the promoters of many genes during normal development, probably through interactions with various transcription factors. Thus, Sicinski and colleagues examining cyclin D1–associated proteins in mouse embryos determined that about one third of the identified proteins were transcription factors (Bienvenu *et al.*, 2010). It is clear that understanding the mediators of PRL/cyclin D1 action in carcinogenesis will reveal potential sites for preventative and therapeutic interventions.

1.3   Serine-Threonine kinase PAK1 is involved in Breast Cancer Progression

We have recently linked PRL signaling to the serine-threonine kinase PAK1 and shown that JAK2 directly phosphorylates PAK1 (Rider *et al.*, 2007) (Figure 1).

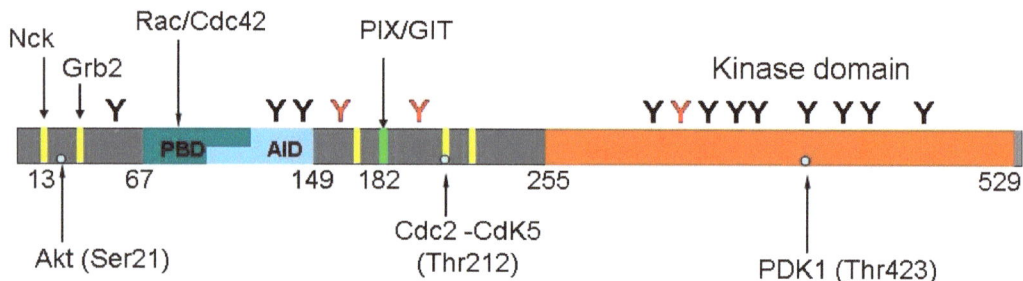

Figure 1: Schematic diagram depicting PAK1. The N-terminus of PAK1 contains five PXXP motifs (yellow bars) of which the first two bind SH2 domain of Nck and Grb2, respectively. PBD (p21-binding domain) domain is responsible for PAK1 activation by Rac1-3, Cdc42, Chp, TC-10 and Wrch-1 (dark-green box, amino acids 67-113). The autoinhibitory domain (AID, blue box, amino acids 87-149) overlaps with PBD, it associates in trans with the kinase domain of PAK1 (orange box, amino acids 255-529). Non-classical proline-rich domain (light-green box, amino acids 182-203) associates with PAX/GIT proteins. Forteen tyrosines of PAK1 and their sequences are shown below. Tyrosines 153, 201 and 285 (shown in red) are sites of JAK2 phopshorylation.

PAK1 is a member of a conserved family of p21-activated serine-threonine kinases, and is important for a variety of cellular functions, including cell morphogenesis, motility, survival, mitosis and malignant transformation (for review Kumar *et al.*, 2006; Zhao and Manser, 2005; Bokoch, 2003). The emerging roles of PAK1 in the regulation of multiple fundamental cellular processes have directed significant attention towards understanding how PAK1 activity is controlled. Autoinhibition of the PAK1 C-terminal catalytic domain by the N-terminal domain is a key mechanism of PAK1 regulation. Several layers of inhibition, involving dimerization and occupation of the catalytic cleft by contact between the N- and C-terminal domains, keep PAK1 kinase activity in check (Lei *et al.*, 2000). Autoinhibition of PAK1 occurs in *trans*, meaning that the inhibitory domain of one PAK1 molecule interacts with the kinase domain of another PAK1 molecule (Parrini *et al.*, 2002). Association of GTP-bound forms of Cdc42 and Rac1 with the PAK1 PBD/CRIB domain induces conformational changes in the N-terminal domain that no longer support its autoinhibitory function. In addition to Cdc42 and Rac1, PAK1 is activated by the binding of small GTPases, Rac2 and Rac3, as well as TC10, CHP and Wrich-1 proteins (Tao *et al.*, 2001; Mira *et al.*, 2000; Aronheim *et al.*, 1998; Knaus and Bokoch, 1998; Neudauer *et al.*, 1998; Manser *et al.*, 1994). PAK1 is a predominantly cytoplasmic protein, but is activated upon recruitment to the cell membrane. PAK1 membrane localization occurs through interaction with adaptor proteins Nck, Grb2 and PIX, all of which are activated by ligation of growth-factor receptors (Zhao *et al.*, 2000b; Daniels *et al.*,

1998; Lu *et al.*, 1997; Bokoch *et al.*, 1996). Membrane recruitment of PAK1 via adapter proteins and subsequent PAK1 activation may involve phosphorylation at Thr 423 (a site that is also autophosphorylated when PAK1 is activated by Rac1 and Cdc42) by PDK1 (King *et al.*, 2000) or interaction with lipids, such as sphingosine, that can activate PAK1 in a GTPase-independent manner (Bokoch *et al.*, 1998). In addition to PDK, several other protein kinases regulate PAK1. Thus, Akt1 phosphorylates PAK1 at Ser 21, decreasing Nck binding to the PAK1 N-terminus and stimulating PAK1 activity (Tang *et al.*, 2000; Zhao *et al.*, 2000a). The p35-bound form of Cdk5, a neuron-specific protein kinase, associates with and phosphorylates PAK1 at Thr 212 and inhibits PAK1 kinase activity (Rashid *et al.*, 2001; Nikolic *et al.*, 1998). The cyclin B-bound form of Cdc2 also phosphorylates PAK1 at Thr 212 (Banerjee *et al.*, 2002; Thiel *et al.*, 2002), affecting PAK1 protein-protein interaction but not PAK1 activation (Thiel *et al.*, 2002).

Accumulating evidence suggests that some PAK1 functions can be kinase-independent. Thus, PAK1 can regulate the actin cytoskeleton in both kinase-dependent and -independent ways (Vadlamudi *et al.*, 2002; Manser *et al.*, 1997). It has been shown that the kinase inhibitory domain of PAK1 (KID) induces cell cycle arrest independently of PAK1 kinase activity (Thullberg *et al.*, 2007). We have previously proposed that tyrosyl phosphorylation of PAK1 by JAK2 creates high-affinity docking sites for binding to SH2-domain-containing proteins and alters the ability of PAK1 to find, bind, and/or phosphorylate intracellular targets, thereby amplifying the effect of PAK1 on cell functions (Rider *et al.*, 2007).

PAK1 is involved in breast cancer progression (for review Gururaj *et al.*, 2005; Kumar and Vadlamudi, 2002). PAK1 is overexpressed (Bekri *et al.*, 1997) or up-regulated (Balasenthil *et al.*, 2004; Salh *et al.*, 2002; Vadlamudi *et al.*, 2000) in some breast cancers. Overexpression of PAK1 was observed in 34 of 60 breast tumor specimens (Balasenthil *et al.*, 2004) and expression of PAK1 in human breast tumors correlates with tumor grade, with higher expression observed in less differentiated ductal breast carcinomas (grade III) than in grade I and II tumors (Salh *et al.*, 2002). Highly proliferating human breast cancer cell lines and tumor tissues express hyperactive PAK1 and its upstream regulator Rac3 (Mira *et al.*, 2000). Activated PAK1 increased cell invasion of breast cancer cells and expression of a kinase-dead PAK1 mutant in the highly invasive breast cancer cell lines led to a reduction in invasiveness (Adam *et al.*, 2000). Conversely, hyperactivation of the PAK1 pathway in the non-invasive breast cancer cell line MCF-7 promotes cell migration and anchorage-independent growth (Vadlamudi *et al.*, 2000). Recently PAK1 has been shown to phosphorylate dynein light chain 1 (DLC1) that plays a critical role in tumorigenic phenotypes of DLC1 in breast cancer cells (Vadlamudi *et al.*, 2004). Thus, PAK1 has become one of the focal points in the investigation into the mechanism and onset of human breast cancer.

PAK1 has also been implicated in regulation of cyclin D1 gene expression. Overexpression of catalytically active PAK1 T423E in MCF7 cells leads to cyclin D1 expression while overexpression of PAK1 lacking the nuclear localization signals does not (Holm *et al.*, 2006; Rayala *et al.*, 2006; Balasenthil *et al.*, 2004). Reducing PAK1 expression by PAK1-siRNA is accompanied by a significant reduction of cyclins D1 and B1 expression (Balasenthil *et al.*, 2004). PAK1 has a well-established role in the nucleus, where it associates with chromatin, phosphorylates histone H3 and several transcription factors and transcriptional coregulators (Park *et al.*, 2007; Singh *et al.*, 2005; Li *et al.*, 2002, for review Rayala and Kumar, 2007).

Understanding the mechanism by which PRL stimulates mitogenesis and how it interacts with other factors important in breast cancer may lead to improved diagnostic assays and therapeutic approaches. In this study we have linked PRL and PAK1 as the JAK2 substrate to the stimulation of cyclin D1 promoter activity. We have proposed two mechanisms by which PRL regulates cyclin D1 promoter activity.

The first is a positive effect that depends on the PRL-dependent phosphorylation of three tyrosines on PAK1 and the presence of PAK1 nuclear localization signals. The second is a counter-regulatory mechanism that involves the interaction between PAK1 and adapter protein Nck, which keeps the Nck-PAK1 complex in the cytoplasm.

2   Results

2.1   Prolactin-activated Tyrosyl Phosphorylated PAK1 Stimulates Cyclin D1 Promoter Activity

Both PAK1 and prolactin have previously been implicated in the regulation of cyclin D1 promoter activity (Balasenthil *et al.*, 2004; Brockman *et al.*, 2002). Since we have recently shown that PRL causes tyrosyl phosphorylation of PAK1 by JAK2 kinase (Rider *et al.*, 2007), we decided to investigate whether tyrosyl phosphorylation of PAK1 is important for cyclin D1 regulation in response to PRL. First, we measured the induction of cyclin D1 promoter activity in T47D cells treated with or without PRL. As shown in Figure 2A, T47D cells transfected with a human cyclin D1 promoter-luciferase construct increased luciferase expression in response to PRL as expected. Second, co-transfection of T47D cells with luciferase construct and PAK1 WT results in a 4.6-fold increase in luciferase expression in the absence of PRL that corresponds to previously published data (white bars in Figure 2B) (Balasenthil *et al.*, 2004). Interestingly, treatment of the PAK1 WT-expressing cells with PRL causes a 14-fold increase in luciferase expression as compared with the cells not expressing PAK1 WT and treated with PRL (black bars in Figure 2B). Overexpression of PAK1 lacking the three phosphorylated tyrosines (PAK1 Y3F) which are sites of JAK2 phosphorylation, reduced PAK1's effect on cyclin D1 promoter activity by 55% compared to PAK1 WT in the presence of PRL. These data suggest that Tyr(s) 153, 201 and 285 of PAK1 are required for maximal cyclin D1 promoter activity in response to PRL.

2.2   PAK1 Shuttles between the Cytoplasm and Nucleus and PRL Promotes PAK1 Nuclear Accumulation

Data from the literature suggest that PAK1 translocates into the nucleus in response to EGF (Singh *et al.*, 2005) and we wished to investigate the potential significance of PAK1 nuclear localization for cyclin D1 regulation. We first studied whether PRL can stimulate nuclear translocation of PAK1. Figure 3 indicates that treatment of T47D cells with PRL for 24h caused nuclear accumulation of endogenous PAK1. Interestingly, extended incubation of T47D cells with PRL up to 48h led to re-distribution of PAK1 back to the cytoplasm. These immunofluorescence data were confirmed by fractionation assay demonstrating the presence of PAK1 in both cytoplasmic and nuclear fractions before PRL treatment, elevated levels of PAK1 in the nuclear fraction 24h after PRL addition and a decrease in nuclear PAK1 after 48h (not shown).

In order to investigate the role of the three sites of JAK2-dependent tyrosyl phosphorylation of the PAK1 molecule in nuclear translocation, we overexpressed either PAK1 WT or PAK1 Y3F in T47D cells, treated them with or without PRL to activate JAK2 and defined the amount of cells with nuclear PAK1 (Figure 4A and B). There were significantly more cells with intranuclear PAK1 WT after PRL treatment than without PRL, while there was no PRL-dependent difference in localization of PAK1 Y3F mutant, suggesting that these three tyrosines may play a role in PAK1 nuclear translocation. We have also seen significant PAK1 translocation into the nucleus when we overexpressed PAK1 WT with JAK2 in COS-7 and MCF-7 cells (Figure 5, left two bars in each plot).

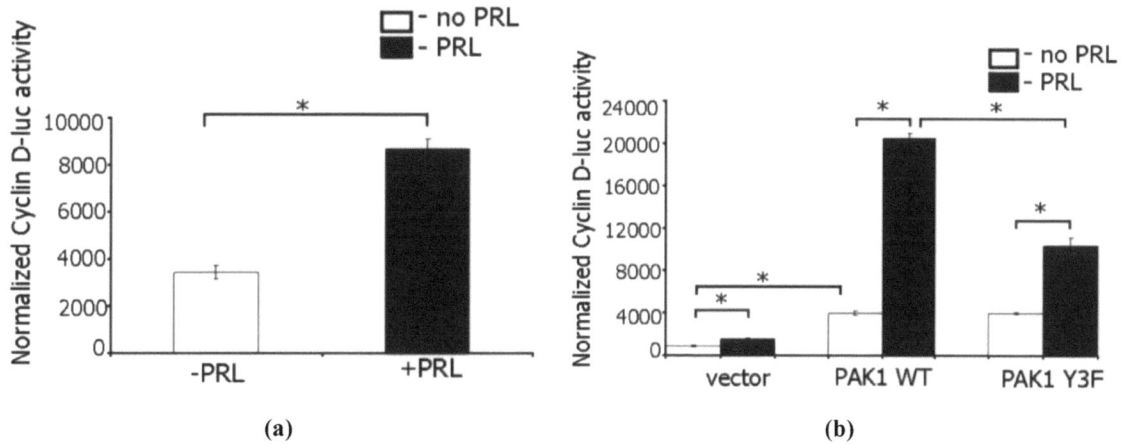

(a)   (b)

Figure 2: Prolactin stimulates cyclin D1 promoter activity through tyrosines 153, 201 and 285 of PAK1. T47D cells were transfected with cyclin D1-luciferase reporter (A) or cotransfected with cyclin D1-luciferase reporter with vector, PAK1 WT or PAK1 Y3F (B). The cells were treated with (black bars) or without (white bars) 500 ng/ml of prolactin for an additional 24h, lysed, and luciferase activity was measured. Luciferase activity was normalized with β-galactosidase activity. Bars represent mean $\pm$S.E., *, p <0.05, n=3.

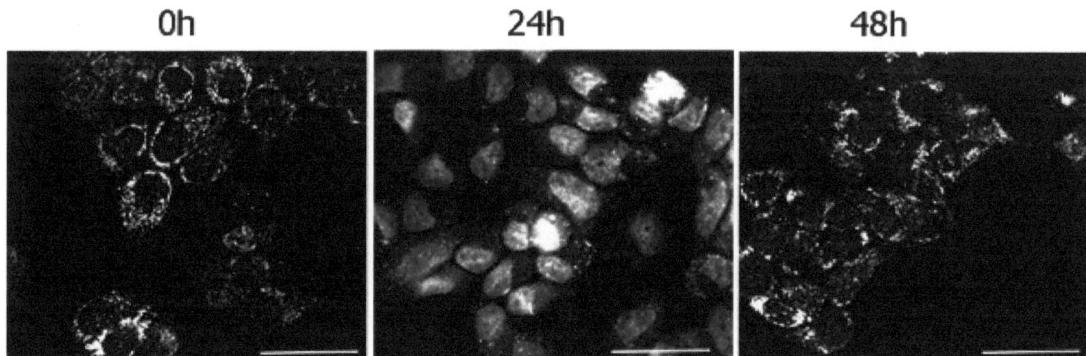

Figure 3: Prolactin causes translocation of endogenous PAK1 into nucleus. T47D cells were deprived of serum for 24h and treated with or without 500 ng/ml PRL for 0, 24 or 48h. Endogenous PAK1 was subjected to confocal immunofluorescence with αPAK1 antibody. *Scale bar*, 50 μm.

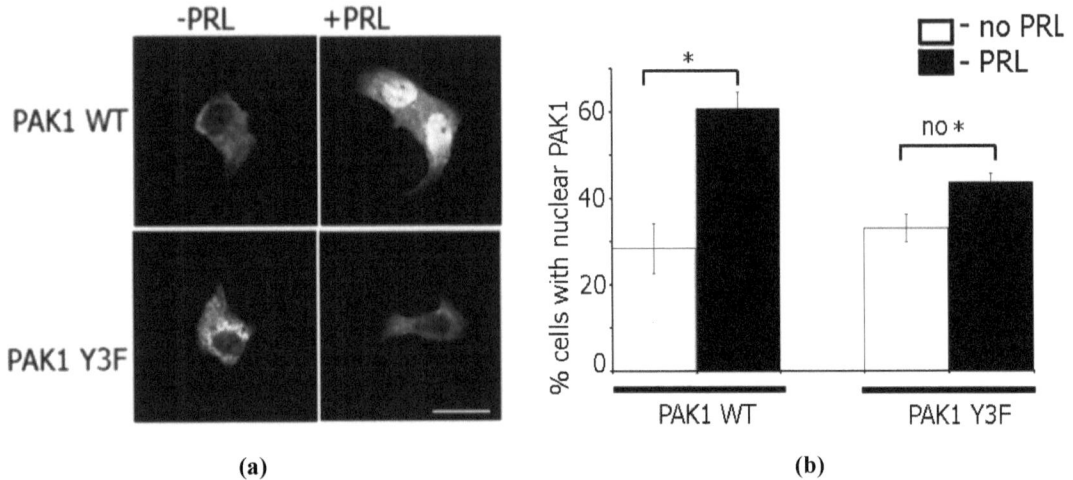

(a)   (b)

Figure 4: Tyrosyl phosphorylation of PAK1 is required for translocation of PAK1 into nucleus in response to PRL. (A) T47D cells were transfected with either PAK1 WT or PAK1 Y3F. The cells were serum deprived for 24h, treated with or without 500 ng/ml of PRL for an additional 24h and PAK1 was immunolocalized with αPAK1 antibody. *Scale bar*, 25 μm. (B) The percentage of cells with PAK1 nuclear localization was counted and plotted. 100 PAK1-expressing cells were assessed for PAK1 or PAK1 Y3F immunolocalization in each experiment for each type of treatment. Bars represent mean ±S.E., *, p<0.05, n=3.

Since the maximal amount of nuclear endogenous PAK1 was observed 24h but not 48h after PRL treatment, we hypothesize that PAK1 may shuttle between the nucleus and the cytoplasm. To test this hypothesis, we treated T47D cells with Leptomycin B (LMB), a specific inhibitor of Crm1-dependent nuclear export. Indeed, LMB treatment lead to nuclear accumulation of overexpressed PAK1 WT in T47D, MCF-7 and COS-7 cells indicating that nucleo-cytoplasmic shuttling of PAK1 was happening and that this occurred in a cell-type independent manner (Figure 5).

2.3   Effect of Nuclear Localization Signals and Tyrosyl Phosphorylation of PAK1 on Cyclin D1 Promoter Activity

To further implicate a regulatory role of PAK1 tyrosyl phosphorylation in nuclear localization and the regulation of cyclin D1 transcription, we used a previously described PAK1 mutant in which three nuclear localization signals (NLS) have been mutated by replacing the three basic lysine residues with alanines (amino acids 48-51 for NLS1, 243-245 for nLS2 and 267-269 for NLS3) (Singh et al., 2005). Because overexpression of this PAK1 mutant lacking the three functional nuclear localization signals (PAK1 mutNLS) decreased but did not eliminate augmentation of cyclin D1 promoter activity compared to PAK1 WT (Holm et al., 2006), we hypothesize that mutation of Tyr(s) 153, 201 and 285 in PAK1 mutNLS will further reduce PRL-induced activation of cyclin D1 promoter. To test this, we transiently expressed PAK1 mutNLS or PAK1 mutNLS Y3F mutants in T47D cells, treated the cells with or without PRL and performed experiments as described above. As shown in Fig.6A, expression of PAK1 mutNLS decreased both PRL-dependent and PRL-independent cyclin D1 transcription activity by 46% i. e. to a similar level caused by expression of PAK1 Y3F mutant (47% inhibition in this experiment). Expression of PAK1 mutNLS Y3F significantly decreased the effect of PRL on cyclin D1 promoter activity by 68%,

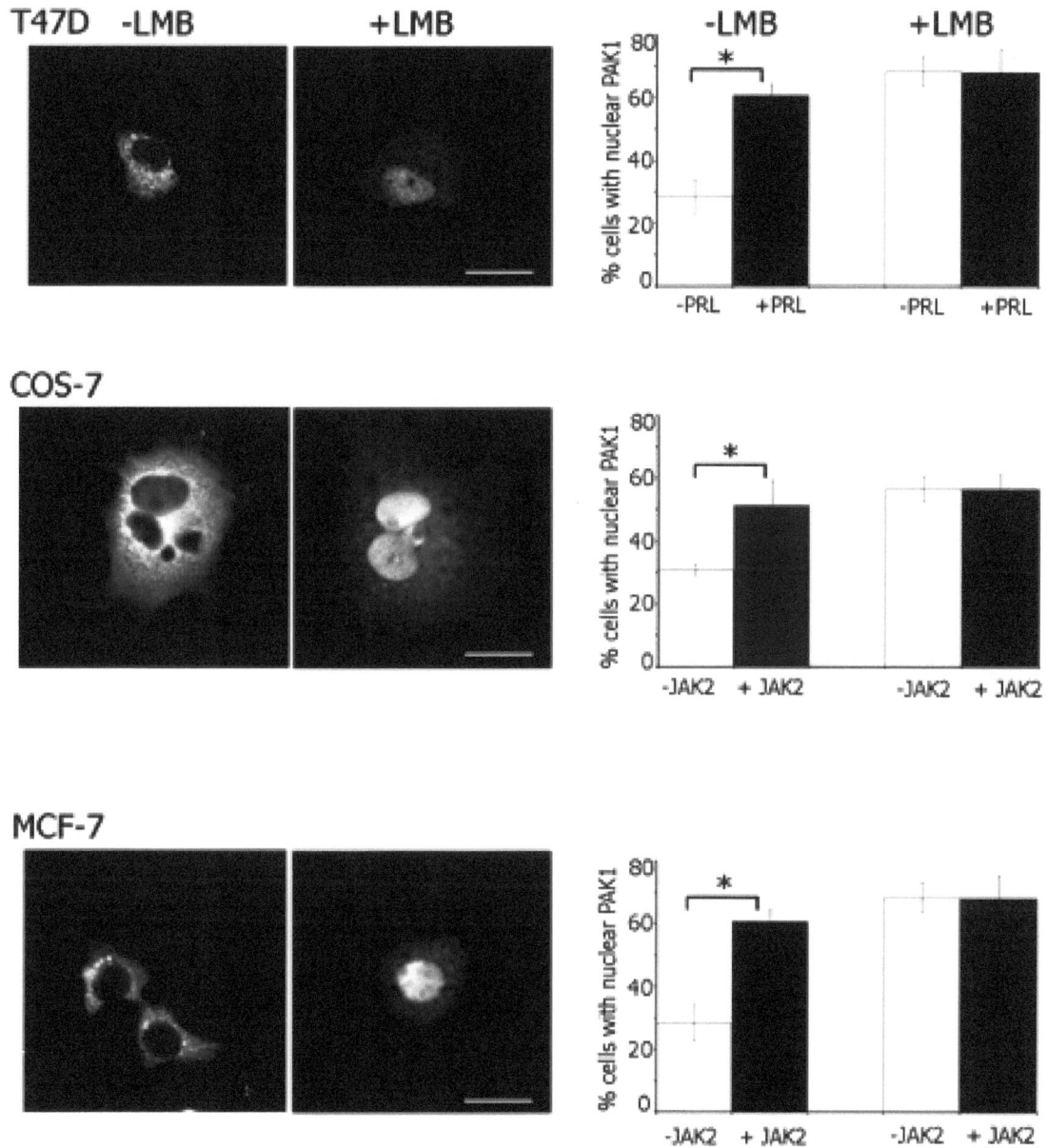

Figure 5: PAK1 shuttles between cytoplasm and nucleus. PAK1 alone (T47D cells) or PAK1 and JAK2 (COS-7 and MCF-7 cells) were overexpressed in the indicated cells. The cells were incubated with Leptomycin B (LMB) for 8h and processed for immunolocalization of PAK1 with αPAK1 antibody. T47D cells were treated with 500 ng/ml of PRL for 48h before LMB was added. The percentage of cells with PAK1 nuclear localization was counted and plotted. 100 PAK1-positive (for T47D cells) and both PAK1- and JAK2-positive (for COS-7 and MCF-7 cells) cells were assessed for PAK1 immunolocalization in each experiment for each type of treatment. *Scale bar*, 25 μm. Bars represent mean ±S.E., *, p<0.05, n=3.

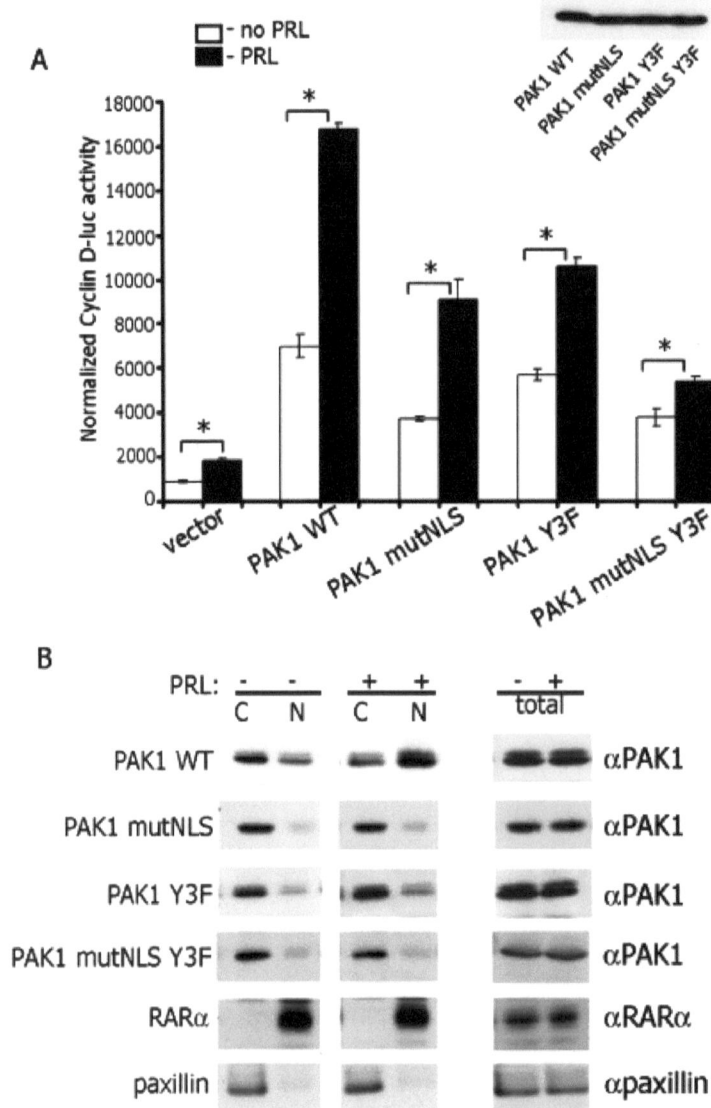

Figure 6: Effect of PAK1 nuclear localization signals and tyrosyl phosphorylation on cyclin D1 promoter activity. T47D cells were cotransfected with cyclin D1-luciferase reporter with either vector, PAK1 WT, PAK1 mutNLS (three nuclear localization signals mutated), PAK1 Y3F or PAK1 mutNLS Y3F. The cells were serum deprived for 24h , treated with (black bars) or without (white bars) 500 ng/ml of prolactin for an additional 24h, lysed, and luciferase activity was measured. Luciferase activity was normalized with β-galactosidase activity. Bars represent mean ±S.E., *, p <0.05, n=3. The expression levels of PAK1 WT and PAK1 mutants are indicated (A). Total cell lysates, cytosolic (C) and nuclear (N) fractions of T47D cells transfected with PAK1 WT or PAK1 mutants and treated with or without PRL were separated by SDS-PAGE, transferred to nitrocellulose and immunoblotted with αPAK1, αpaxillin as a cytosolic marker and αRARα as a nuclear marker (B).

suggesting that both nuclear localization and tyrosyl phosphorylation of PAK1 are required for the maximal effect of PRL on cyclin D1 promoter activity. Figure 6B indicates that treatment of T47D cells with PRL caused nuclear accumulation of overexpressed PAK1 WT but not PAK1 mutNLS, PAK1 Y3F or PAK1 mutNLS Y3F mutants.

2.4   Nck Regulates PAK1 Nuclear Localization and Inhibits PAK1-stimulated Cyclin D1 Promoter Activity

In our search for additional PAK1-dependent mechanisms of cyclin D1 promoter activation, we investigated a role for the adapter protein Nck since Nck is a known binding partner of PAK1 (Bokoch *et al.*, 1996; Galisteo *et al.*, 1996), that is known to shuttle between the cytoplasm and nucleus (Kremer *et al.*, 2007). We first investigated the effect of Nck expression on PAK1 nuclear relocation in response to PRL by overexpressing PAK1 WT alone, Nck alone or PAK1 with Nck together and treating T47D cells with or without PRL. The number of the cells with nuclear PAK1 and the number of cells with nuclear Nck were counted and plotted (Figure 7 B, C). As illustrated in Figure 7A-C, Nck retained PAK1 in the cytoplasm (2 left white bars in Figure 7B) and inhibited PAK1 nuclear translocation in response to PRL (2 left black bars in Figure 7B). This effect was partially inhibited by expressing PAK1 Y3F instead of PAK1 WT, but only for PRL-untreated cells (PAK1 WT+Nck vs. PAK1 Y3F +Nck without PRL, white bars in Figure 7B). We did not see a significant difference between the cells expressing the same constructs but treated with PRL (PAK1 WT+Nck vs. PAK1 Y3F-Nck with PRL, black bars in Figure 7B). These data suggest that the three tyrosines on PAK1 may play a role in localization of the PAK1-Nck complex, but this effect is not affected by PRL-dependent tyrosyl phosphorylation. Interestingly, the percentage of cells in which Nck localized to both the cytoplasmic and nuclear compartments was decreased by up to 45% when it was co-expressed with PAK1 (Figure 7A and C). This effect was independent of PRL treatment (Figure 7A and C). These data suggest that Nck sequesters PAK1 in the cytoplasm and that it stays in the cytoplasm itself when complexed with PAK1. Tyrosyl phosphorylation of PAK1 on the three tyrosines assessed does not play a role in this process (Figure 7A and C, last two bars).

Data from the experiments with the luciferase-cyclin D1 promoter construct demonstrated that co-expression of Nck with PAK1 WT strongly inhibited (by 95%) the impact of PAK1 on cyclin D1 promoter activity both in the presence and absence of PRL (Figure 8A). This inhibition was much stronger than that caused by expression of PAK1 Y3F (by 60%).

To study further whether the inhibitory effect of Nck on PAK1-induced cyclin D1 promoter activity was relieved by disruption of Nck-PAK1 binding, we used two mutants: Nck W143R mutant has a mutation in the second SH3 domain and fails to bind to PAK (Zhu *et al.*, 2010), and PAK1 P13A mutant, a mutant that is unable to interact with Nck (Bokoch *et al.*, 1996; Galisteo *et al.*, 1996). Our co-immunoprecipitation experiments confirmed that only PAK1 WT and Nck WT bound to each other *in vivo* while PAK1 P13A and Nck W143R did not (Figure 9B). Data in Fig. 9A demonstrate that PAK1 P13A and PAK1 WT augment cyclin D1 promoter activity. Mutation of tryptophan 143 to arginine in Nck had no effect on cyclin D1 promoter activity as compared with Nck WT. Expression of both PAK WT and Nck WT strongly inhibited cyclin D1 promoter activity as described before. However, disruption of Nck-PAK1 binding by expression of mutated PAK1 and Nck partially but significantly relieved the repression of PRL-dependent stimulation, induced by Nck WT (Figure 9A). These data confirm that a functional Nck-PAK1 complex is required for optimal regulation of cyclin D1 promoter activity.

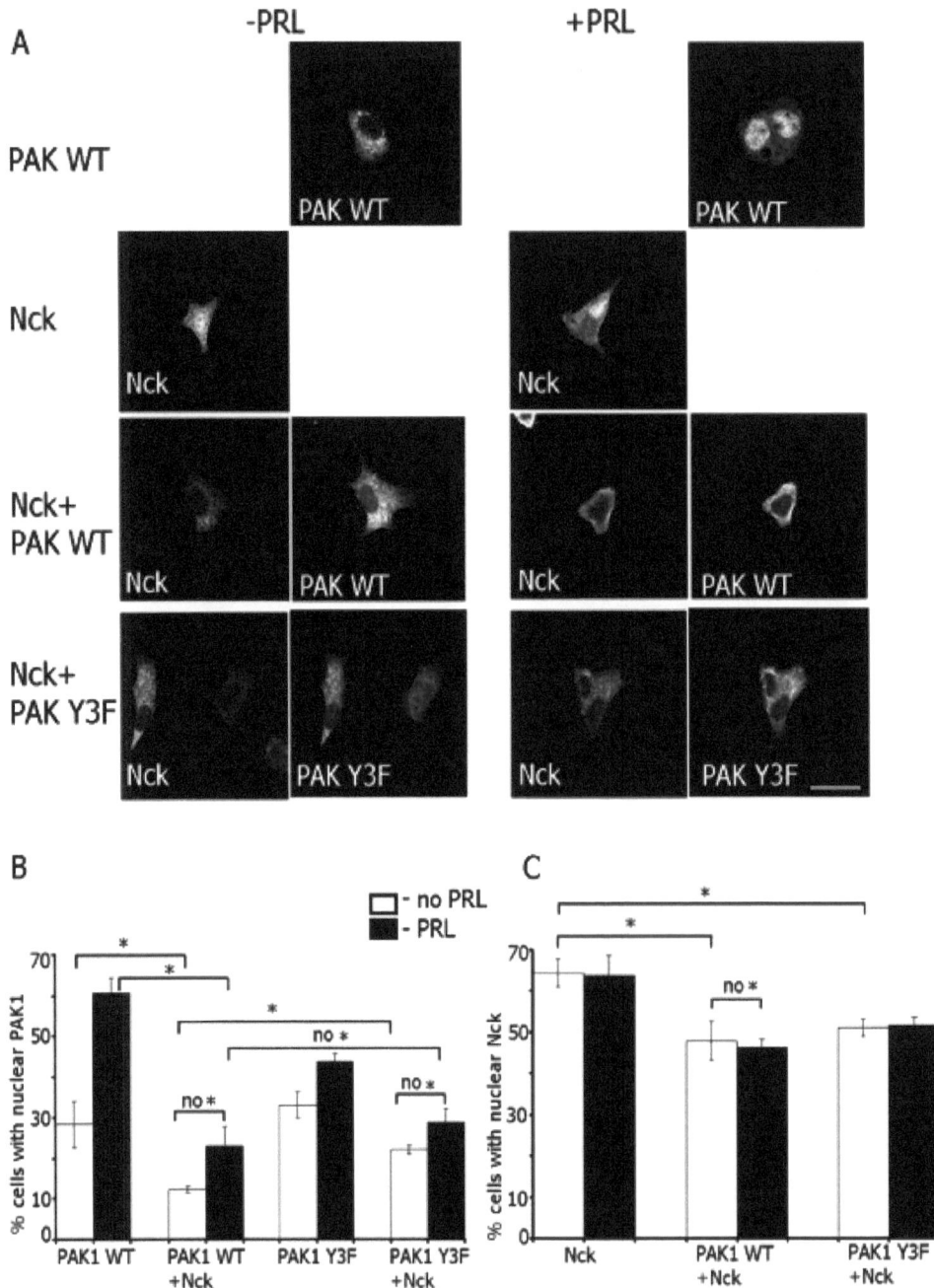

Figure 7: Nck retains PAK1 in the cytoplasm. T47D cells were either transfected with PAK1 WT or Nck, or co-transfected with Nck and either PAK1 WT or PAK1 Y3F, serum deprived for 24h, treated with or without 500 ng/ml of PRL for an additional 24h. PAK1 and Nck were immunolocalized with αPAK1 or αNck correspondingly. *Scale bar*, 25 μm. (A). The percentage of cells with PAK1 (B) or Nck (C) nuclear localization was counted and plotted. 100 PAK1-expressing or both PAK1- and Nck-expressing cells were assessed for PAK1 or Nck immunolocalization in each experiment for each type of treatment. Bars represent mean ±S.E., *, $p<0.05$, n=3.

A

B

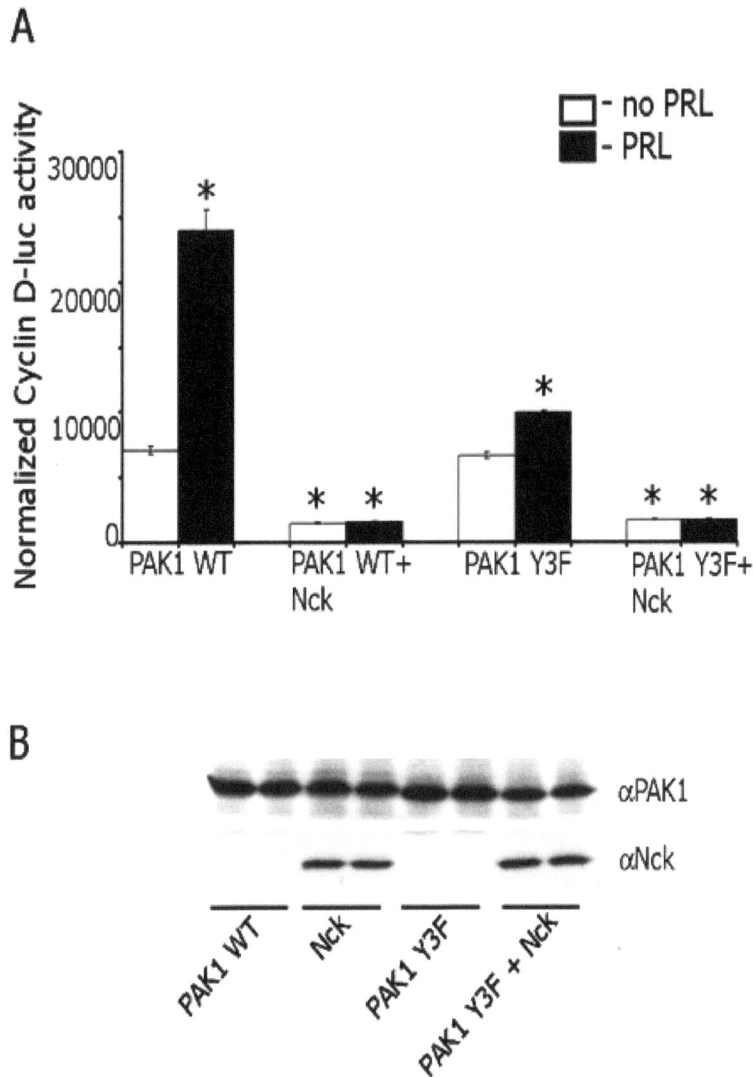

Figure 8: Nck blocks the amplifying effect of PAK1 on cyclin D1 promoter activity. (A) T47D cells were cotransfected with cyclin D1-luciferase reporter, and either PAK1 WT, PAK1 and Nck, PAK1 Y3F or PAK1 Y3F and Nck. The cells were serum deprived for 24h, treated with (black bars) or without (white bars) 500 ng/ml of PRL for an additional 24h, lysed, and luciferase activity was measured. Luciferase activity was normalized with β-galactosidase activity. Bars represent mean ±S.E., *, p <0.05 compared with cells expressing PAK1 WT and untreated with PRL, n=3. (B) Whole-cell lysates of T47D cells transfected with PAK1 WT, PAK1 Y3F and Nck were subjected to αPAK1 and αNck Western blotting. The expression levels of PAK1 WT, PAK1 Y3F and Nck are indicated.

3   Discussion

The effect of PRL on regulation of the cell cycle progression increases our understanding of the mechanism by which PRL may stimulate growth during mammary development. Furthermore, in an abnormal genetic or environmental context, this action may contribute to mammary carcinogenesis and may point toward potential targets for pharmacological intervention in this process. Here we introduce the serine-threonine kinase PAK1 as a possible target in the PRL-dependent signaling pathway leading to cyclin D1 activation.

PAK1 has been suggested to serve as the key effector for Rac1 activation of cyclin D1 (Westwick *et al.*, 1997). Later, PAK1 was shown to activate cyclin D1 *in vivo* and *in vitro* (Balasenthil *et al.*, 2004). Overexpression of both wild type and catalytically active PAK1 T423E in different cell lines led to increased cyclin D1 promoter activity, and the overexpression of PAK1 T423E in MCF-7 cells also elevated levels of cyclin D1 mRNA, protein and nuclear accumulation of cyclin D1. Reducing PAK1 expression by PAK1-siRNA or overexpression of dominant negative PAK1 were accompanied by a significant reduction of cyclin D1 expression (Balasenthil *et al.*, 2004). The same authors demonstrated that hyperplastic mammary glands from PAK1 T423E transgenic mice exhibited increased expression of cyclin D1 as compared to the wild type mice. The authors proposed a model wherein PAK1 regulation of cyclin D1 expression involves an NFkB-dependent pathway (Balasenthil *et al.*, 2004). Merlin, the NF2 tumor suppressor gene product, has been proposed as a negative regulator of PAK1-stmulated cyclin D1 promoter activity by inhibition of PAK1 activity (Xiao *et al.*, 2005). Nheu et al. (2004) demonstrated that PAK activity is essential for rennin-angiotensin system-induced upregulation of cyclin D1 (Nheu *et al.*, 2004). All of the aforementioned studies explained the effect of PAK1 on cyclin D1 activity by the serine-threonine kinase activity of PAK1.

However, many of the effects of PAK1 seem to be independent of its kinase activity but dependent on protein-protein interaction. Thus, the kinase inhibitory domain of PAK1 (KID) induced a cell cycle arrest and inhibition of cyclin D1 and D2 expression. More importantly, this arrest could not be rescued by the expression of activated PAK1 T423E demonstrating that KID-induced cell cycle arrest occurs independently of PAK1 kinase activity (Thullberg *et al.*, 2007).

Here we linked upstream PRL-triggered signaling via JAK2 tyrosine kinase to downstream PAK1 which is a JAK2 target. We have previously demonstrated that PAK1 is a novel binding partner and a substrate of JAK2 in response to PRL activation, and identified three tyrosines (Tyr(s) 153, 201 and 285) of PAK1 that are phosphorylated by JAK2 (Rider *et al.*, 2007). Here we have shown that PAK1, in response to PRL, causes an increase of cyclin D1 promoter activity and mutation of three tyrosines (Tyrs 153, 201, 285) inhibit this amplifying effect by 55%. In an attempt to find a mechanism of this pTyr-PAK1 action, we noticed that PRL causes translocation of PAK1 into the nuclei. Nuclear translocation of PAK1 in response to EGF has been previously described (Singh *et al.*, 2005; for review Rayala and Kumar, 2007). Thus, endogenous PAK1 localizes in the nucleus in 18-24% of the interphase MCF-7 cells and directly phosphorylates histone H3 (Li *et al.*, 2002). PAK1 associates with the promoter of PFK-M gene and stimulates PFK-M expression, and also with a portion of the NFAT1 gene and represses expression of this gene (Singh *et al.*, 2005). In addition, increased levels of nuclear PAK1 were linked to intrinsic tamoxifen resistance of breast cancer cells (Holm *et al.*, 2006; Li *et al.*, 2002). We extended these findings and demonstrated that PAK1 shuttles between the cytoplasm and the nucleus in different cell lines including T47D, COS-7 and MCF-7. Furthermore, we have shown that PRL-dependent PAK1 nuclear translocation depends on Tyrs 153, 201 and 285 since the PAK1 Y3F mutant does not translocate into the nucleus in response to PRL. Three nuclear localization signals have been mapped on PAK1, and PAK1 lacking these three functional NLS (PAK1 mutNLS) fails to translocate into the nucleus in response to EGF (Singh *et al.*, 2005). We have shown here that PAK1 mutNLS exhibited 46% less impact on cyclin D promoter activity as compared to PAK1 WT. We hypothesized that by eliminating both PAK1 tyrosine phosphorylation and functional NLSs, we would completely inhibit PRL-dependent amplification of cyclin D1 promoter activity. However, PAK1 mutNLS Y3F exhibited only 68% inhibition, suggesting that both the three nuclear localization signals and three tyrosines which are phosporylated by JAK2 in response to PRL contribute to but are not exclusively required for the PRL-dependent induction of cyclin D1 promoter activity. Why do PAK1 mutNLS and PAK1 mutNLS Y3F, which both retain in the cytoplasm, still have an amplifying effect on cyclin D1 activity? PAK1 may activate cyclin D1 promoter activity in response to PRL via multiple mechanisms. For example, PAK1 phosphorylates specific cytoplasmic proteins that can directly or indirectly regulate cyclin D1 promoter activity. In this context it is interesting to note that, although PRL signals via STAT5 to the distal GAS1 binding sites in the cyclin D1 promoter, co-expression of dominant negative STAT5A and PAK1 WT showed no effect on cyclin D1 promoter activity (Brockman and Schuler, 2005; Balasenthil *et al.*, 2004; Brockman *et al.*, 2002). We are currently investigating which regulatory elements of cyclin D1 promoter are affected by PRL-dependent PAK1 tyrosyl phosphorylation.

In attempt to find another mechanism that can regulate the action of PRL on the cyclin D1, we focused on Nck for several reasons. First, adapter protein Nck is a binding partner of PAK1 (Bokoch *et al.*, 1996; Galisteo *et al.*, 1996). Nck W143R mutant with a mutation in the second SH3 domain, fails to bind to PAK (Zhu *et al.*, 2010) and the PAK1 P13A mutant is unable to interact with Nck (Bokoch *et al.*, 1996; Galisteo *et al.*, 1996). Second, Nck is present in both the cytoplasm and the nucleus (Lawe *et al.*, 1997). Nck rapidly accumulates in the nucleus after the introduction of DNA damage (Kremer *et al.*, 2007). In agreement with Lawe et.al., who showed that nuclear localization of Nck does not depend on growth factor stimulation (Lawe *et al.*, 1997), we have shown here that PRL also does not cause Nck nuclear translocation and that around 65% of cells contain nuclear Nck regardless of PRL treatment. However, when we co-expressed both Nck and PAK1, both molecules were mostly retained in the cytoplasm. This effect was especially dramatic for PAK1, since 3-fold fewer cells had nuclear PAK1 as compared with cells without Nck co-expression. More importantly, Nck abolished the ability of PRL to induce PAK1 nuclear translocation. These data suggest that Nck can sequester PAK1 in the cytoplasm. This sequestering has a physiological role since co-expression of both PAK1 and Nck inhibits the amplifying effect of PRL-induced PAK1 on cyclin D1 promoter activity (95% inhibition). This inhibition was partially abolished by disruption of the PAK1-Nck binding by using either PAK1 P13A mutant, Nck W143R mutant, or both. This partial inhibition implies the presence of Nck-PAK1-interaction-independent mechanisms that affect cyclin D1 promoter activity. Nck is a common target for a variety of growth factor receptors and becomes phosphorylated on serine, threonine and tyrosine residues after growth factor stimulation (Chou *et al.*, 1992; Li *et al.*, 1992; Park and Rhee, 1992). Nck is implicated in the regulation of different signal transduction pathways including c-Jun N-terminal kinase (JNK) and mixed lineage kinase 2 (MLK2) pathways (Miyamoto *et al.*, 2004; Poitras *et al.*, 2003; Murakami *et al.*, 2002; Becker *et al.*, 2000; Stein *et al.*, 1998; Su *et al.*, 1997). Furthermore, nuclear Nck is essential for activation of p53 in response to UV-induced DNA damage (Kremer *et al.*, 2007). Transcriptional regulation of the cyclin D1 gene as a complex and many different transcription factors have been identified that regulate the cyclin D1 promoter (reviewed in Wang *et al.*, 2004). The regulation of cyclin D1 by integrin signaling is well-documented (reviewed in Musgrove, 2006) and Nck is an important member of focal adhesions and integrin-dependent pathway (reviewed in Buday *et al.*, 2002).

It is possible that there are mechanisms other than retention of Nck-pTyr-PAK1 complex in the cytoplasm, to regulate the cyclin D1 promoter activity. Nck is a binding partner of PTP-PEST (a cytosolic protein tyrosine phosphatase) (Zhao *et al.*, 2000a). PTP-PEST has been shown to dephosphorylate PRL-activated JAK2 *in vitro* (Horsch *et al.*, 2001). We can speculate that Nck brings PTP-PEST to the PRL-induced JAK2-PAK1 complex that may lead to dephosphorylation and inactivation of JAK2. Inactive JAK2 cannot tyrosyl phosphorylate PAK1 which leads to inability of PAK1 to enhance cyclin D1 activation. Another possible common target which binds to both Nck and JAK2 is the ubiquitin ligase c-Cbl, which is a negative regulator of various signaling pathways. C-Cbl becomes tyrosyl-phosphorylated after stimulation of a wide variety of receptors including the PRL receptor (Hunter *et al.*, 1997). The negative regulation of PRL signaling by c-Cbl is confirmed by observations that c-Cbl repression leads to enhanced JAK2/STAT activation while c-Cbl overexpression results in increased ubiquitination and proteosomal degradation of STAT5 (Goh *et al.*, 2002; Wang *et al.*, 2002). Since c-Cbl binds to Nck (Wunderlich *et al.*, 1999; Rivero-Lezcano *et al.*, 1994), we can speculate that Nck may bring c-Cbl to the PRL-induced JAK2-PAK1 complex, thus leading to proteosomal degradation of JAK2 followed by attenuation of pTyr-PAK1's effect on cyclin D1 promoter activity. Nck also binds to SOCS-3 and recruits Nck to the plasma membrane (Sitko *et al.*, 2004). SOCS-3 negatively regulates PRL signaling by interacting with phosphorylated PRLR leading to JAK2 supression and, probably, by directly interacting with JAK2 which has been shown for the erythropoietin receptor (Dif *et al.*, 2001; Sasaki *et al.*, 2000; Tomic *et al.*, 1999). It would be attractive to speculate that Nck-SOCS-3 complex is recruited to the plasma membrane to bind to the PRLR leading to inactivation of JAK2 and decreased pTyr-PAK1's activity toward cyclin D1 promoter. We should, however, note that we have not seen relocation of Nck to the plasma membrane in response to PRL. It is possible that the redistribution of Nck to the plasma membrane occurs shortly after ligand treatment (for example, in 30 min as it was described for PDGF treatment (Sitko *et al.*, 2004)) while long-term treatment of PRL (24 h in the current research) has no effect on the predominantly intranuclear localization of Nck (Figure 7).

To summarize, Figure 10 shows an overall view of mechanisms of cyclin D1 promoter activity regulation by tyrosyl phosphorylated PAK1 in response to PRL. First, PRL binds to the PRL receptor and activates JAK2 which tyrosyl phosphorylates PAK1 on three tyrosines. Tyrosyl phosphorylated PAK1 translocates into the nucleus where it stimulates cyclin D1 promoter activity. Both tyrosyl phosphorylation of PAK1 and the three intact NLSs are required for this maximal effect of PRL on cyclin D1 because PAK1 mutNLS Y3F mutant has 68% reduced ability to activate the cyclin D1 promoter. However, the more critical mechanism for PAK1-dependent regulation of cyclin D1 activation is the formation of the PAK1-Nck complex in the cytoplasm. This complex retains PAK1 in the cytoplasm which leads to the inhibition of the amplifying effect of PAK1 on cyclin D1 promoter activity in response to PRL. Which protein(s) can regulate the formation of the Nck-PAK1 complex and what kind of role the phosphorylated tyrosines on PAK1 play are currently under our investigation.

It is of note that both PRL and PAK1 are oncogenic. Considering that cyclin D1 promoter activity is positively regulated by tyrosyl phosphorylated PAK1 in a PRL-dependent manner, we may speculate that the PRL-activated JAK2/PAK1 axis plays a role in breast cancer promotion. Whether JAK2-dependent phosphorylation of PAK1 plays a role in normal cells and in other types of cancer requires future investigation.

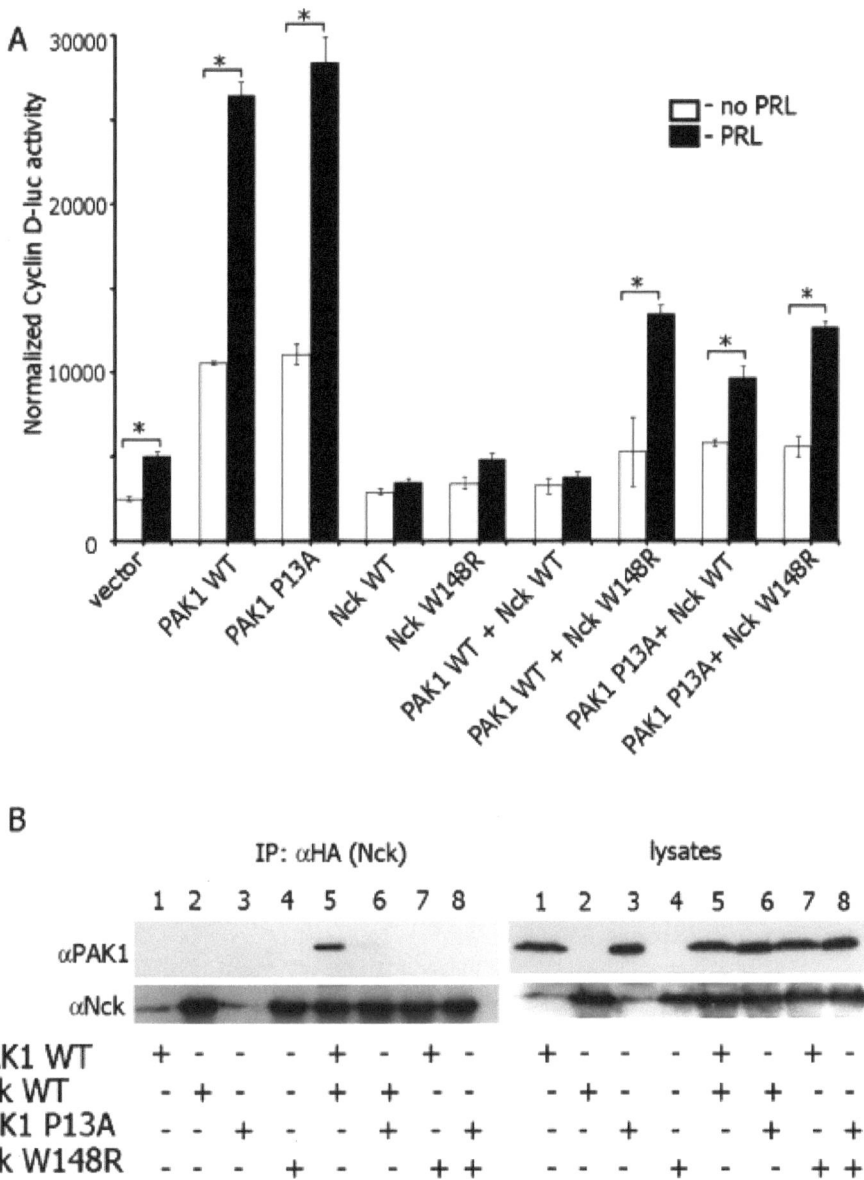

Figure 9: PAK1-Nck binding is required for the effect of Nck on cyclin D1 promoter activity.
(A) T47D cells were cotransfected with cyclin D1-luciferase reporter and cDNAs encoding the indicated proteins and treated as in Figure 7A. Luciferase activity was normalized with β-galactosidase activity. Bars represent mean ±S.E., *, p <0.05 compared with cells expressing PAK1 WT and untreated with PRL, n=3. (B) Nck WT is co-immunoprecipitated with PAK1 WT (lane 5) but not with PAK1 P13A (lane 6). Nck W148R is co-immunoprecipitated neither with PAK1 WT (lane 7) nor with PAK1 P13A (lane 8). HA-tagged Nck was immunoprecipitated with αHA from T47D cells overexpressing the indicated proteins and immunoblotted with the indicated antibodies. The light bands in lanes 1 and 3 in the αNck blot represent endogenous Nck.

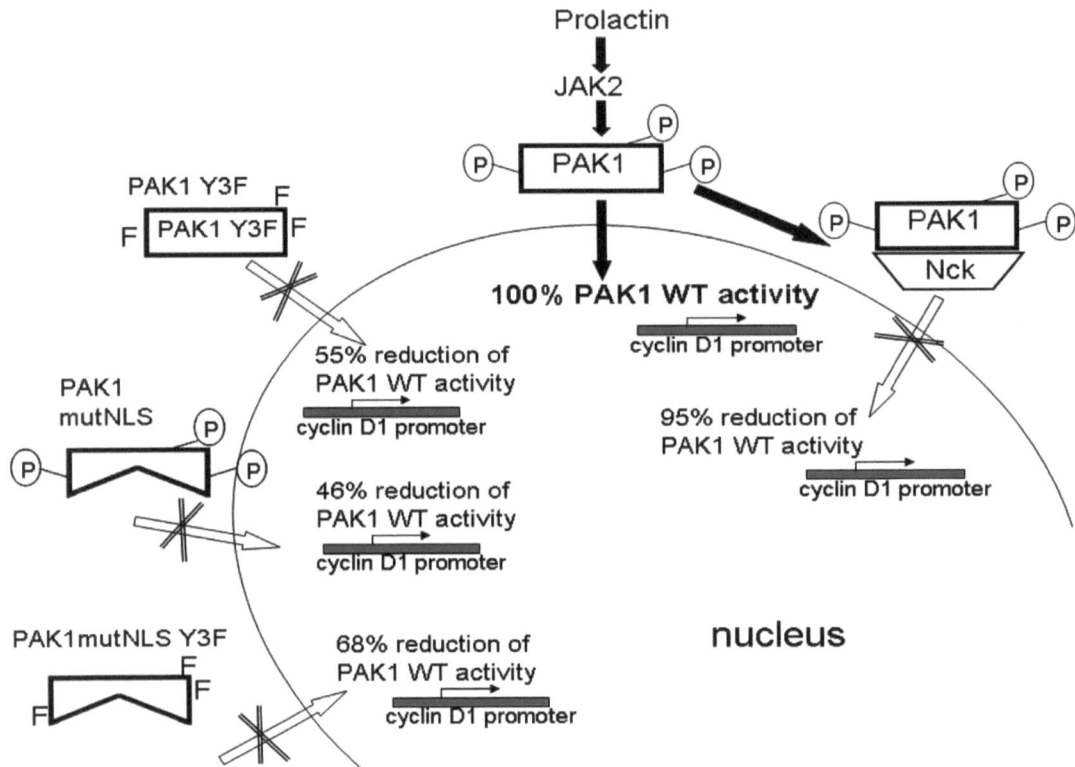

Figure 10: PAK1 regulates prolactin-dependent cyclin D1 promoter activity by two distinct mechanisms. In response to cytokines such as prolactin, PAK1 is tyrosyl phosphorylated by JAK2 and translocates into the nucleus where it stimulates cyclin D1 promoter activity. The nuclear localization signals (NLS) and the three tyrosines of PAK1 are sufficient but not required for this PAK1 function since deletion of these three phosphorylated tyrosines (PAK1 Y3F) and mutation of the three NLSs (PAK1 mutNLS) decreased PAK1 WT activity on cyclin D1 promoter activity by 55% and 46%, respectively. The double mutant of PAK1 (mutNLS Y3F) decreased PAK1 WT activity on cyclin D1 promoter activity by 68%. Another mechanism regulating the PAK1 function is Nck-PAK1 binding, since co-expression of PAK1 and Nck inhibited PAK1-dependent stimulation of cyclin D1 promoter activity by 95%. We propose that the Nck-PAK1 complex sequesters both molecules in the cytoplasm, thereby abolishing the amplifying effect of PAK1 on the prolactin-induced activation of cyclin D1.

Acknowledgement

The article has been adapted from the journal "Molecular Endocrinology" ("PAK1-Nck Regulates Cyclin D1 Promoter Activity in Response to Prolactin", v. 25, 9, 2011, p. 1565-1578; doi:10.1210/me.2011-0062)

References

Adam, L., Vadlamudi, R., Mandal, M., Chernoff, J. and Kumar, R. (2000) Regulation of microfilament reorganization and invasiveness of breast cancer cells by kinase dead p21-activated kinase-1. J Biol Chem. 275: 12041-12050.

Arnold, A. and Papanikolaou, A. (2005) Cyclin D1 in breast cancer pathogenesis. J Clin Oncol. 23: 4215-4224.

Aronheim, A., Broder, Y.C., Cohen, A., Fritsch, A., Belisle, B. and Abo, A. (1998) Chp, a homologue of the GTPase Cdc42Hs, activates the JNK pathway and is implicated in reorganizing the actin cytoskeleton. Curr Biol. 8: 1125-1128.

Asher, J.M., O'Leary, K.A., Rugowski, D.E., Arendt, L.M. and Schuler, L.A. (2012) Prolactin promotes mammary pathogenesis independently from cyclin D1. Am J Pathol. 181: 294-302.

Balasenthil, S., Sahin, A.A., Barnes, C.J., Wang, R.A., Pestell, R.G., Vadlamudi, R.K. and Kumar, R. (2004) p21-activated kinase-1 signaling mediates cyclin D1 expression in mammary epithelial and cancer cells. J Biol Chem. 279: 1422-1428.

Ball, R.K., Friis, R.R., Schoenenberger, C.A., Doppler, W. and Groner, B. (1988) Prolactin regulation of beta-casein gene expression and of a cytosolic 120-kd protein in a cloned mouse mammary epithelial cell line. Embo J. 7: 2089-2095.

Banerjee, M., Worth, D., Prowse, D.M. and Nikolic, M. (2002) Pak1 phosphorylation on t212 affects microtubules in cells undergoing mitosis. Curr Biol. 12: 1233-1239.

Becker, E., Huynh-Do, U., Holland, S., Pawson, T., Daniel, T.O. and Skolnik, E.Y. (2000) Nck-interacting Ste20 kinase couples Eph receptors to c-Jun N-terminal kinase and integrin activation. Mol Cell Biol. 20: 1537-1545.

Bekri, S., Adelaide, J., Merscher, S., Grosgeorge, J., Caroli-Bosc, F., Perucca-Lostanlen, D., et al (1997) Detailed map of a region commonly amplified at 11q13-->q14 in human breast carcinoma. Cytogenet Cell Genet. 79: 125-131.

Ben-Jonathan, N., LaPensee, C.R. and LaPensee, E.W. (2008) What can we learn from rodents about prolactin in humans? Endocr Rev. 29: 1-41.

Bernichtein, S., Touraine, P. and Goffin, V. (2010) New concepts in prolactin biology. J Endocrinol. 206: 1-11.

Bienvenu, F., Jirawatnotai, S., Elias, J.E., Meyer, C.A., Mizeracka, K., Marson, A., et al (2010) Transcriptional role of cyclin D1 in development revealed by a genetic-proteomic screen. Nature. 463: 374-378.

Bokoch, G.M. (2003) Biology of the p21-activated kinases. Annu Rev Biochem. 72: 743-781.

Bokoch, G.M., Wang, Y., Bohl, B.P., Sells, M.A., Quilliam, L.A. and Knaus, U.G. (1996) Interaction of the Nck adapter protein with p21-activated kinase (PAK1). J Biol Chem. 271: 25746-25749.

Bokoch, G.M., Reilly, A.M., Daniels, R.H., King, C.C., Olivera, A., Spiegel, S. and Knaus, U.G. (1998) A GTPase-independent mechanism of p21-activated kinase activation. Regulation by sphingosine and other biologically active lipids. J Biol Chem. 273: 8137-8144.

Brockman, J.L. and Schuler, L.A. (2005) Prolactin signals via Stat5 and Oct-1 to the proximal cyclin D1 promoter. Mol Cell Endocrinol. 239: 45-53.

Brockman, J.L., Schroeder, M.D. and Schuler, L.A. (2002) PRL activates the cyclin D1 promoter via the Jak2/Stat pathway. Mol Endocrinol. 16: 774-784.

Buday, L., Wunderlich, L. and Tamas, P. (2002) The Nck family of adapter proteins: regulators of actin cytoskeleton. Cell Signal. 14: 723-731.

Chou, M.M., Fajardo, J.E. and Hanafusa, H. (1992) The SH2- and SH3-containing Nck protein transforms mammalian fibroblasts in the absence of elevated phosphotyrosine levels. Mol Cell Biol. 12: 5834-5842.

Clevenger, C.V. (2003) Role of prolactin/prolactin receptor signaling in human breast cancer. Breast Dis. 18: 75-86.

Clevenger, C.V., Chang, W.P., Ngo, W., Pasha, T.L., Montone, K.T. and Tomaszewski, J.E. (1995) *Expression of prolactin and prolactin receptor in human breast carcinoma. Evidence for an autocrine/paracrine loop. Am J Pathol. 146: 695-705.*

Coqueret, O. (2002) *Linking cyclins to transcriptional control. Gene. 299: 35-55.*

Daniels, R.H., Hall, P.S. and Bokoch, G.M. (1998) *Membrane targeting of p21-activated kinase 1 (PAK1) induces neurite outgrowth from PC12 cells. Embo J. 17: 754-764.*

DaSilva, L., Rui, H., Erwin, R.A., Howard, O.M., Kirken, R.A., Malabarba, M.G., et al (1996) *Prolactin recruits STAT1, STAT3 and STAT5 independent of conserved receptor tyrosines TYR402, TYR479, TYR515 and TYR580. Mol Cell Endocrinol. 117: 131-140.*

Dickson, C., Fantl, V., Gillett, C., Brookes, S., Bartek, J., Smith, R., et al (1995) *Amplification of chromosome band 11q13 and a role for cyclin D1 in human breast cancer. Cancer Lett. 90: 43-50.*

Diehl, J.A. (2002) *Cycling to cancer with cyclin D1. Cancer Biol Ther. 1: 226-231.*

Dif, F., Saunier, E., Demeneix, B., Kelly, P.A. and Edery, M. (2001) *Cytokine-inducible SH2-containing protein suppresses PRL signaling by binding the PRL receptor. Endocrinology. 142: 5286-5293.*

Fantl, V., Stamp, G., Andrews, A., Rosewell, I. and Dickson, C. (1995) *Mice lacking cyclin D1 are small and show defects in eye and mammary gland development. Genes Dev. 9: 2364-2372.*

Fu, M., Wang, C., Li, Z., Sakamaki, T. and Pestell, R.G. (2004) *Minireview: Cyclin D1: normal and abnormal functions. Endocrinology. 145: 5439-5447.*

Galisteo, M.L., Chernoff, J., Su, Y.C., Skolnik, E.Y. and Schlessinger, J. (1996) *The adaptor protein Nck links receptor tyrosine kinases with the serine-threonine kinase Pak1. J Biol Chem. 271: 20997-21000.*

Ginsburg, E. and Vonderhaar, B.K. (1995) *Prolactin synthesis and secretion by human breast cancer cells. Cancer Res. 55: 2591-2595.*

Goh, E.L., Zhu, T., Leong, W.Y. and Lobie, P.E. (2002) *c-Cbl is a negative regulator of GH-stimulated STAT5-mediated transcription. Endocrinology. 143: 3590-3603.*

Gururaj, A.E., Rayala, S.K. and Kumar, R. (2005) *p21-activated kinase signaling in breast cancer. Breast Cancer Res. 7: 5-12.*

Hankinson, S.E., Willett, W.C., Michaud, D.S., Manson, J.E., Colditz, G.A., Longcope, C., et al (1999) *Plasma prolactin levels and subsequent risk of breast cancer in postmenopausal women. J Natl Cancer Inst. 91: 629-634.*

Holm, C., Rayala, S., Jirstrom, K., Stal, O., Kumar, R. and Landberg, G. (2006) *Association between Pak1 expression and subcellular localization and tamoxifen resistance in breast cancer patients. J Natl Cancer Inst. 98: 671-680.*

Horsch, K., Schaller, M.D. and Hynes, N.E. (2001) *The protein tyrosine phosphatase-PEST is implicated in the negative regulation of epidermal growth factor on PRL signaling in mammary epithelial cells. Mol Endocrinol. 15: 2182-2196.*

Hunter, S., Koch, B.L. and Anderson, S.M. (1997) *Phosphorylation of cbl after stimulation of Nb2 cells with prolactin and its association with phosphatidylinositol 3-kinase. Mol Endocrinol. 11: 1213-1222.*

Jeselsohn, R., Brown, N.E., Arendt, L., Klebba, I., Hu, M.G., Kuperwasser, C. and Hinds, P.W. (2010) *Cyclin D1 kinase activity is required for the self-renewal of mammary stem and progenitor cells that are targets of MMTV-ErbB2 tumorigenesis. Cancer Cell. 17: 65-76.*

Keyomarsi, K. and Pardee, A.B. (1993) *Redundant cyclin overexpression and gene amplification in breast cancer cells. Proc Natl Acad Sci U S A. 90: 1112-1116.*

Khaled, W.T., Read, E.K., Nicholson, S.E., Baxter, F.O., Brennan, A.J., Came, P.J., et al (2007) *The IL-4/IL-13/Stat6 signalling pathway promotes luminal mammary epithelial cell development. Development. 134: 2739-2750.*

King, C.C., Gardiner, E.M., Zenke, F.T., Bohl, B.P., Newton, A.C., Hemmings, B.A. and Bokoch, G.M. (2000) p21-activated kinase (PAK1) is phosphorylated and activated by 3-phosphoinositide-dependent kinase-1 (PDK1). J Biol Chem. 275: 41201-41209.

Knaus, U.G. and Bokoch, G.M. (1998) The p21Rac/Cdc42-activated kinases (PAKs). Int J Biochem Cell Biol. 30: 857-862.

Knudsen, K.E., Diehl, J.A., Haiman, C.A. and Knudsen, E.S. (2006) Cyclin D1: polymorphism, aberrant splicing and cancer risk. Oncogene. 25: 1620-1628.

Kremer, B.E., Adang, L.A. and Macara, I.G. (2007) Septins regulate actin organization and cell-cycle arrest through nuclear accumulation of NCK mediated by SOCS7. Cell. 130: 837-850.

Kumar, R. and Vadlamudi, R.K. (2002) Emerging functions of p21-activated kinases in human cancer cells. J Cell Physiol. 193: 133-144.

Kumar, R., Gururaj, A.E. and Barnes, C.J. (2006) p21-activated kinases in cancer. Nat Rev Cancer. 6: 459-471.

Landis, M.W., Pawlyk, B.S., Li, T., Sicinski, P. and Hinds, P.W. (2006) Cyclin D1-dependent kinase activity in murine development and mammary tumorigenesis. Cancer Cell. 9: 13-22.

Lawe, D.C., Hahn, C. and Wong, A.J. (1997) The Nck SH2/SH3 adaptor protein is present in the nucleus and associates with the nuclear protein SAM68. Oncogene. 14: 223-231.

Lee, Y.M. and Sicinski, P. (2006) Targeting cyclins and cyclin-dependent kinases in cancer: lessons from mice, hopes for therapeutic applications in human. Cell Cycle. 5: 2110-2114.

Lei, M., Lu, W., Meng, W., Parrini, M.C., Eck, M.J., Mayer, B.J. and Harrison, S.C. (2000) Structure of PAK1 in an auto-inhibited conformation reveals a multistage activation switch. Cell. 102: 387-397.

Li, F., Adam, L., Vadlamudi, R.K., Zhou, H., Sen, S., Chernoff, J., et al (2002) p21-activated kinase 1 interacts with and phosphorylates histone H3 in breast cancer cells. EMBO Rep. 3: 767-773.

Li, W., Hu, P., Skolnik, E.Y., Ullrich, A. and Schlessinger, J. (1992) The SH2 and SH3 domain-containing Nck protein is oncogenic and a common target for phosphorylation by different surface receptors. Mol Cell Biol. 12: 5824-5833.

Lim, C.P. and Cao, X. (2006) Structure, function, and regulation of STAT proteins. Mol Biosyst. 2: 536-550.

Lin, D.I., Lessie, M.D., Gladden, A.B., Bassing, C.H., Wagner, K.U. and Diehl, J.A. (2008) Disruption of cyclin D1 nuclear export and proteolysis accelerates mammary carcinogenesis. Oncogene. 27: 1231-1242.

Lu, W., Katz, S., Gupta, R. and Mayer, B.J. (1997) Activation of Pak by membrane localization mediated by an SH3 domain from the adaptor protein Nck. Curr Biol. 7: 85-94.

Manser, E., Leung, T., Salihuddin, H., Zhao, Z.S. and Lim, L. (1994) A brain serine/threonine protein kinase activated by Cdc42 and Rac1. Nature. 367: 40-46.

Manser, E., Huang, H.Y., Loo, T.H., Chen, X.Q., Dong, J.M., Leung, T. and Lim, L. (1997) Expression of constitutively active alpha-PAK reveals effects of the kinase on actin and focal complexes. Mol Cell Biol. 17: 1129-1143.

McIntosh, G.G., Anderson, J.J., Milton, I., Steward, M., Parr, A.H., Thomas, M.D., et al (1995) Determination of the prognostic value of cyclin D1 overexpression in breast cancer. Oncogene. 11: 885-891.

Megha, T., Lazzi, S., Ferrari, F., Vatti, R., Howard, C.M., Cevenini, G., et al (1999) Expression of the G2-M checkpoint regulators cyclin B1 and P34CDC2 in breast cancer: a correlation with cellular kinetics. Anticancer Res. 19: 163-169.

Meng, J., Tsai-Morris, C.H. and Dufau, M.L. (2004) Human prolactin receptor variants in breast cancer: low ratio of short forms to the long-form human prolactin receptor associated with mammary carcinoma. Cancer Res. 64: 5677-5682.

Mira, J.P., Benard, V., Groffen, J., Sanders, L.C. and Knaus, U.G. (2000) Endogenous, hyperactive Rac3 controls proliferation of breast cancer cells by a p21-activated kinase-dependent pathway. Proc Natl Acad Sci U S A. 97: 185-189.

Miyamoto, Y., Yamauchi, J., Mizuno, N. and Itoh, H. (2004) The adaptor protein Nck1 mediates endothelin A receptor-regulated cell migration through the Cdc42-dependent c-Jun N-terminal kinase pathway. J Biol Chem. 279: 34336-34342.

Murakami, H., Yamamura, Y., Shimono, Y., Kawai, K., Kurokawa, K. and Takahashi, M. (2002) Role of Dok1 in cell signaling mediated by RET tyrosine kinase. J Biol Chem. 277: 32781-32790.

Musgrove, E.A. (2006) Cyclins: roles in mitogenic signaling and oncogenic transformation. Growth Factors. 24: 13-19.

Musgrove, E.A., Caldon, C.E., Barraclough, J., Stone, A. and Sutherland, R.L. (2011) Cyclin D as a therapeutic target in cancer. Nat Rev Cancer. 11: 558-572.

Neudauer, C.L., Joberty, G., Tatsis, N. and Macara, I.G. (1998) Distinct cellular effects and interactions of the Rho-family GTPase TC10. Curr Biol. 8: 1151-1160.

Nheu, T., He, H., Hirokawa, Y., Walker, F., Wood, J. and Maruta, H. (2004) PAK is essential for RAS-induced upregulation of cyclin D1 during the G1 to S transition. Cell Cycle. 3: 71-74.

Nikolic, M., Chou, M.M., Lu, W., Mayer, B.J. and Tsai, L.H. (1998) The p35/Cdk5 kinase is a neuron-specific Rac effector that inhibits Pak1 activity. Nature. 395: 194-198.

Park, D. and Rhee, S.G. (1992) Phosphorylation of Nck in response to a variety of receptors, phorbol myristate acetate, and cyclic AMP. Mol Cell Biol. 12: 5816-5823.

Park, J.B., Kim, E.J., Yang, E.J., Seo, S.R. and Chung, K.C. (2007) JNK- and Rac1-dependent induction of immediate early gene pip92 suppresses neuronal differentiation. J Neurochem. 100: 555-566.

Parrini, M.C., Lei, M., Harrison, S.C. and Mayer, B.J. (2002) Pak1 kinase homodimers are autoinhibited in trans and dissociated upon activation by Cdc42 and Rac1. Mol Cell. 9: 73-83.

Poitras, L., Jean, S., Islam, N. and Moss, T. (2003) PAK interacts with NCK and MLK2 to regulate the activation of jun N-terminal kinase. FEBS Lett. 543: 129-135.

Rashid, T., Banerjee, M. and Nikolic, M. (2001) Phosphorylation of Pak1 by the p35/Cdk5 kinase affects neuronal morphology. J Biol Chem. 276: 49043-49052.

Rayala, S.K. and Kumar, R. (2007) Sliding p21-activated kinase 1 to nucleus impacts tamoxifen sensitivity. Biomed Pharmacother.

Rayala, S.K., Talukder, A.H., Balasenthil, S., Tharakan, R., Barnes, C.J., Wang, R.A., et al (2006) P21-activated kinase 1 regulation of estrogen receptor-alpha activation involves serine 305 activation linked with serine 118 phosphorylation. Cancer Res. 66: 1694-1701.

Reich, N.C. (2007) STAT dynamics. Cytokine Growth Factor Rev. 18: 511-518.

Rider, L., Shatrova, A., Feener, E.P., Webb, L. and Diakonova, M. (2007) JAK2 tyrosine kinase phosphorylates PAK1 and regulates PAK1 activity and functions. J Biol Chem. 282: 30985-30996.

Rivero-Lezcano, O.M., Sameshima, J.H., Marcilla, A. and Robbins, K.C. (1994) Physical association between Src homology 3 elements and the protein product of the c-cbl proto-oncogene. J Biol Chem. 269: 17363-17366.

Sakamoto, K., Creamer, B.A., Triplett, A.A. and Wagner, K.U. (2007) The Janus kinase 2 is required for expression and nuclear accumulation of cyclin D1 in proliferating mammary epithelial cells. Mol Endocrinol. 21: 1877-1892.

Salh, B., Marotta, A., Wagey, R., Sayed, M. and Pelech, S. (2002) Dysregulation of phosphatidylinositol 3-kinase and downstream effectors in human breast cancer. Int J Cancer. 98: 148-154.

Sasaki, A., Yasukawa, H., Shouda, T., Kitamura, T., Dikic, I. and Yoshimura, A. (2000) CIS3/SOCS-3 suppresses erythropoietin (EPO) signaling by binding the EPO receptor and JAK2. J Biol Chem. 275: 29338-29347.

Schaber, J.D., Fang, H., Xu, J., Grimley, P.M. and Rui, H. (1998) Prolactin activates Stat1 but does not antagonize Stat1 activation and growth inhibition by type I interferons in human breast cancer cells. Cancer Res. 58: 1914-1919.

Schindler, C., Levy, D.E. and Decker, T. (2007) JAK-STAT signaling: from interferons to cytokines. J Biol Chem. 282: 20059-20063.

Schroeder, M.D., Symowicz, J. and Schuler, L.A. (2002) PRL modulates cell cycle regulators in mammary tumor epithelial cells. Mol Endocrinol. 16: 45-57.

Sherr, C.J. (1995) D-type cyclins. Trends Biochem Sci. 20: 187-190.

Sicinski, P., Donaher, J.L., Parker, S.B., Li, T., Fazeli, A., Gardner, H., et al (1995) Cyclin D1 provides a link between development and oncogenesis in the retina and breast. Cell. 82: 621-630.

Singh, R.R., Song, C., Yang, Z. and Kumar, R. (2005) Nuclear localization and chromatin targets of p21-activated kinase 1. J Biol Chem. 280: 18130-18137.

Sitko, J.C., Guevara, C.I. and Cacalano, N.A. (2004) Tyrosine-phosphorylated SOCS3 interacts with the Nck and Crk-L adapter proteins and regulates Nck activation. J Biol Chem. 279: 37662-37669.

Stein, E., Huynh-Do, U., Lane, A.A., Cerretti, D.P. and Daniel, T.O. (1998) Nck recruitment to Eph receptor, EphB1/ELK, couples ligand activation to c-Jun kinase. J Biol Chem. 273: 1303-1308.

Su, Y.C., Han, J., Xu, S., Cobb, M. and Skolnik, E.Y. (1997) NIK is a new Ste20-related kinase that binds NCK and MEKK1 and activates the SAPK/JNK cascade via a conserved regulatory domain. Embo J. 16: 1279-1290.

Sutherland, R.L. and Musgrove, E.A. (2004) Cyclins and breast cancer. J Mammary Gland Biol Neoplasia. 9: 95-104.

Suzuki, R., Kuroda, H., Komatsu, H., Hosokawa, Y., Kagami, Y., Ogura, M., et al (1999) Selective usage of D-type cyclins in lymphoid malignancies. Leukemia. 13: 1335-1342.

Swaminathan, G., Varghese, B. and Fuchs, S.Y. (2008) Regulation of prolactin receptor levels and activity in breast cancer. J Mammary Gland Biol Neoplasia. 13: 81-91.

Tan, S.H. and Nevalainen, M.T. (2008) Signal transducer and activator of transcription 5A/B in prostate and breast cancers. Endocr Relat Cancer. 15: 367-390.

Tang, Y., Zhou, H., Chen, A., Pittman, R.N. and Field, J. (2000) The Akt proto-oncogene links Ras to Pak and cell survival signals. J Biol Chem. 275: 9106-9109.

Tao, W., Pennica, D., Xu, L., Kalejta, R.F. and Levine, A.J. (2001) Wrch-1, a novel member of the Rho gene family that is regulated by Wnt-1. Genes Dev. 15: 1796-1807.

Thiel, D.A., Reeder, M.K., Pfaff, A., Coleman, T.R., Sells, M.A. and Chernoff, J. (2002) Cell cycle-regulated phosphorylation of p21-activated kinase 1. Curr Biol. 12: 1227-1232.

Thullberg, M., Gad, A., Beeser, A., Chernoff, J. and Stromblad, S. (2007) The kinase-inhibitory domain of p21-activated kinase 1 (PAK1) inhibits cell cycle progression independent of PAK1 kinase activity. Oncogene. 26: 1820-1828.

Tomic, S., Chughtai, N. and Ali, S. (1999) SOCS-1, -2, -3: selective targets and functions downstream of the prolactin receptor. Mol Cell Endocrinol. 158: 45-54.

Tornell, J., Rymo, L. and Isaksson, O.G. (1991) Induction of mammary adenocarcinomas in metallothionein promoter-human growth hormone transgenic mice. Int J Cancer. 49: 114-117.

Touraine, P., Martini, J.F., Zafrani, B., Durand, J.C., Labaille, F., Malet, C., et al (1998) Increased expression of prolactin receptor gene assessed by quantitative polymerase chain reaction in human breast tumors versus normal breast tissues. J Clin Endocrinol Metab. 83: 667-674.

Tworoger, S.S. and Hankinson, S.E. (2006) Prolactin and breast cancer risk. Cancer Lett. 243: 160-169.

Vadlamudi, R.K., Li, F., Adam, L., Nguyen, D., Ohta, Y., Stossel, T.P. and Kumar, R. (2002) Filamin is essential in actin cytoskeletal assembly mediated by p21-activated kinase 1. Nat Cell Biol. 4: 681-690.

Vadlamudi, R.K., Bagheri-Yarmand, R., Yang, Z., Balasenthil, S., Nguyen, D., Sahin, A.A., et al (2004) Dynein light chain 1, a p21-activated kinase 1-interacting substrate, promotes cancerous phenotypes. Cancer Cell. 5: 575-585.

Vadlamudi, R.K., Adam, L., Wang, R.A., Mandal, M., Nguyen, D., Sahin, A., et al (2000) Regulatable expression of p21-activated kinase-1 promotes anchorage-independent growth and abnormal organization of mitotic spindles in human epithelial breast cancer cells. J Biol Chem. 275: 36238-36244.

Wagner, K.U. and Rui, H. (2008) Jak2/Stat5 signaling in mammogenesis, breast cancer initiation and progression. J Mammary Gland Biol Neoplasia. 13: 93-103.

Wakao, H., Gouilleux, F. and Groner, B. (1994) Mammary gland factor (MGF) is a novel member of the cytokine regulated transcription factor gene family and confers the prolactin response. Embo J. 13: 2182-2191.

Wang, C., Li, Z., Fu, M., Bouras, T. and Pestell, R.G. (2004) Signal transduction mediated by cyclin D1: from mitogens to cell proliferation: a molecular target with therapeutic potential. Cancer Treat Res. 119: 217-237.

Wang, L., Rudert, W.A., Loutaev, I., Roginskaya, V. and Corey, S.J. (2002) Repression of c-Cbl leads to enhanced G-CSF Jak-STAT signaling without increased cell proliferation. Oncogene. 21: 5346-5355.

Wang, T.C., Cardiff, R.D., Zukerberg, L., Lees, E., Arnold, A. and Schmidt, E.V. (1994) Mammary hyperplasia and carcinoma in MMTV-cyclin D1 transgenic mice. Nature. 369: 669-671.

Wennbo, H., Gebre-Medhin, M., Gritli-Linde, A., Ohlsson, C., Isaksson, O.G. and Tornell, J. (1997) Activation of the prolactin receptor but not the growth hormone receptor is important for induction of mammary tumors in transgenic mice. J Clin Invest. 100: 2744-2751.

Westwick, J.K., Lambert, Q.T., Clark, G.J., Symons, M., Van Aelst, L., Pestell, R.G. and Der, C.J. (1997) Rac regulation of transformation, gene expression, and actin organization by multiple, PAK-independent pathways. Mol Cell Biol. 17: 1324-1335.

Wunderlich, L., Goher, A., Farago, A., Downward, J. and Buday, L. (1999) Requirement of multiple SH3 domains of Nck for ligand binding. Cell Signal. 11: 253-262.

Xiao, G.H., Gallagher, R., Shetler, J., Skele, K., Altomare, D.A., Pestell, R.G., et al (2005) The NF2 tumor suppressor gene product, merlin, inhibits cell proliferation and cell cycle progression by repressing cyclin D1 expression. Mol Cell Biol. 25: 2384-2394.

Yu, Q., Geng, Y. and Sicinski, P. (2001) Specific protection against breast cancers by cyclin D1 ablation. Nature. 411: 1017-1021.

Zhang, Q., Sakamoto, K., Liu, C., Triplett, A.A., Lin, W.C., Rui, H. and Wagner, K.U. (2011) Cyclin D3 compensates for the loss of cyclin D1 during ErbB2-induced mammary tumor initiation and progression. Cancer Res. 71: 7513-7524.

Zhao, Z.S. and Manser, E. (2005) PAK and other Rho-associated kinases--effectors with surprisingly diverse mechanisms of regulation. Biochem J. 386: 201-214.

Zhao, Z.S., Manser, E. and Lim, L. (2000a) Interaction between PAK and nck: a template for Nck targets and role of PAK autophosphorylation. Mol Cell Biol. 20: 3906-3917.

Zhao, Z.S., Manser, E., Loo, T.H. and Lim, L. (2000b) Coupling of PAK-interacting exchange factor PIX to GIT1 promotes focal complex disassembly. Mol Cell Biol. 20: 6354-6363.

Zhu, J., Attias, O., Aoudjit, L., Jiang, R., Kawachi, H. and Takano, T. (2010) p21-activated kinases regulate actin remodeling in glomerular podocytes. Am J Physiol Renal Physiol. 298: F951-961.

Evaluation of Methods of Adrenalectomy

Virgilijus Beiša

Vilnius University, Faculty of Medicine
Vilnius University Hospital Santariskiu Clinics, Lithuania

1   Introduction

Gagner *et al.* has reported laparoscopic adrenalectomy in 1992 (Fernandez-Cruz *et al.*, 1996) and it has become a "golden standard" for adrenal surgery soon, due to various benefits this methods, in comparison with conventional surgery (Smith *et al.*, 1999; Gagner *et al.*, 1997; Higashihara *et al.*, 1992; Jacobs *et al.*, 1997; Kebebew et al., 2001). In 1995, S. Mercan and M. K. Walz published an article about the first endoscopic retroperitoneal adrenalectomy (Walz *et al.*, 1995). Minimally invasive adrenalectomy is associated with lower morbidity rates, reduced postoperative pain, shorter hospital stay, a more rapid postoperative recovery and economic cost reduction than conventional open surgery (Brunt *et al.*, 1996; Rubinstein *et al.*, 2005; Thompson *et al.*, 1997; Hallfeldt *et al.*, 2003). Indications for conventional open surgery include large adrenal tumors (> 10 cm) and adrenal cancer involving adjacent tissues and organs. The group of tumors with the size ranging from 3 to 7 cm that are operated on most frequently include incidentalomas (incidentally diagnosed, hormone non-producing tumors), hormone producing tumors (aldosteronoma, corticosteroma, pheochromocytoma), non-primary adrenal cancer pathology (metastases). These tumors are removed using lateral transabdominal adrenalectomy (LTA) or posterior retroperitoneoscopic adrenalectomy (PRA) techniques. The laparoscopic approach is reported most often in the literature because it offers simple identifying, dissecting, and mobilizing of intra-abdominal structures. The posterior retroperitoneoscpic approach has the following advantages: it is a minimally invasive procedure and allows direct access to the adrenal gland without affecting intra peritoneal organs (Mercan *et al.*, 1995; Walz *et al.*, 1996). However, further studies showed that posterior retroperitoneoscpic adrenalectomies had no advantages when compared with lateral transabdominal adrenalectomy (Duh *et al.*, 1996; Kebebew *et al.*, 2001), except in patients with bilateral lesions of the adrenal glands, obese patients and patients with peritoneal adhesions (Gockel *et al.*, 2005; Lezoche *et al.*, 2002; Walz *et al.*, 2001). Which approach, transabdominal or retroperitoneal, is the best, is not determined yet and there are supporters of both methods. The adrenal tumors, smaller than 3 cm, are being removed in event they have hormone activity or a metastasis is present. Among small (< 3 cm) hormone active tumors, aldosteronoma (Conn's adenoma) is found most frequently (Johnson *et al.*, 2009). All methods of minimally invasive surgery, including laparoscopic, posterior retroperitoneoscpic, single incision laparoscopic surgery (SILS), single access retroperitoneoscopic adrenalectomy (SARA) may be used to remove small (<3 cm) tumors. Good cosmetic result is an advantage of SILS and SARA, in comparison with other endoscopic methods. We have performed two retrospective studies and compared the results of LTA and PRA for the patients who underwent removal of adrenal gland tumors ranging from 3 – 7 cm (group I A and I B) and results of LTA, PRA, SILS and SARA technique for the patients who underwent removal of adrenal gland tumors < 3 cm (groups II A, II B, II C). We had an aim to analyse which method of operation was the most suitable for surgery of tumors ranging from 3 – 7 cm and small tumours (less than 3 cm).

2   Patients and Methods

Seventy patients with adrenal tumors (Group I) operated on at Vilnius University Hospital Santariškių Clinics were included in this retrospective study: 40 patients underwent LTA (Group I A) and 30 patients (1 patient had bilateral lesion of adrenals) underwent PRA (Group I B). The patients of IA and IB group were distributed, according cohort principle: till 2008, all the patients with adrenal gland tumours < 7 cm large (Group I A) were operated on using lateral transabdominal method. Since 2008, all the patients with tumours of the same size were operated on using posterior retroperitoneoscopic mode (Group I B). The same surgeon had operated on 49 patients (70%) (22/40 in group I A, and 27/30 in group I B). All patients with adrenal gland lesions were thoroughly examined by endocrinologist using ultrasound and CT scans. Blood and urine levels of electrolytes and catecholamines and blood levels of aldosterone and cortisol were evaluated in patients with elevated arterial blood pressure.

The size of a tumour was < 3 cm in all patients of groups II A, II B, II C ($n = 31$). The indications for removal of such tumours include metastasis in the adrenal gland and aldosteronoma. All patients in the second group underwent surgery for aldosteronoma. Group II A ($n = 6$) patients had undergone the LTA, group II B ($n = 20$) – the PRA and group II C ($n = 5$) – the posterior retroperitoneoscopic approach via single incision (1 SILS and 4 SARA adrenalectomies). The same surgeon had operated on 70% patients of groups II A and II B and all the patients of group II C.

3   Surgical Methods

3.1   Lateral Transabdominal Adrenalectomy (LTA)

The surgery is performed under general anesthesia. The patient is positioned on one side, bent at the waist at 30° angle with a roller below. The surgeon and the first assistant stands in front of the patient. *Veress* needle is inserted into abdominal cavity 2 cm below the costal margin, along *l. medioclavicularis*. Pneumoperitoneum (12 mmHg) is created by insufflation of carbon dioxide. After that, if the surgery is being done on the right side, four 10 mm-diameter trocars are introduced 2 cm below the costal margin, along *l. medioclavicularis, l. axillaris anterior, l. axilaris medialis* and *l. axilaris posterior* into abdominal cavity. A liver retractor is inserted into the first trocar, the second one is used for the scissors or ultrasound scalpel, the third one – for 30° optics and the fourth trocar is used for forceps. The liver retractor is held by the second assistant who stands on the opposite side (behind the back of the patient) (Figure 1).

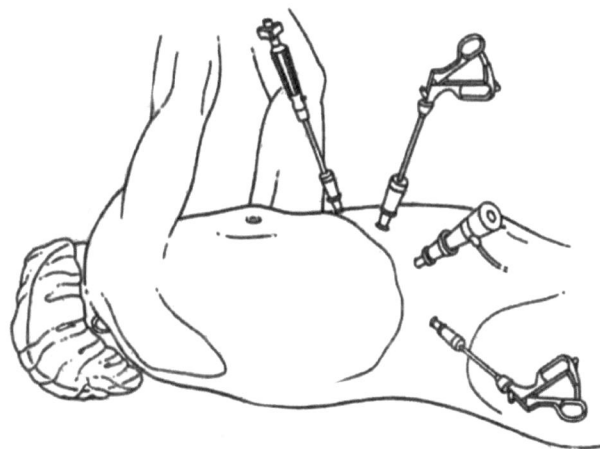

Figure 1: Right lateral transabdominal adrenalectomy. Positions of the patient and trocars.

Lig. triangulare hepatis dex. is cut and the peritoneum is incised along the inferior margin of the right liver lobe. The right lobe of the liver is retracted superomedially. A *Kocher's* maneuver is performed to realease duodenum. *V. cava inferior* and the upper pole of the right kidney are mobilized. The right adrenal gland is prepared between *v. cava inferior* and the upper pole of the kidney. The separation is started from the medial margin. Small vessels are coagulated or transected with the ultrasound scalpel, *v. centralis* above conjunction with *v. cava inferior* is clamped with 2 metal clips and transected. The upper and lower adrenal poles are mobilized. The separated adrenal gland is placed into retrieval bag and extracted through the expanded opening of insertion of the second trocar.

In event the surgery is being done on the left side, the patient is placed on the right side. The operation is being performed using three trocars, as the retractor is not required. The first trocar used for forceps, the second – for 30° optics and the third trocar is used for ultrasound scalpel or scissors.

Lig. phrenicocolicum is cut and the left colic flexure is mobilized. After that, the large intestine is retracted downwards. The peritoneum and *lig. phrenicolienale* are cut from the lower to the upper spleen pole laterally. The tail of pancreas is also mobilized along with the spleen. Then, the spleen is rotated medially. The left adrenal gland is separated under the tail of the pancreas more medially from the upper pole of the left kidney. At the inferomedial margin, *v. centralis* is clamped with two metal clips before conjunction with *v. renalis sin.* The vein is transected between the clips. The superomedial margin of the left adrenal gland is mobilized. Small vessels are coagulated or transected with ultrasound scalpel. The lateral margin of adrenal gland is mobilized. The separated adrenal gland is placed into a retrieval bag and extracted through the expanded opening of insertion of the third trocar.

The latter opening is sutured with double stitch: the muscles and the aponeurosis of the external oblique muscle are sutured with two separate absorbable 3/0 stitches and the skin is sutured with 1 or 2 separate stitches. The drain is not inserted. The openings of the other trocars insertions are sutured only with separate skin stitches.

3.2   Posterior Retroperitoneoscopic Adrenalectomy (PRA)

The surgery is performed under general anaesthesia. The patient is placed in the prone jack-knife position or above-mentioned lateral decubitus position 45° angle (Figure 2).

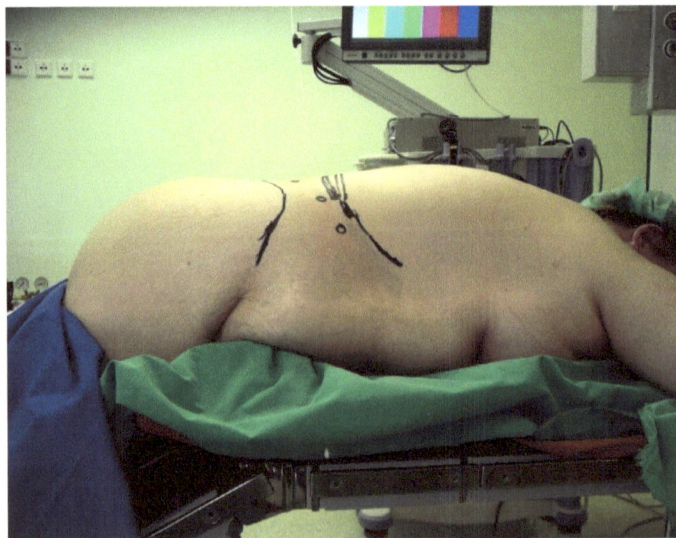

Figure 2: Posterior retroperitoneoscopic adrenalectomy. Placing of trocars. The surgeon and assistant stand on the side of the adrenal gland to be removed.

A 1.5 cm transverse incision is made at the tip of XII rib. After preparing the subcutaneous and muscular layers, *fascia thoracolumbalis* is dissected. Following these steps, the retroperitoneal space is accessed and a small cavity is prepared digitally (Figure 3).

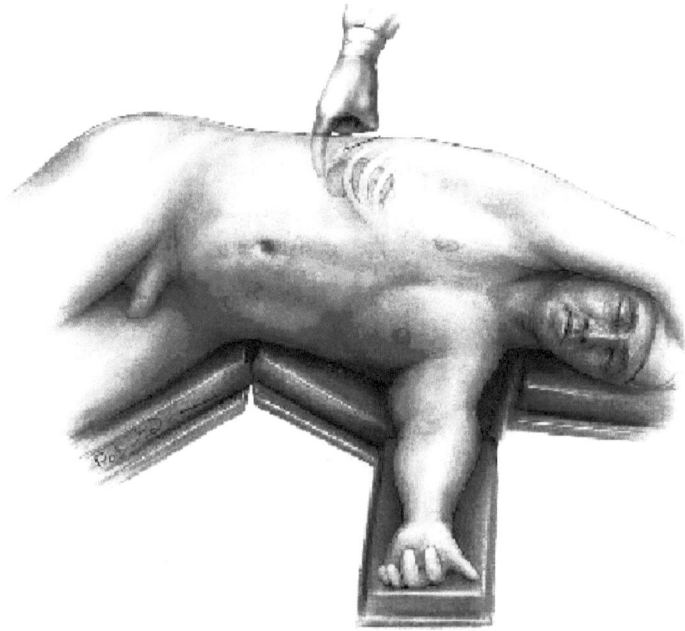

Figure 3: Creation of a cavity using finger in the retroperitoneal space.

While removing the left adrenal gland a 10 mm trocar for forceps under finger guidance is placed at the tip of XI rib. In the same way, a 10 mm trocar for ultrasound scalpel is introduced 4-5 cm medially and 2 cm below the tip of XII rib. When removing the right adrenal gland the positions of forceps and ultrasound scalpel are switched. A 10 mm trocar for 30° optics is placed through the first incision at the tip of XII rib, and the skin incision is diminished with 1-2 skin stitches. The capnoretroperitoneum is created by insufflating CO_2 until the pressure gradient reaches 20 mmHg.

The upper renal pole is mobilized and the kidney is drawn down; the adrenal gland is uncovered by preparation of tissues in the retroperitoneal space and the adipose capsule of the kidney using ultrasound scalpel and forceps. The mobilization of the adrenal gland is started from the inferior pole, *v. centralis* which connects *v. cava inferior* is also mobilized on the right side. When operating on the left side, the upper renal pole is mobilized and the kidney is pulled down. The left adrenal gland and its *v. centralis* connecting *v. renalis sinistra* are also mobilized *V. centralis* is clamped with two clips and transected. The adrenal gland is separated from the surrounding tissues and placed in a retrieval bag. The optic equipment is re-inserted through the second or third trocar and the retrieval bag is extracted through the largest first trocar opening. The drain is not inserted. The incisions are sutured with separate skin stitches.

3.3   Single Incision Laparoscopic Surgery (SILS) Adrenalectomy

The ports for single incision laparocopic surgery are being used in retroperitonescopic operations, also. This type of surgery is similar to the above-mentioned posterior retroperitoneoscopic approach, but it is performed through a single 3 cm incision at the tip of XII rib. The muscles of the waist are perforated with a straight clamp, opened and an instrument with three working channels – TriPort® (Olimpus, Europe Holding GmbH, Hamburg, Germany) or SILS Port® (Covidien, Gosport, UK) – is inserted through the wound opening. 5 or 10 mm 30° optic equipment is inserted in one channel and a 5 mm-diameter ultrasound scalpel and forceps are placed in two other (Figure 4).

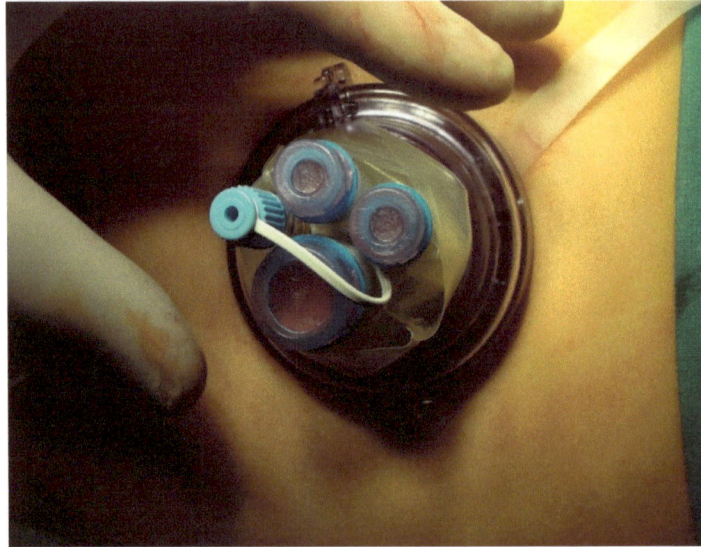

(a)

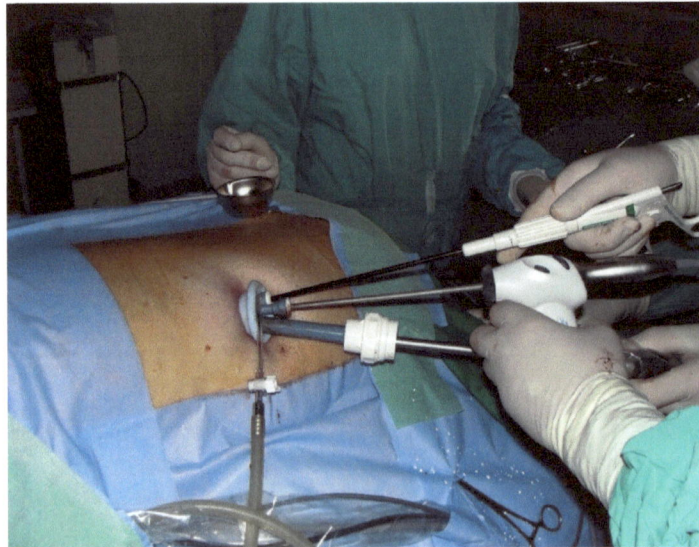

(b)

Figure 4: Single incision retroperitoneoscopic adrenalectomy. (a) TriPort® (Olimpus). (b) SILS Port® (Covidien).

Usual instruments for laparoscopic surgery are used. Curved instruments that were specially designed for this surgical approach are adapted for surgery in the abdominal cavity. They are not intended for manipulations in a small retroperitoneal space. The process of surgery is similar to the usual posterior retroperitoneoscopic adrenalectomy. The mobilized adrenal gland is placed in a retrieval bag and extracted along with a single port device. The drain is not inserted. The muscles of the waist are sutured with absorbable 3/0 stitches and the skin incision is closed with separate stitches.

3.4 Single Access Retroperitoneoscopic Adrenalectomy (SARA)

After induction of general anesthesia, the patient is placed in the above-mentioned prone jack-knife position. A 2.5 cm transverse skin incision is made at the tip of XII rib. The muscles of the waist are perforated and the retroperitoneal space is accessed using a 10 mm cutting optical trocar under the endoscopic view with 10 mm 30° endoscope (Karl Storz Endoskope, Tuttlingen, Germany). The latter endoscope or a 10 mm-diameter metal rod allows to create a cavity in the retroperitoneal space by performing piston movements. The 10 mm-diameter optical trocar is replaced with a 5 mm-diameter trocar for the same diameter 30° optics. The second 5 mm trocar is introduced through the same skin incision for the ultrasound scalpel and for insufflation of carbon dioxide to create the cavity. Intraperitoneal pressure should reach 20 mmHg. The surgeon holds the optics in the left hand and the ultrasound dissector – in the right one and prepares the adrenal gland by manipulating it (Figure 5).

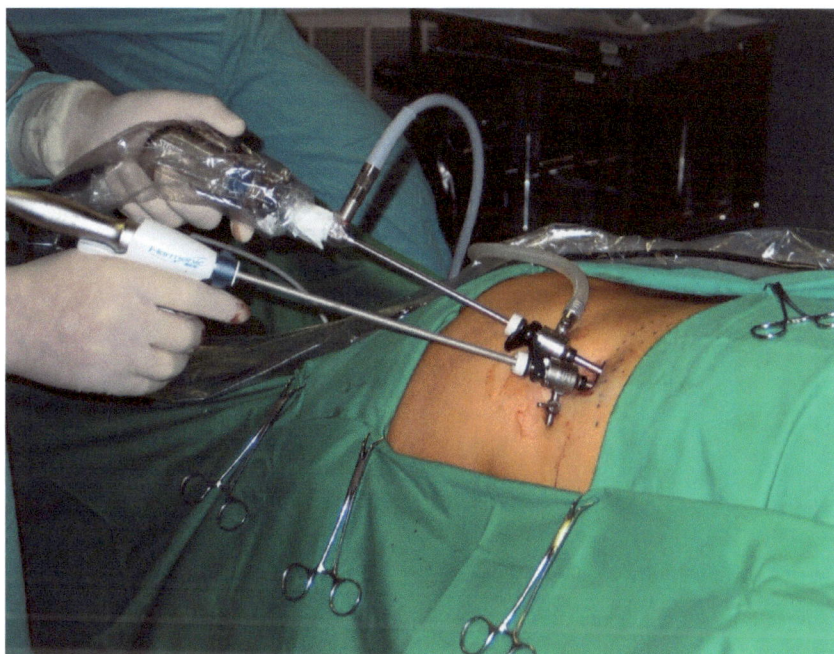

Figure 5: SARA adrenalectomy.

V. centralis is coagulated and transected with a bipolar dissector. One of the 5 mm trocars is replaced with a 10 mm-diameter trocar again after separation of the adrenal gland from the surrounding tissues. The adrenal gland is grasped with wide *Babcock* forceps and extracted along with the trocar. The drain is not inserted. The skin incision is closed with separate stitches.

4   Statistical Analysis

Data was analyzed using SPSS software for Windows (version 11.5.0). All data are presented as mean ± SD. Student's t - test was used for the comparison of two groups of independent samples. Proportions were compared using Fisher's Exact Test. Statistical significance was set at $p < 0.05$.

5   Results

The patients of group I A (n = 40) and I B (n = 30) were classified in accordance to American Society of Anesthesiology (ASA) classification. Patient characteristics (age, gender, ASA grade, tumor size and side, body mass index, indications) were summarized. Both groups were comparable regarding age, sex, risk of surgery in accordance with ASA and tumor parameters (Table 1).

Characteristic	Group I A (n = 40)		Group I B (n = 30)[*]		P
Age	53.7 ± 13.2		50.7 ± 13.5		0.40
ASA grade	2.2 ± 0.5		2.1 ± 0.05		0.45
Gender (m/f)	9 / 31		4 / 30		0.16[**]
Side (left/right)	11 / 29		11 / 20		0.20[**]
Tumor diameter cm.	3.49 ± 1.28		3.9 ± 1,38		0.24
BMI kg/m^2					
≤ 30	14 (35%)		12 (40%)		
> 30,1	26 (65%)		18 (60%)		
Character of lesion of adrenal glands (symptoms, pathology)					
Nonfunctional adrenal tumors (incidentaloma > 3.5 cm.)					
Adrenal adenoma	24	60%	14	45.2%	
Nodal hyperplasia	4	10%	10	32.2%	
Cyst	5	12.5%	2	6.5%	
Lymphangioma	-	-	1	3.2%	
Myelolipoma	1	2.5%	1	3.2%	
Functional adrenal tumors					
Corticosteroma	1	2.5%	2	6.5%	
Pheochromocytoma	3	7.5%	1	3.2%	
Aldosteronoma	2	5%	-	-	

Table 1: Characteristics of the patients undergoing lateral transabdominal and posterior retro-peritoneoscopic adrenalectomy.

---

[*] Bilateral endoscopic adrenalectomy was performed in one patient

[**] Fischer exact test

There were no statistically significant differences between the duration of LTA and PRA (p = 0.26). The first 20 LTA were performed in 133.00 ± 24.14 min.; the duration of 21 - 40 LTA was 111.25 ± 32.68 min. (Table 2).

Patient groups	Right adrenalectomy (min.)	Left adrenalectomy (min.)	p
Group I A (n =40)	123.3 ± 26.50 (n = 29)	119 ± 40.46 (n = 11)	0.38
Group I B (n =30)*	122.8 ± 42.04 (n = 20)	157.3 ± 74.6 (n = 11)	0.35
Group I A / Group I B (n = 40 / n = 30)	122.1 ± 30.42 / 135.00 ± 57.05		0.26

Table 2: Technique and duration of endoscopic adrenalectomy.

The increasing experience of the surgeon had a significant influence on duration of the LTA operation (p = 0.01). The first 20 PRA were performed in 122.25 ± 47.75 min.; the mean duration of the next 11 operations was even longer (158.18 ± 67.20 min.) (p = 0.15). As the majority of the patients had only slight overweight, we distributed all the patients into two groups: patients with slight overweight (BMI < 30) and obese patients (BMI > 30). Tumor size and the BMI of patients did not have a statistically significant influence on the duration of LTA and PRA (Table 3, Table 4).

Tumor size (cm.)	Lateral transabdominal adrenalectomy (min.) (n = 40)	Posterior retroperitoneoscopic adrenalectomy (min.) (n = 31)	p
≤ 5	122.7 ± 31.6 (n = 36)	136.9 ± 63.0 (n = 24)	0.32
> 5.1	118.8 ± 22.5 (n = 4)	131.4 ± 38.0 (n = 7)	0.50

Table 3: Duration of endoscopic adrenalectomy and its dependence on tumor size.

BMI	Lateral transabdominal adrenalectomy (min.) (n = 40)	Posterior retroperitoneoscopic adrenalectomy (min.) (n = 31)	p
≤ 30 (n = 26)	112.9 ± 33.3 (n = 14)	111.2 ± 25.6 (n = 12)	0.88
> 30,1 (n = 45)	127.1 ± 24.4 (n = 26)	112.9 ± 65.1 (n = 19)	0.38

Table 4: Duration of endoscopic adrenalectomy and its dependence on patient's body mass index.

Considerable blood loss was observed in 5 out of the 40 patients (12.5%) who underwent LTA. Lesion of v. cava inferior occurred in one patient. Diffuse bleeding from the dense, adherent perinephric fat during dissection and from the adrenal gland parenchyma because of fracture of the adrenal gland capsule occurred in three and one patients, respectively. None of the patients required a blood transfusion, except one patient in group I A, who had undergone conversion for bleeding due to lesion of v.cava inferior.

There were 2 complications (6.4%) out of the 30 patients who underwent PRA (31 adrenal glands were removed): in 1 patient the v. cava inferior was injured and in 1 patient wide subcutaneous emphysema extending up to the patient's head occurred. The incidence of intraoperative complications was similar (p = 0.23) with both techniques.

There were no statistically significant differences in blood loss between the two techniques (p = 0.18) but in all cases with intraoperative complications and bleeding we had to convert to an open approach.

Postoperative complications occurred in 6 (15%) out of 40 patients in group I A: pneumonia was diagnosed in 2 patients; subhepatic hematoma due to bleeding into the peritoneal cavity in 1 patient; pancreatic fistula persisting for 2 months after operation in 1 patient; left retroperitoneal abscess in 1 patient; and pulmonary artery embolism in 1 patient. This patient died.

There was only 1 postoperative complication in group I B. An abdominal wall muscle relaxation occurred after 1 month. There was no significant difference in the rate of complications and conversion between the two groups of patients (Table 5).

	Group I A (n = 40)		Group I B (n = 30)[*]		p
	right	left	right	left	
Operations (n)	29	11	20	11	
Conversions (n)	5	-	1	-	0.14[**]
Blood loss (ml)	58.5 ± 82.4		37.2 ± 29.3		0.18[***]
Intraoperative complications	n = 5		n = 2		0.23[**]
V. cava inferior lesion	1	-	1	-	
Diffuse bleeding (n)	4	-	-	-	
Subcutaneous emphysema (n)	-	-	-	1	
Postoperative complications	n = 6		n = 1		0.09[**]
Pneumonia (n)	2	-	-	-	
Bleeding (n)	1	-	-	-	
Pancreatic fistula (n)	-	1	-	-	
Retroperitoneal abscess (n)	-	1	-	-	
Pulmonary artery embolism	1	-	-	-	
Relaxation of abdominal wall muscles	-	-	-	1	
Mortality (n)	1	-	-	-	

Table 5: Conversions, blood loss and complications in endoscopic adrenalectomies.

The group II patients operated on for aldosteronoma (n = 31) were distributed into 3 groups according to the method of surgery: group II A (n = 6) patients had undergone the LTA, group II B (n = 20) – the PRA and group II C (n = 5) – the posterior retroperitoneoscopic approach through single incision (1 SILS and 4 SARA adrenalectomies). The means of age, size of aldosteronoma and body mass index (BMI) of the patients of all 3 groups were similar (Table 6).

---

[*] Bilateral endoscopic adrenalectomy was performed in one patient

	Group II A (n = 6)	Group II B (n = 20)	Group II C (n = 5)	p value
Age (years)	55 ± 18	56 ± 10	58 ± 11	0.911
Male (m/f)	1/5	7/13	1/4	0.610
Side (left/right)	3/3	10/10	2/3	0.919
Tumor diameter (mm)	20 ± 4	21 ± 10	14 ± 3	0.292
BMI (kg/m^2)	29 ± 3.7	28 ± 3.4	30 ± 2.7	0.429
Characteristics of histological examination				
Conn's adenoma	5	16	4	
Nodal hyperplasia	1	3	1	
Carcinoma	---	1	---	
Average duration of surgery (min)	91 ± 23	118 ± 57	144 ± 88	0.205
Duration of left adrenalectomy (min)	77 ± 6	126 ± 57	240 ± 0	0.023
Duration of right adrenalectomy (min)	105 ± 26	109 ± 50	80 ± 0	0.604
Blood loss (ml)	40 ± 15	30 ± 9	13 ± 7	0.003[*]

Table 6: Characteristics of the patients (Group II).

The average size of the adrenal tumor for groups II A, II B and II C found on CT and MRI was 19 ± 9 mm (Figure 6).

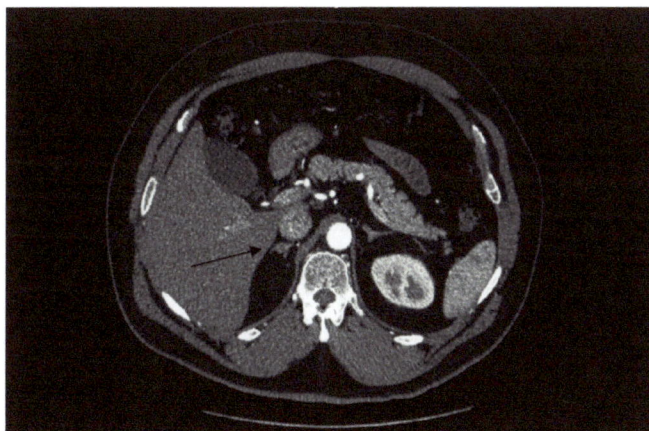

Figure 6: Abdominal CT scan with aldosteronoma of the right adrenal gland.

The average duration of surgery in group II A was shorter than in groups II B and II C (91 ± 23 vs. 118 ± 57 vs. 144 ± 88 min). The right laparoscopic adrenalectomy was longer than the left one (105 ± 26 vs. 77 ± 6 min), whereas the right PRA was shorter than the left (109 ± 50 vs. 126 ± 57 min). The best cosmetic result (because of single incision) was present in group II C.

There were no "major complications" during the intraoperative (bleeding, injuries of other organs) and postoperative (bleeding, hematoma in the abdominal cavity or retroperitoneal space, abscesses, disorders of the cardiovascular system) periods in groups II A, II B and II C.

Double conversion was performed for one patient of group II C. SARA method was converted into the PRA (by using three trocars), and then into the LTA. The surgery lasted 240 minutes. The other three SARA surgeries lasted 80 minutes each (Table 7).

Patient	Age/sex	BMI	Site	Size (mm)	Method	Operative time (min)	Blood loss (ml)
1	46/F	32	R	12	SARA	80	10
2*	65/M	32	L	13	SARA	240	20
3	45/F	27	R	12	SARA	80	20
4	66/F	33	R	20	SARA	80	5
5	67/F	28	L	12	SILS	240	10

Table 7: Characteristics of patients undergoing SARA and SILS adrenalectomy (Group II C).

Case report. Patient Č. K., 65 years-old, BMI – 32, was examined at the department of endocrinology for hypertension (arterial blood pressure – 170/100 mmHg). The plasma concentration of catecholamines was normal; potassium – 3 mmol/l; sodium – 146 mmol/l; aldosterone in the recumbency – 490 ng/l, in the standing position 494.5 ng/l; rennin at rest and after load – 1 ng/l. According to the data of CT scan, the 13 mm large adenoma of the left adrenal gland was present (Figure 6). The aldosteronoma of the left adrenal gland was diagnosed.

The patient was operated on. The surgery was started using SARA method by making a 2.5 cm transverse incision at the tip of XII rib on the left side. However, it was impossible to prepare the adrenal gland because of abundant fatty tissue in the renal capsule, a short waist of the patient, difficulty to perform the movements of the instruments and minor anatomic alterations of the left adrenal gland. Two additional 10 mm-diameter trocars were introduced into the retroperitoneal space and the surgery was continued by means of the posterior retroperitoneoscopic approach. Because of the reasons mentioned above and impossibility to find the adrenal gland within 1 hour, the surgery was converted into lateral laparoscopic approach by turning the patient on the right side. The left adrenal gland with a 13 mm-diameter aldosteronoma was removed.

There were no intraoperative and postoperative complications and due to this the patient was discharged from the hospital two days after the surgery.

6   Discussion

Several different approaches for minimal invasive adrenalectomy are currently available, including the anterior transabdominal, lateral transabdominal, posterior retroperitoneoscopic approach. Although the transperitoneal techniques remain more popular and widely reported, the retroperitoneal approach to the adrenal gland has several distinct advantages, which make it an attractive alternative for removal of adrenal tumors (Fernandez-Cruz et al., 1996).

The advantages and disadvantages of transperitoneal and retroperitoneal approaches have been reported (Chiu, 2003; Del Pizzo, 2003; Fernandez-Cruz et al., 1999). The transperitoneal approach provides a larger working space, better visibility and anatomic familiarity for most surgeons. It provides greater exposure for larger adrenal tumors (> 7 cm) and for pheochromocytomas requiring minimal manipulation prior to vascular control. However, the transperitoneal approach requires mobilization of intra-abdominal structures and has a higher risk of vascular and intra-abdominal organ injury, prolonged ileus, diaphragmatic irritation, and adhesion formation (Fernandez-Cruz et al., 1996). This approach is especially difficult and challenging in patients who have had previous abdominal surgery and intra-abdominal adhesions.

The retroperitoneal approach has the distinct advantage of offering a more direct route to the adrenal gland without affecting intra-abdominal organs. It does not require mobilizing of intraperitoneal structures, releasing adhesions, and hepatic retraction. As a result, several journals report shorter operative duration with the retroperitoneal approach (Bonjer et al., 2000; Chiu, 2003). The retroperitoneal approach has its limitations. It has a restricted working space that can make dissection more cumbersome for an inexperienced surgeon. Another essential drawback of this approach is the limited number of usable trocar sites that are in close proximity to one another. The small space limits instrument placement and crossing of instruments can easily occur. In order to overcome this shortcoming partially, full medial mobilization of the peritoneum is necessary. Typically, this method is not suitable for removal of large tumors (> 7 cm), because the working space is too limited. Although larger tumors have been removed using this approach, it was associated with longer operative times and higher open conversion rates (Chiu, 2003).

In our patient population, the transperitoneal approach was used primarily in the early phase of the study, whereas the retroperitoneal technique was selected later because of the shorter operating times reported (Bonjer et al., 1997; Walz et al., 2001). This does not exclude the possibility that the experience gained in performing of the transperitoneal procedure had exerted an influence on the results of the retroperitoneal approach.

In a case control study of open, lateral transabdominal and posterior retroperitoneoscopic adrenalectomies, operating times were the longest for lateral transabdominal adrenalectomy (Bonjer et al., 1997). Longer operating times for retroperitoneal endoscopic adrenalectomy were reported in a prospective follow-up study by Gockel et al. (Gockel et al., 2005), but two randomized clinical trials have compared transperitoneal and retroperitoneal approaches to adrenal pathology and neither found significant differences in operating time, blood transfusions or hospital stays (Fernandez-Cruz et al., 1996; Rubinstein et al., 2005).

The results of our own study demonstrated shorter operation duration for the transperitoneal approach than for the retroperitoneal procedure. However, there were no statistically significant differences. It should be mentioned that it is more convenient to remove the right adrenal gland while using endoscopic retroperitoneal method; on the other hand, the lateral transperitoneal method is more convenient for removal of the left gland. In order to clamp and cut the vein of the left adrenal gland, while using PRA method, one should properly mobilize the left kidney and push it downwards, as the vein of the left adrenal gland joins the vein of the left kidney from the inferior pole of the adrenal gland medially from the kidney. While using LTA method, the vein of the left adrenal gland and kidney are exposed more easily after mobilization of the left flexure of the large intestine and spleen. The vein of the right adrenal gland is exposed more easily while using PRA method, as mobilization of the superior pole of the right kidney is required, only. Short vein of the right adrenal gland connects the inferior v. cava at the level of the middle part of adrenal gland. While using LTA method, mobilisation of the liver is required, in order to expose the vein of the right adrenal gland.

Obesity is a problem in laparoscopic surgery, but it can be overcome by improving surgical technique. With obese patients, choosing of the approach is a dilemma. Dissection via retroperitoneal approach in obese patients with large amounts of retroperitoneal fat can be very challenging. Conversely, when using the transperitoneal approach, the instruments are sometimes not long enough to reach the adrenal gland, because it sits at the very back of the retroperitoneum.

Naya *et al.* found a correlation between BMI and the duration of operation in patients undergoing adrenal surgery (Naya *et al.*, 2002). As the patient's BMI increased, the duration of surgery increased for both retroperitoneal and transperitoneal approaches. However Lezoche *et al.* reported that in both of the transperitoneal approaches (lateral and anterior) operative time correlated with patient's BMI, this was not the case with the retroperitoneal approach (Lezoche *et al.*, 2002). In the present study, the mean duration of surgery in obese patients (BMI > 30.1) was shorter for the retroperitoneal adrenalectomies, but we found no statistically significant differences in operating time and BMI between the retroperitoneal and transperitoneal approaches.

In 2008, M. K. Walz performed the first adrenalectomy using SARA approach – through a single 1.5 cm transverse incision from the back side using only two trocars: one for optics and another for bipolar scissors (Walz & Alesina, 2009). The adrenal gland was mobilized with one instrument; therefore, only one surgeon was required to perform the surgery. The main advantage of this method is a well-looking cosmetic view of the surgical wound. However, it is impossible to remove tumors larger than 3 cm in size using this method. As a matter of fact, it is perfect for removing Conn's adenomas with the diameter that in the majority of the cases does not exceed 2.5 cm. The advantages of SILS include: (1) a good cosmetic result, (2) a well-sealed retroperitoneal space and (3) mobilization of the adrenal gland using two instruments. On the other hand, instrumental manipulations in the retroperitoneal space are very limited because of the restricted working space. For this reason, special curved instruments used for SILS in the abdominal cavity are not intended for surgeries in the retroperitoneal space (Beiša *et al.*, 2011). The movements of instruments are limited, while using SILS port. The range of the movements is highly dependent on the diameter of the head of a troacar. The smaller diameter of the head determines the higher range of the movements of troacars with instruments inserted. We are using trocars manufactured by Karl Storz Company. Besides, this method requires using of the port and this increases financial costs of the operation (Beiša *et al.*, 2012). SARA is performed via a single incision with two trocars. In case of removing of small adrenal tumors using SARA approach; it is easy to convert it into the posterior retroperitoneoscopic method by inserting two more trocars without any extra financial costs. It is the main advantage of SARA method over SILS method. The diameter of the heads of trocars and the connection between the optical fibre and optics are very important in SARA method. It is easier to avoid "crossing" of instruments in the retroperitoneal space with optical fibre at the end of optical equipment with trocars with the heads of small diameter.

In conclusion, the training period is shorter for lateral transabdominal adrenalectomies in comparison with posterior retroperitoneoscopic adrenalectomies. Lateral transabdominal and posterior retroperitoneoscopic adrenalectomies are similar in terms of duration of operation, blood loss, and incidence of complications. The tumours with the size 3 – 7 cm may be removed using laparoscopic transabdominal method or endoscopic retroperitoneal approach, in accordance with surgeon's choice. Taking into account the minimal invasiveness and advantages of the method, simplicity to be converted into another type of endoscopic approach, SARA approach should be the first option for removing of small (< 3 cm) tumors of adrenal glands.

References

Beiša, V., Kildušis, E., & Strupas, K. (2012). Single access retroperitoneoscopic adrenalectomy: initial experience. Videochir Inne Tech Malo Inwazyjne, 7, 45-49.

Beiša, V., Simutis, G., Lagunavičius, K., & Strupas, K. (2011). Single-port endoscopic retroperitoneal adrenalectomy: initial experience. Videochir Inne Tech Malo Inwazyjne, 6, 103-107.

Bonjer, H. J., Lange, J. F., Kazemier, G., de Herder, W. W., Steyerberg, E. W., & Bruining, H. A. (1997). Comparison of three techniques for adrenalectomy. Br J Surg, 84, 679-682.

Bonjer, H. J., Sorm, V., Berends, F. J., Kazemier, G., Steyerberg, E. W., de Herder, W. W., & Bruining, H. A. (2000). Endoscopic retroperitoneal adrenalectomy: lessons learned from 111 consecutive cases. Ann Surg, 232, 796–803.

Brunt, L. M., Doherty, G. M., Norton, J. A., Soper, N. J., Quasebarth, M. A., & Moley, J. F. (1996). Laparoscopic adrenalectomy compared to open adrenalectomy for benign adrenal neoplasms. J Am Coll Surg, 183, 1-10.

Chiu, A. W. (2003). Laparoscopic retroperitoneal adrenalectomy: clinical experience with 120 consecutive cases. Asian J Surg, 26, 139-144.

Del Pizzo, J. J. (2003). Transabdominal laparoscopic adrenalectomy. Curr Urol Rep, 4, 81-86.

Duh, Q. Y., Siperstein, A. E., Clark, O. H., Schester, W. P., Horn, J. K., Harisson, M. R., Hunt, T. K., & Way, L. W. (1996).

Laparoscopic adrenalectomy: comparison of the lateral and posterior approaches. Arch Surg, 131, 870-875.

Fernandez-Cruz, L., Saenz, A., Benarroch, G., Astudillo, E., Taura, P., & Sabater, L. (1996). Laparoscopic unilateral and bilateral adrenalectomy for Cushing's syndrome: transperitonel and retroperitoneal approaches. Ann Surg, 224, 727-734.

Fernandez-Cruz, L., Saenz, A., Taura, P., Benarroch, G., Astudillo, E., & Sabater L. (1999). Retroperitoneal approach in laparoscopic adrenalectomy: is it advantageous? Surg Endosc, 13, 86-90.

Gagner, M., Lacroix, A., & Bolte, E. (1992). Laparoscopic adrenalectomy in Cushing's syndrome and pheochromocytoma. N Engl J Med, 327, 1033.

Gagner, M., Pomp, A., Heniford, B.T., Pharand, D., & Lacroix, A. (1997). Laparoscopic adrenalectomy: lessons learned from 100 consecutive procedures. Ann Surg, 226, 238-247.

Gockel, J., Kneist, W., Hentz, A., Beyer, J., & Junginger, T. (2005). Endoscopic adrenalectomy. An analysis of the transperitoneal and retroperitoneal approaches and results of a prospective following study. Surg Endosc, 19, 569-573.

Hallfeldt, K. K., Mussack, T., Trupka, A., Hohenbleicher, F., & Schmidbauer, S. (2003). Laparoscopic lateral adrenalectomy versus open posterior adrenalectomy for the treatment of benign adrenal tumors. Surg Endosc, 17, 264-267.

Higashihara, E., Tanaka, Y., Horie, S., Aruga, S., Nutahara, K., Homma, Y., Minowada, S., & Aso, Y. (1992). A case report of laparoscopic adrenalectomy. Nihon Hinyokika Gakkai Zasshi, 83, 1130–1133.

Jacobs, J. K., Goldstein, R. E., & Geer, R. J. (1997). Laparoscopic adrenalectomy: a new standard of care. Ann Surg, 225, 495-501.

Johnson, P. T., Horton, K. M., & Fishman, E. K. (2009). Adrenal mass imaging with multidetector CT: pathologic conditions, pearls, and pitfalls. Radiographics, 29, 1333–1351.

Kebebew, E., Siperstein, A. E., & Duh, Q. Y. (2001). Laparoscopic adrenalectomy: the optimal surgical approach. J. Laparoendosc Adv Surg Tech, 11, 409-413.

Lezoche, E., Guerrieri, M., Feliciotti, F., Paganini, A. M., Perretta, S., Baldarelli, M., Bonjer, J., & Miccoli, P. (2002). Anterior, lateral, and posterior retroperitoneal approaches in endoscopic adrenalectomy. Surg Endosc, 16, 96-99.

Mercan, S., Seven, R., Ozarmagan, S., & Tezelman, S. (1995). Endoscopic retroperitoneal adrenalectomy. Surgery, 118, 1071-1076.

Naya, Y., Nagata, M., Ichikawa, T., Amakasu, M., Omura, M., Nishikawa, T., Yamaguchi, K., & Ito, H. (2002). Laparo-scopic adrenalectomy: comparison of transperitoneal and retroperitoneal approaches. BJU Int, 90, 199-204.

Rubinstein, M., Gill, I. S., Aron, M., Kilciler, M., Meraney, A. M., Finelli, A., Moinzadeh, A., Ukimura, O., Desai, M. M., Kaouk, J., & Bravo, E. (2005). Prospective, randomized comparison of transperitoneal versus retroperitoneal adrenalectomy. J Urol, 174, 442-445.

Smith, C. D., Weber, C. J., & Amerson, J. R. (1999). Laparoscopic adrenalectomy: new gold standard. World J Surg, 23, 389–396.

Thompson, G. B., Grant, C. S., van Heerden, J. A., Schlinker, R. T., Young, W. F. Jr., Farley, D. R., & Ilstrup, D. M. (1997). Laparoscopic versus open posterior adrenalectomy: a case – control study of 100 patients. Surgery, 122, 1132-1136.

Walz, M. K., & Alesina, P. F. (2009). Single access retroperitoneoscopic adrenalectomy (SARA) – one step beyond in en-docrine surgery. Langenbecks Arch Surg, 394, 447–450.

Walz, M. K., Peitgen, K., Hoermann, R., Giebler, R.M., Mann, K., & Eigler, F. W. (1996). Posterior retroperitoneoscopy as a new minimally invasive approach for adrenalectomy: results of 30 adrenalectomies in 27 patients. World J Surg, 20,

769-774.

Walz, M. K., Peitgen, K., Krause, U., & Eigler, F. W. (1995). Die dorsale Adrenalektomie- eine operative Technik. Zent-ralbl Chir, 120, 53-58.

Walz, M. K., Peitgen, K., Walz, M. V., Hoermann, R., Saller, B., Giebler, R. M., Jockenhovel, F., Philipp, T., Broelsch, C. E., Eigler, F. W., & Mann, K. (2001). Posterior retroperitoneoscopic adrenalectomy: lessons learned within five years. World J Surg, 25, 728-734.

Czajkowski, K., Fitzgerald, S., Foster, I., & Kesselman, C. (2001). Grid information services for distributed resource shar-ing. In 10th IEEE International Symposium on High Performance Distributed Computing (pp. 181–184).

Foster, I., Kesselman, C., Nick, J., & Tuecke, S. (2002). The Physiology of the Grid: an Open Grid Services Architecture for Distributed Systems Integration. Technical report, Global Grid Forum.

Gusfield, D. (1997). Algorithms on Strings, Trees and Sequences: Computer Science and Computational Biology. Cam-bridge: Cambridge University Press.

Hern'andez, M. A. & Stolfo, S. J. (1995). The merge/purge problem for large databases. SIGMOD Record, 24(2), 127–138.

Smith, T. F. & Waterman, M. S. (1981). Identification of common molecular subsequences. Journal of Molecular Biology, 147, 195–197.